Hyperglycemia, Diabetes, and Vascular Disease

CLINICAL PHYSIOLOGY SERIES

HYPERGLYCEMIA, DIABETES, AND VASCULAR DISEASE
Edited by Neil Ruderman, Joseph Williamson, and Michael Brownlee

ENDOTHELIN
Edited by Gabor M. Rubanyi

HYPOXIA, METABOLIC ACIDOSIS, AND THE CIRCULATION
Edited by Allen I. Arieff

RESPONSE AND ADAPTATION TO HYPOXIA: ORGAN
TO ORGANELLE
Edited by Sukhamay Lahiri, Neil S. Cherniack, and Robert S. Fitzgerald

CLINICAL PHYSIOLOGY OF SLEEP
Edited by Ralph Lydic and Julien F. Biebuyck

ATRIAL HORMONES AND OTHER NATRIURETIC FACTORS
Edited by Patrick J. Mulrow and Robert Schrier

PHYSIOLOGY OF OXYGEN RADICALS
Edited by Aubrey E. Taylor, Sadis Matalon, and Peter A. Ward

EFFECTS OF ANESTHESIA
Edited by Benjamin G. Covino, Harry A. Fozzard, Kai Rehder, and Gary Strichartz

INTERACTION OF PLATELETS WITH THE VESSEL WALL
Edited by John A. Oates, Jacek Hawiger, and Russell Ross

HIGH ALTITUDE AND MAN
Edited by John B. West and Sukhamay Lahiri

DISTURBANCES IN NEUROGENIC CONTROL
OF THE CIRCULATION
Edited by Francois M. Abboud, Harry A. Fozzard, Joseph P. Gilmore,
and Donald J. Reis

NEW PERSPECTIVES ON CALCIUM ANTAGONISTS
Edited by George B. Weiss

SECRETORY DIARRHEA
Edited by Michael Field, John S. Fordtran, and Stanley G. Schultz

PULMONARY EDEMA
Edited by Alfred P. Fishman and Eugene M. Renkin

DISTURBANCES IN LIPID AND LIPOPROTEIN METABOLISM
Edited by John M. Dietschy, Antonio M. Gotto, Jr., and Joseph A. Ontko

DISTURBANCES IN BODY FLUID OSMOLALITY
Edited by Thomas E. Andreoli, Jared J. Grantham, and Floyd C. Rector, Jr.

Hyperglycemia, Diabetes, and Vascular Disease

EDITED BY

NEIL RUDERMAN

Diabetes and Metabolism Unit,
Evans Memorial Department of Clinical Research
and Department of Physiology
Boston University School of Medicine
Boston, Massachusetts

JOSEPH WILLIAMSON

Department of Pathology
Washington University School of Medicine
St. Louis, Missouri

MICHAEL BROWNLEE

Diabetes Research Center
and Departments of Medicine and Pathology
Albert Einstein College of Medicine
Bronx, New York

New York   Oxford

Published for the American Physiological Society by
OXFORD UNIVERSITY PRESS

1992

Oxford University Press

Oxford   New York   Toronto
Delhi   Bombay   Calcutta   Madras   Karachi
Kuala Lumpur   Singapore   Hong Kong   Tokyo
Nairobi   Dar es Salaam   Cape Town
Melbourne   Auckland

and associated companies in
Berlin   Ibadan

Library of Congress Cataloging-in-Publication Data
Hyperglycemia, diabetes, and vascular disease / edited by
Neil Ruderman, Joseph Williamson, Michael Brownlee.
p. cm.   (Clinical physiology series)
Includes bibliographical references and index.
ISBN 0-19-506773-8
1. Diabetic angiopathies—Pathogenesis.
2. Diabetes—Complications and sequelae.
3. Hyperglycemia—Pathophysiology.
I. Ruderman, Neil.
II. Williamson, J. R. (Joseph R.)
III. Brownlee, Michael, 1948–   .
IV. American Physiological Society (1887–)   V. Series
[DNLM: 1. Diabetes Mellitus—complications.
2. Hyperglycemia—complications.
3. Vascular Diseases—complications.
WK 880 H9975]   RC700.D5H96   1992
616.4′62—dc20   DNLM/DLC   for Library of Congress
91-32160

1 3 5 7 9 8 6 4 2

Printed in the United States of America
on acid-free paper

Preface

It is estimated that 1–5% of the world's population is affected by some form of diabetes. Patients with these disorders are highly likely to develop microvascular pathology in the retina and glomerulus and they are at a 2–6-fold greater risk for atherosclerotic vascular disease than individuals without diabetes. In addition, hypertension is far more prevalent in patients with diabetes than in the general population. As a consequence of these complications, diabetes is a leading cause of blindness and renal failure in young and middle-aged adults and it is a major risk factor for coronary heart disease, stroke and peripheral vascular disease in the Western world.

An understanding of the relationship of these vascular complications to diabetic hyperglycemia has become a critical issue for clinicians in recent years, since the prevalence of diabetes appears to be increasing dramatically world-wide. In addition, it is now possible to achieve improved glycemic control in many patients—although not without incurring other risks. This volume explores two principal hypotheses concerning these complications. One is that hyperglycemia underlies or at least contributes to the pathogenesis of both micro- and macrovascular disease in patients with diabetes. The other is that it does so by producing specific metabolic and biochemical alterations in the vascular wall that lead to abnormalities in its function and ultimately its structure.

The authors include epidemiologists, clinicians and biochemists, many of whom have made pioneering contributions in this area. Key chapters describe how hyperglycemia initiates signal transduction mechanisms that can alter vascular function, and how it causes the glycation of proteins, which in turn can cause such diverse events as enhanced binding of low density lipoproteins to vascular collagen, altered macrophage function and hemostasis, and changes in the structure of extracellular matrix molecules such as type IV collagen. Also discussed are the effects of hyperglycemia on the synthesis of proteoglycans and the hypothesis that protein glycation contributes to the pathophysiological alterations associated with aging. Other chapters discuss the epidemiological evidence for an association of hyperglycemia and coronary heart disease based on the data from the Framingham Heart Project, and the effects of hyperglycemia on the brain and on the blood-brain-barrier.

This volume evolved from a symposium sponsored by the American Physiological Society at the 74th Annual Meeting of the American Societies for Experimental Biology in April 1990. The chapters were written over the following six months and then revised and edited. The editors gratefully acknowledge the assistance of some of the people and organizations that made this book and the symposium possible. These include the American Physiological Society; Nordisk and Upjohn, which generously provided financial support; Maryse Roudier and Heather Adams at Boston University, who provided administrative and secretarial assistance; and at Oxford University Press, Susan Hannan who expertly edited the manuscript, Stan George who guided it through publication, and Edith Barry. Finally our thanks to Dr. Julien Biebuyck, the Chairman of the APS Clinical Sciences Subcommittee, who coaxed us into initiating this project and, together with Martin Frank of the APS, assisted us greatly in its initial organization.

November 1991   N.R.
                                                                  J.W.
                                                                  M.B.

Contents

Contributors

JOHN W. BAYNES, Ph. D.
Department of Chemistry
University of South Carolina
Columbia, South Carolina

MICHAEL L. BROWN, Ph.D.
Hemostasis Research
Boston Veterans Administration
    Medical Center
Boston, Massachusetts

MICHAEL BROWNLEE, M.D.
Diabetes Research Center and
    Departments of Medicine and
    Pathology
Albert Einstein College of Medicine
Bronx, New York

ARISTIDIS S. CHARONIS, M.D.,
    Ph.D.
Department of Laboratory Medicine
    and Pathology
University of Minnesota Medical School
Minneapolis, Minnesota

RICHARD A. COHEN, M.D.
Vascular Biology Unit
Evans Memorial Department
    of Clinical Research
Boston University School of Medicine
Boston, Massachusetts

JOHN A. COLWELL, M.D., Ph.D.
Research Service
Veterans Administration Medical Center
    and Endocrinology, Metabolism and
    Nutrition Division
Department of Medicine
Medical College of South Carolina
Charleston, South Carolina

RONALD L. ENGERMAN, Ph.D.
Department of Ophthalmology
University of Wisconsin Medical School
Madison, Wisconsin

EDWARD P. FEENER, Ph.D.
Joslin Diabetes Center
Boston, Massachusetts

LEO T. FURCHT, M.D.
Department of Laboratory Medicine
    and Pathology
University of Minnesota Medical School
Minneapolis, Minnesota

CHRISTOPH GISINGER, M.D.
Research Service
Veterans Administration Medical Center
    and Endocrinology, Metabolism and
    Nutrition Division
Department of Medicine
Medical College of South Carolina
Charleston, South Carolina

SANDEEP GUPTA, Ph.D.
Diabetes and Metabolism Unit
Evans Memorial Department
    of Clinical Research and
    Department of Physiology
Boston University School of Medicine
Boston, Massachusetts

HANS-PETER HAMMES, M.D.
Center for Internal Medicine
Justus-Liebig University
Giessen, Germany

WILLIAM B. KANNEL, M.D.
Department of Medicine
Boston University School of Medicine
Boston, Massachusetts

TIMOTHY S. KERN, Ph.D.
Department of Ophthalmology
University of Wisconsin Medical School
Madison, Wisconsin

CHARLES KILO, M.D.
Department of Medicine
Washington University School
    of Medicine
St. Louis, Missouri

GEORGE L. KING, M.D.
Joslin Diabetes Center
Boston, Massachusetts

DAVID J. KLEIN, M.D., Ph.D.
Department of Pediatrics
University of Minnesota Medical School
Minneapolis, Minnesota

RICHARD KLEIN, Ph.D.
Veterans Administration Medical Center
    and Endocrine, Metabolism and
    Nutrition Division
Department of Medicine
Medical College of South Carolina
Charleston, South Carolina

TIMOTHY J. LYONS, Ph.D.
Research Service
Veterans Administration Medical Center
    and Endocrine, Metabolism and
    Nutrition Division
Department of Medicine
Medical University of South Carolina
Charleston, South Carolina

ANTHONY L. McCALL, M.D., Ph.D.
Diabetes Program
Portland Veterans Administration
    Medical Center
Portland, Oregon

RAMESH NAYAK, Ph.D.
Joslin Diabetes Center
Boston, Massachusetts

NEIL B. RUDERMAN, M.D., D.Phil.
Diabetes and Metabolism Unit
Evans Memorial Department of Clinical
    Research and Department of
    Physiology
Boston University School of Medicine
Boston, Massachusetts

TERUO SHIBA, M.D., Ph.D.
Joslin Diabetes Center
Boston, Massachusetts

DAVID A. SIMMONS, M.D.
Department of Medicine
University of Pennsylvania
School of Medicine
Philadelphia, Pennsylvania

ILENE SUSSMAN, Ph.D.
Diabetes and Metabolism Unit
Evans Memorial Department
    of Clinical Research
Boston University School of Medicine
Boston, Massachusetts

BELAY TESFAMARIAM, Ph.D.
Vascular Biology Unit
Evans Memorial Department
    of Clinical Research
Boston University School of Medicine
Boston, Massachusetts

SUZANNE R. THORPE, Ph.D.
Department of Chemistry
University of South Carolina
Columbia, South Carolina

RONALD G. TILTON, Ph.D.
Department of Pathology
Washington University School
    of Medicine
St. Louis, Missouri

EFFIE C. TSILIBARY, M.D., Ph.D.
Department of Laboratory Medicine
    and Pathology
University of Minnesota Medical School
Minneapolis, Minnesota

HELEN VLASSARA, M.D.
Picower Institute for Medical Research
Manhasset, New York

JOSEPH R. WILLIAMSON, M.D.
Department of Pathology
Washington University School
   of Medicine
St. Louis, Missouri

PETER W. F. WILSON, M.D.
Framingham Heart Study
Framingham, Massachusetts

ALBERT I. WINEGRAD, M.D.
Department of Medicine
University of Pennsylvania
School of Medicine
Philadelphia, Pennsylvania

I

EPIDEMIOLOGY AND PHYSIOLOGY

1

Hyperglycemia, Diabetes, and Vascular Disease: An Overview

NEIL B. RUDERMAN, SANDEEP GUPTA, AND ILENE SUSSMAN

VASCULAR DISEASE IN DIABETES

Diabetes is a disease, or group of diseases, characterized by hyperglycemia, a relative or absolute lack of insulin, and a propensity to vascular disease and neuropathy. Two types of vascular disease have been described: a microangiopathy that affects capillaries and arterioles in the eye and kidney and other organs and is relatively unique to diabetes, and a macroangiopathy that is morphologically very similar to atherosclerosis in nondiabetics, but is more extensive and occurs at an earlier age (72). In addition, alterations in vascular reactivity have been observed that could hypothetically play a role in the pathogenesis of vasospastic angina (Chapter 4), hypertension (81) and an impaired response of diabetics to ischemia. Patients with primary diabetes are classified as insulin-dependent (type I) or non-insulin-dependent (type II), based on differences in etiology and clinical characteristics. Micro- and macrovascular disease are more common among patients with both subtypes of diabetes than in the general population (Table 1.1).

The clinical significance of diabetic vascular disease resides in the fact that diabetes is a common disorder: there are estimated to be over 12 million people with diabetes in the United States. Also, patients with diabetes are many times more likely to develop blindness (42,43,46) and renal failure (24,31), and they are at 2–6-fold greater risk for atherosclerotic vascular disease (38,72). In addition, hypertension is far more prevalent among patients with diabetes than in the general population (18,32). As a consequence of these complications, diabetes is perhaps the leading cause of blindness (46,52) and renal failure (24,31,42) in young and middle-aged adults and is a major risk factor for coronary heart disease, stroke, and peripheral vascular disease (38,72) in the Western world.

The central theme of this and the other chapters in this volume is the link between hyperglycemia and vascular disease in diabetes. Two hypotheses will be addressed: first, that hyperglycemia underlies, or at least contributes to, the pathogenesis of both micro- and macrovascular disease in patients with diabetes; and second, that it does so by producing metabolic and biochemical alterations in the vascular wall that lead to abnormalities in its function and, ultimately, its structure. The evidence for these hypotheses will be examined

TABLE 1.1. Characteristics of types I and II diabetes

	Type I	Type II
Synonym	Insulin-dependent (IDD)	Non-insulin-dependent (NIDD)
Old name	Juvenile-onset	Maturity-onset
Usual age of onset (years)	<35	>35
Estimated prevalence (%)	0.5	5.0
Insulin deficiency	Absolute	Variable
Etiology	Autoimmune	Unknown
Microvascular disease	+ + + +	+ + +
Macrovascular disease	+ + +	+ + + +

at clinical, epidemiological, and biochemical levels, and their therapeutic implications will be discussed. The emphasis will be on the common mechanisms by which hyperglycemia produces changes in large and small blood vessels; however, this is done with the understanding that there are also distinct differences in the pathogenesis of the two forms of vascular disease and possibly even in the pathogenesis of each type of vascular disease at different sites.

HYPERGLYCEMIA AND MICROVASCULAR DISEASE

Clinical Pathology and Physiology

Kidney
The dominant structural change in the renal microvasculature in a patient with advanced diabetic renal disease is diffuse glomerulosclerosis. Glomerular capillaries are compressed by periodic acid–Schiff (PAS)-positive material composed of thickened basement membrane, transudated protein, and most importantly, an expanded mesangium (extracellular matrix). In addition, the efferent and afferent glomerular arterioles are sclerotic. Patients with this picture usually are hypertensive and they have severe albuminuria, a diminished glomerular filtration rate, and azotemia. Many of them are candidates for dialysis or renal transplantation (33,56).

In type I diabetes, significant renal disease typically emerges after 20–30 years, and it occurs in about 40% of all patients (47). Early in the course of diabetes, there generally are minimal changes in kidney morphology (61), but there may be functional changes such as increased glomerular filtration rate (56,63). Likewise, renal mass is increased and microalbuminuria, an early indication of altered glomerular permeability and/or vascular damage may be present (82). Based on studies in experimental animals and in humans, such functional abnormalities can be reversed by weeks-months-years of tight glycemic control. (10,24,55,56,70,82). On the other hand, intensive insulin therapy appears to have little effect on the clinical course of patients in whom the nephropathy is advanced (56,82).

Eye

The earliest morphological changes in the eye of a patient with diabetes include capillary basement membrane thickening, degeneration of intramural pericytes, and microaneurysm formation (14,46). These changes are the hallmarks of nonproliferative diabetic retinopathy and they eventually occur in nearly all patients with type I diabetes and the majority of type II subjects. Such nonproliferative retinopathy is benign and has no visual consequences. In a substantial number of patients, however, it progresses to a phase characterized by capillary closure and increases in vascular permeability leading to retinal edema and hard exudate formation. When the latter involve the macula, moderate impairment of vision may occur. In some patients the vaso-occlusive process worsens and, possibly because of the elaboration of growth factors from the ischemic tissue, proliferation of new vessels and accompanying fibrous tissue occurs on the surface of the retina and optic disc. In this phase, which is referred to as proliferative retinopathy, hemorrhage from the fragile new vessels, and contraction of the fibrous proliferations and new vessels can lead to retinal distortion or detachment and visual loss (14). Over 95% of type I diabetics of 20 years duration have some form of retinopathy; however, in only 50% of them is the retinopathy proliferative. The difference in prevalence of proliferative and nonproliferative retinopathy is even greater among type II diabetics; indeed, 20 years after diagnosis 50% of type II diabetics treated with diet or oral agents have some form of retinopathy, but less than 5% of such patients progress to the proliferative phase (43). The reason for the differences in the prevalence of background and proliferative retinopathy is not known. Available evidence suggests that several months-years of intensive insulin therapy may arrest the progression of nonproliferative retinopathy and reverse increases in vascular permeability in some people (14,70). At what stage such intensive therapy is no longer efficacious remains to be determined.

Association of Hyperglycemia and Microvascular Disease in Humans and Experimental Animals

Human Studies

The first substantive evidence linking hyperglycemia and microvascular disease in diabetes was obtained in clinical studies. A number of earlier reports had suggested that patients under better glycemic control developed fewer eye and/or renal complications; however, most of the earlier studies aimed at examining these interrelations were inconclusive (44,70,77). In 1977, Pirart (65) reported his landmark study in which the association between glycemic status and the development of nephropathy and retinopathy was conclusively demonstrated. Over 4,000 patients with both types I and II diabetes were followed. Glycemic status was quantitated on the basis of serial blood glucose measurements, glycosuria, and episodes of ketoacidosis. Retinopathy and nephropathy were gauged by standard clinical parameters. As shown in Figure 1.1, patients in the good control group ($c < 1.5$ = glucose determinations less than 200 mg/dl) had less retinopathy than the intermediate control group ($1.5 < c < 2$), and

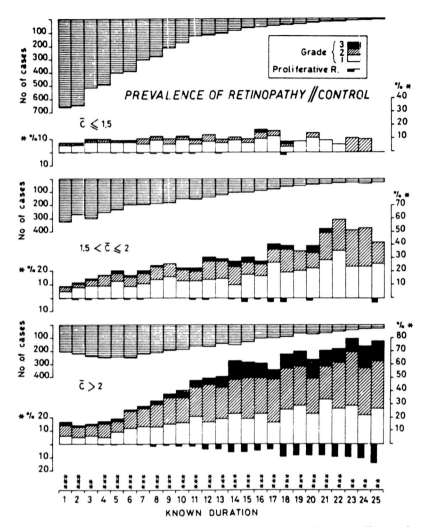

FIGURE 1.1. Increasing prevalence of each grade of retinopathy, as a function of known duration of diabetes, compared in three groups with various degrees of glycemic control from good (top) to poor (bottom). The accumulation of severe cases is striking in the group with poorest control. The significant differences, *p<0.05, **p<0.01, ***p<0.001) between the poorest and the good control groups relate both to numbers of cases and to grade of retinopathy. [Reproduced with permission from 65.]

they in turn had less than the poor control group (c > 2). A nearly identical relationship was shown between the magnitude of hyperglycemia and the incidence of nephropathy. The Pirart study also demonstrated that the relationship between glycemic status and complications applies to both types I and II diabetes, and that the correlation is closest to overall glycemic control over many years, and not the severity of diabetes at the time of onset. As pointed out by the authors, the principal limitation of this trial was that patients were not randomized when they entered the study. Thus the possibility that those who achieved better glycemic control were intrinsically less susceptible to complications was not excluded.

Since the completion of Pirart's study the association between hyperglycemia and microvascular complications has been strengthened by the conclusive demonstration that complications of diabetes develop in humans with secondary forms of the disease (23). The results of several small randomized prospective trials in which tight glycemic control was achieved and of studies in which the development of complications was followed in patients in whom glucose homeostasis was normalized by a pancreatic transplant are not definitive. In the prospective trials, intensive insulin therapy for 2–3 years appeared to stabilize retinopathy and nephropathy in some patients with type I diabetes; however, in other patients these complications clearly progressed (14,70,77). Likewise, pancreas transplantation has been reported to arrest the progression of nephropathy (4) but to have no effect on retinopathy (66). It must be emphasized that the follow-up periods in all of these studies have been brief and the numbers of patients evaluated were small. In addition, many of the patients already had established microvascular disease. For the most part these limitations are specifically addressed in the Diabetes Control and Complications Trial [DCCT; (15,16)].

Studies in Experimental Animals
A second line of evidence supporting a linkage between hyperglycemia and microvascular disease derives from animal studies. Lesions in the eye (24) and kidney (20,54,67) similar to those in humans have been described in dogs (20,40), and rodents (54,67) with experimental diabetes. In a seminal series of studies, Engerman et al. [(21); Chapter 8] demonstrated that dogs with alloxan-induced diabetes of several years duration develop retinal microaneurysms, pericyte degeneration, and other changes comparable to those observed in humans with diabetic retinopathy. They further showed that intensive insulin therapy, when initiated shortly after alloxan administration, both markedly improved the glycemic status of the dogs and prevented the appearance of significant retinopathic changes. When therapy was initiated 2.5 years after alloxan administration, however, the dogs developed the same retinopathic changes as did dogs that were in poor glycemic control throughout the study (19,40). Engerman and Kern (20,40) have also demonstrated that early insulin therapy prevents the nephropathic changes that follow induction of alloxan-diabetes in the dog. Interestingly, in contrast to its lack of effect on retinopathy, intensive insulin therapy instituted 30 months after the induction of diabetes prevented the progression of these changes in the kidney (40). These studies underscore the possibility that there may be a limited period after the onset of diabetes during which improved glycemic control can prevent or reverse microvascular complications and that this time may differ for the eye and kidney. They also underscore the fact that the effect of improved glycemic control on microvascular disease will need to be examined in both primary and secondary prevention trials.

Metabolic and Biochemical Abnormalities Associated with Hyperglycemia

Additional evidence linking hyperglycemia and microvascular disease derives from studies showing that hyperglycemia per se produces many of the metabolic, biochemical, and functional abnormalities seen in diabetes. The putative interrelationships between hyperglycemia and these abnormalities and diabetic vascular disease is presented in Figure 1.2 and will be discussed in depth elsewhere in this volume. They will be mentioned here, primarily to provide a historical perspective and to give the reader a frame of reference for later chapters.

Polyol Pathway
The first of the metabolic abnormalities linking hyperglycemia with vascular and other complications of diabetes was an increase in the formation of the polyol sorbitol (Fig. 1.3). The first enzyme in the polyol pathway, aldose reductase, has a low affinity for glucose (K_m), and its activity increases as cell glucose levels increase even to very high physiological concentrations. The second enzyme in the pathway, sorbitol dehydrogenase, catalyzes the formation of fructose from sorbitol with the generation of NADH. Aldose reductase (polyol pathway), is ubiquitous and therefore polyols accumulate in nearly all tissues of diabetic animals. Likewise, the concentrations of sorbitol and fructose increase when tissues are incubated in vitro with a high concentration of glucose (Chapters 6 and 7). The importance of increased polyol formation in the pathogenesis of diabetic microvascular disease is supported by the following observations: (*1*) certain metabolic, functional, and structural abnormalities in the microvasculature of diabetic rats are prevented by administration of an inhibitor of aldose reductase (3,11,13,41,69,80,83); (*2*) polyol formation has been linked to functional and metabolic alterations analogous to those produced in diabetes in cultured vascular cells grown in an hyperglycemic medium [(50); Chapter 9]; and (*3*) chronic administration of galactose to the dog causes polyol accumulation without attendant hyperglycemia and leads to a morphological

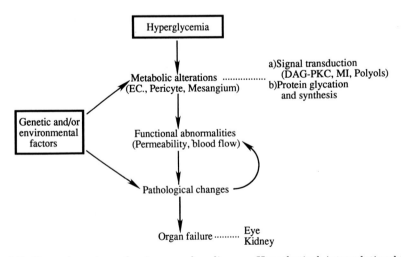

FIGURE 1.2. Hyperglycemia and microvascular disease. Hypothetical interrelationship between chronic hyperglycemia and metabolic, functional, and pathological changes in the microvasculature. EC, endothelial cell; DAG, diacylglycerol; PKC, protein kinase C; MI, *myo*-inositol.

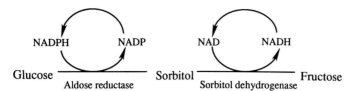

FIGURE 1.3. Aldose reductase pathway. Aldose reductase has a low affinity for glucose, and its activity increases as cell glucose levels increase to high physiological concentrations. In the lens, when flux through this pathway is increased by hyperglycemia, increases occur in intracellular sorbitol and fructose, NADH generation, and flux through the pentose shunt to regenerate NADPH [From 26 with permission.]

picture in the eye similar to that of diabetic retinopathy [(22); Chapter 8]. Interestingly, in the latter studies, galactose administration failed to produce changes in the kidney analogous to those of diabetic nephropathy, suggesting that factors in addition to an increase in polyol formation are needed for nephropathy to occur (see below). In this context several groups have pointed out the potential importance of specific hemodynamic alterations in the kidney in the pathogenesis of diabetic nephropathy (2,56,63). Whether the failure of certain of these alterations to occur accounts for the absence of nephropathy in galactose-treated dogs remains to be determined.

myo-inositol Depletion
Another metabolic abnormality linked to hyperglycemia and diabetic vascular disease is a depletion of *myo*-inositol [(85); Chapter 7]. *myo*-inositol is a normal constituent of the diet and it is also synthesized by many cells (27). It appears to play an important role in signal transduction, by virtue of the fact it is needed for the synthesis of phosphoinositides. In keeping with this notion, myo-inositol administration has been shown to diminish increases in vascular permeability, blood flow [(84); Chapter 6], and glomerular filtration (25) in diabetic rats. Winegrad and co-workers [(76,85); Chapter 7] have presented evidence that a small intracellular pool of *myo*-inositol is depleted in neural and vascular tissue as a consequence of diabetes and/or hyperglycemia. Their data suggest that this pool of *myo*-inositol is derived from extracellular *myo*-inositol and that it is specifically utilized for the synthesis of a rapidly turning over pool of phosphoinositide that is not on the classic pathway leading to PI-4,5-P_2. They have also found that the turnover of this PI pool is governed by adenosine released from the endothelium (76). According to their hypothesis, adenosine-mediated hydrolysis of this PI leads to the release of a mediator that activates $Na^+ K^+$-ATPase and thereby regulates many cell functions. Depletion of this pool of PI and a decrease in its response to adenosine both occur in diabetes, and they can be prevented by aldose reductase inhibitors [(64,85); Fig. 1.4].

Diacylglycerol, Protein Kinase C, and $Na^+ K^+$-ATPase
Most recently, hyperglycemia has been linked to alterations in the diacylglycerol–protein kinase C signaling system in the microvasculature. Studies in cultured vascular cells by King and co-workers (50,51), in rat granulation tissue

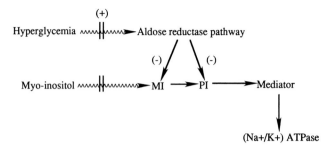

FIGURE 1.4. The *myo*-inositol depletion hypothesis. According to Winegrad [85, see also Chapter 7], an intracellular pool of *myo*-inositol derived from extracellular *myo*-inositol is utilized for the synthesis of a rapidly turning over pool of phosphatidylinositol. Adenosine-mediated hydrolysis of the phosphatidylinositol leads to the release of a mediator that activates Na^+K^+-ATPase. Hyperglycemia, by virtue of its effects on the aldose reductase pathway, is thought to inhibit this signaling mechanism by impairing *myo*-inositol transport into the cell and/or inhibiting adenosine stimulation of phosphatidylinositol hydrolysis.

by Williamson and co-workers [(89); Chapter 6] and in the glomerulus by Craven et al. (12) indicate that hyperglycemia causes an increase in diacylglycerol mass and, presumably secondary to this, an increase in protein kinase C activity (Fig. 1.5). Protein kinase C affects a variety of cell processes, including ion transport, DNA synthesis, receptor function, and smooth muscle contraction (60,90); therefore, alterations in its activity would be expected to have a significant impact. Whether alterations in protein kinase C in diabetes are linked to alterations in polyol and *myo*-inositol metabolism secondary to hyperglycemia is unclear [Chapters 6 and 9; (11,50,51,84)]. Also unclear is how changes

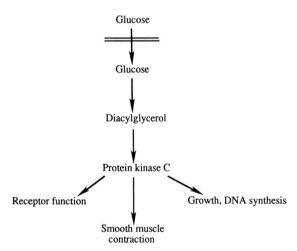

FIGURE 1.5. Hyperglycemia and the DAG-PKC signaling system. Hyperglycemia causes an increase in diacylglycerol content in many cells, probably by enhancing its de novo synthesis. In vascular cells this is associated with an increase in membrane-associated (activated) protein kinase C (51). The precise metabolic effects of such an increase in protein kinase C remain to be determined.

in protein kinase C relate to the decrease in Na^+K^+-ATPase found in various tissues of diabetic animals (27) and in cells grown in a hyperglycemic milieu (50). As reviewed elsewhere in this volume (Chapter 9), protein kinase C activity appears to be increased under these conditions. However, addition of a phorbol ester to activate protein kinase C further, restores Na^+K^+-ATPase activity to control values (27).

Protein Glycation
Abnormalities in polyol metabolism, *myo*-inositol transport, and diacylglycerol formation presumably would affect vascular function due to their effects on signal transduction. A second mechanism by which hyperglycemia could alter vascular structure and function is by increasing protein glycation. The studies of Cerami and Gallop and co-workers established that glucose slowly interacts with free amino groups on proteins to form Schiff bases, which can then undergo an Amadori rearrangement to yield fructosamine [(5); Fig. 1.6]. Similar reactions have been shown to occur when proteins interact with other hexoses, e.g. fructose, or with various hexose and triose phosphates. In the case of glucose, the extent to which the Amadori product forms appears to be a function of the ambient concentration of glucose and the life-span of a protein in the circulation or tissue. Based on this phenomenon, an assay for glycosylated hemoglobin (HbAic) has been developed to provide physicians with a quantitative measure of the average blood glucose concentration over the preceding 8–12 weeks (59).

Recently a number of investigators have shown that the reaction leading to the formation of Amadori products is slowly reversible [(5); Chapter 12]. In addition, it has been shown that in the presence of O_2 (Chapter 11), the Amadori products can themselves undergo further irreversible changes to form molecules able to cause cross-linking of proteins (Maillard reaction) [(8); Chapters 11 and 12]. Such molecules are commonly referred to as advanced glycosylation end products (AGE), and they have been implicated in the development of diabetic complications in many tissues (5). Long-lived proteins such as collagen are most affected by AGE and develop multiple cross-links due to their presence. The increased stiffness and diminished digestibility of arterial collagen in diabetes has been attributed to AGE (Chapters 12 and 14). Likewise, AGE have been shown to alter the structure of basement membrane collagen so that its ability to self-associate and to interact with other basement membrane components (eg. heparan SO_4) is impaired (Chapter 14). The association of such cross-linked collagen with a variety of other proteins, including circulating immunoglobulins and lipoproteins, appears to be quite different

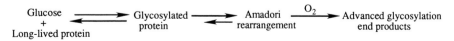

FIGURE 1.6. Formation of advanced glycosylation end products (AGE). The magnitude of AGE formation appears to be a function of the ambient glucose concentration and the half-life of the protein or DNA molecule that is glycated [5,6, Chapter 12]. Macrophages possess specific receptors for AGE and may be involved in their removal from tissues (Chapter 13).

from that of normal collagen [(5); Chapter 12]. The metabolism of AGE is not well understood; however, recent investigations by Vlassara and co-workers suggest that the macrophage possesses specific receptors for AGE and may be involved in their removal from tissues (Chapter 13).

Hyperglycemia and Microvascular Disease: Current Perspectives

The available clinical, metabolic, and biochemical evidence provides a compelling case for an etiological role of hyperglycemia in the pathogenesis of diabetic microvascular disease. This view is widely held in the diabetes community, although it is recognized that definitive proof is still lacking. In keeping with this assessment, the Diabetes Control and Complications Trial was initiated in 1983 (15,16). To date, over 1,400 patients in 28 centers have been enrolled in the study. Patients with type I diabetes were randomly divided into groups receiving standard (1–2 injections of insulin/day), and intensive (multiple blood glucose determinations and 3 or more injections/day or insulin by infusion pump) insulin therapy. To determine the impact of tight glycemic control on both primary and secondary prevention, the patients were further subdivided into those in whom diabetes was diagnosed within the preceding month and those in whom it was known to be present for several years. The four groups are being followed closely for early clinical manifestations of retinopathy and nephropathy, and the results will be correlated with serial measurements of glycosylated hemoglobin and other indices of long-term glycemic control. This randomized prospective trial will be completed in 1993.

Studies such as the DCCT may establish more conclusively the connection between hyperglycemia and microvascular disease and whether tight glycemic control should be initiated near the time of onset of diabetes for maximal benefit. At the same time, such studies will leave numerous questions unanswered. For instance, why are certain microvascular beds such as those in the retina and kidney subject to diabetic complications when to our knowledge the cerebral microvasculature is relatively unaffected [(85); Chapter 5]? Likewise, why are 20% of patients with type I diabetes spared from microvascular complications despite poor glycemic control over many years, whereas others with relatively mild-modest hyperglycemia may develop severe retinopathy or nephropathy within a few years (reviews in 70, 77)? Such findings suggest that important environmental influences, e.g. dietary protein, as well as genetic factors could interact with hyperglycemia to cause microvascular complications. Of interest in this regard are recent reports suggesting that nephropathy develops predominantly in those patients with diabetes who have a family history of hypertension (47,73). Whether the requirement of an inherited predisposition to hypertension for it to develop accounts for the lower incidence of nephropathy than of retinopathy in patients with type I diabetes (see above) remains to be determined.

HYPERGLYCEMIA AND MACROVASCULAR DISEASE

Clinical and Epidemiological Studies

The relationship between hyperglycemia and macrovascular disease in patients with diabetes is complex. An association between asymptomatic hyperglycemia and coronary heart disease has been demonstrated in both middle-aged (36) and elderly (17,58) people. However, interpretation of the data is confounded by the fact that patients with even mild diabetes often have hypertension, dyslipoproteinemias, and other factors that put them at risk for coronary heart disease. That hyperglycemia may not by itself be the cause of atherosclerosis is suggested by data from population studies indicating that diabetes increases atherosclerosis primarily in populations in which its prevalence is already high (68,72). In keeping with this notion, Pirart found that no clear-cut relationship could be established between the average magnitude of hyperglycemia (as far as this could be ascertained) and the prevalence of atherosclerotic vascular disease in his patient population (65). Because of such findings, the clinical and epidemiological data linking hyperglycemia to macrovascular disease in diabetes cannot be considered compelling [(1); Chapter 2]. Nevertheless the data are consistent with the possibility that hyperglycemia accelerates atherosclerosis in patients who are already at some risk. Thus, in a number of studies, when the effect of most standard risk factors is taken into account, patients with hyperglycemia are still at greater risk for coronary heart disease [(17,45,77); Chapter 2].

Additional insight into whether hyperglycemia is a risk factor for atherosclerosis in an intact organism will require both the development of animal models (9) and studies in subgroups of diabetic patients in whom other risk factors are no different from those of the general population. With respect to the latter, it is of interest that Krolewski et al. (48) have observed that type I diabetics without renal disease or significant dyslipoproteinemia have at least a 3–4-fold greater incidence of coronary heart disease than the general population. Whether subtle disturbances in lipoproteins (3,28,34) or an as yet unidentified risk factor accounts for this remains to be determined. Nevertheless, these findings raise the possibility that hyperglycemia may be a more dominant risk factor in this subgroup of patients with diabetes. They also suggest that such type I diabetics without renal disease may be the optimal target population for examining the role of hyperglycemia in the pathogenesis of diabetic macrovascular disease.

Parallel Changes in the Micro- and Macrovasculature

Perhaps the strongest evidence that hyperglycemia plays a role on the pathogenesis of macrovascular disease in diabetes are the numerous parallelisms between changes in arteries and renal and retinal microvessels in this disorder. Shared pathological features include extravasation of plasma proteins, expanded extracellular matrix, and cellular hyperplasia (Chapter 12). Even more impressive are the shared metabolic features. Essentially all the metabolic alterations and a number of the functional abnormalities in the microvasculature attributed to hyperglycemia have also been observed in arteries (Fig. 1.7).

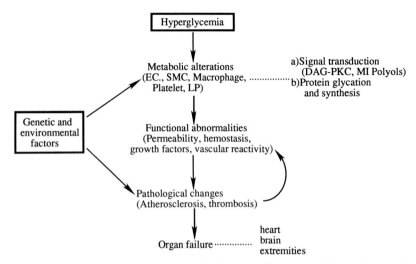

FIGURE 1.7. Hyperglycemia and macrovascular disease. Hypothetical interrelationships between metabolic, functional, and pathological changes. According to proposed schema, early
metabolic and biochemical alterations secondary to hyperglycemia are similar in the micro-
and macrovasculature. SMC, smooth muscle cells; LP, lipoproteins; EC, endothelial cell; DAG,
diacylglycerol; PKC, protein kinase C; MI, *myo*-inositol.

Furthermore, these metabolic alterations cause changes in vascular function
that could easily be atherogenic. Thus, alterations in polyol and *myo*-inositol
metabolism have been implicated both in the increased permeability and decreased Na^+K^+-ATPase activity in the aortas of diabetic animals [(84,85);
Chapters 6 and 7]. Likewise, a myriad of potentially atherogenic effects of protein glycation have been described. These include alterations in the function
of platelets (Chapter 3), smooth muscle cells (Chapter 9), endothelial cells
(Chapters 9 and 13), and macrophages (Chapter 13), and changes in the structure of arterial collagen that enhance its affinity for low density lipoproteins
and other circulating proteins [(5,6); Chapter 12]. As mentioned earlier, glycation leading to cross-linking of collagen also appears to alter the association
of collagen with heparan SO_4 and other substances in the vascular wall (Chapters 14 and 15). In addition, protein glycation has been shown to alter the
metabolism and immnogenecity of low-density lipoproteins (88). Recent studies demonstrating that hexoses, hexose phosphate, and triose phosphate can
cause cross-linking of nuclear DNA suggest yet another mechanism by which
hyperglycemia could alter cell structure and function (8). The relationship of
such AGE-induced cross-linking of DNA to increases in the mRNA and synthesis of type IV collagen, fibronectin, and other molecules by diabetes and
hyperglycemia [(71); Chapters 9 and 12] remains to be determined.

Hyperglycemia and Macrovascular Disease: Current Perspectives

Nearly every known component of the atherogenic process can be affected by
hyperglycemia. Despite this fact, the relationship between hyperglycemia and
the development of macrovascular disease in patients with diabetes remains

uncertain. As noted earlier, the presence of other risk factors for atherosclerosis in many patients with diabetes and the lack of a suitable animal model in which diabetes accelerates atherosclerosis account for this difficulty. Nephropathy is closely associated with accelerated atherosclerosis in the diabetic (37,49). It is unclear, however, whether the nephropathy accelerates atherosclerosis or is simply a consequence of the same causal factor, e.g. injury to the vascular wall. Whatever the interrelationship, to the extent that control of hyperglycemia prevents or retards the development of nephropathy, it would be expected to diminish the large blood vessel consequences of diabetes.

Vascular Reactivity and Endothelial Cell–Derived Vasoactive Factors (EDRF)

The discussion till now has focused on the possible contribution of hyperglycemia to the pathogenesis of premature atherosclerotic vascular disease in diabetes. In addition, Cohen and co-workers (Chapter 4) have shown that hyperglycemia stimulates the production of vasoconstrictor prostanoids by the rabbit aorta and may concurrently inhibit the generation of an endothelial cell–derived relaxation factor (EDRF). Similar changes were observed in aortas from diabetic rabbits. Preliminary data suggest that these effects may be related to alterations in myo-inositol and polyol metabolism (Chapter 4) and Na^+K^+-ATPase (29). Whatever the mechanism, the contribution of altered vascular relaxation to vasospasm-induced ischemia in patients with diabetes is clearly a subject for further study.

Also warranting attention is the possibility that hyperglycemia, by altering the release of endothelial-derived relaxation or constrictive factors, contributes to the pathogenesis of hypertension in patients with diabetes. In this context, inhibition of endothelium-induced relaxation by specific agents has been shown to cause hypertension in experimental animals (81). Likewise, abnormalities in endothelium-dependent vascular relaxation have been observed in patients with essential hypertension (62). The relationship of endothelium-dependent relaxation and constriction factors to hypertension in diabetes has not been specifically studied; however, abnormalities have been noted in arteries of diabetic rats (28,30,39) and in penile smooth muscle of diabetic men with impotence (74). In addition, quenching of the endothelium-derived relaxation factor, nitric oxide, by advanced glycosylation end-products has recently been described (7). Studies of the generation of relaxation and constriction factors by microvascular endothelium, and the effect on it of diabetes and hyperglycemia will be of considerable interest.

CONCLUDING REMARKS

The evidence linking hyperglycemia to micro- and macrovascular disease in patients with diabetes has been examined. From our perspective, the data are consistent with the view that hyperglycemia can produce metabolic biochemical and functional alterations in both the micro- and macrovasculature. A reasonable case can also be made to show that these alterations play a role in the pathogenesis of diabetic microvascular disease. The concurrence of the diabetes community with this perception is perhaps most evident by its initiation of the ongoing Diabetes Control and Complications Trial (15).

The relationship between hyperglycemia and atherosclerosis is less clear. Similar biochemical and metabolic abnormalities occur in the macro- and microvasculature in diabetes. Nevertheless, the presence of other risk factors, the lack of an animal model in which diabetes accelerates atherosclerosis, and the greater complexity of atherosclerosis than microvascular disease have made the relationship more difficult to evaluate. Perhaps what is most clear is that establishing such a linkage, and explaining its metabolic and biochemical basis would have a profound impact on our therapeutic approaches to diabetes.

ACKNOWLEDGMENTS

This work was supported in part by U.S.P.H.S. grant AM-39814, a mentor-based training grant from the American Diabetes Association, and a donation from the Cogan Trust.

REFERENCES

1. AMERICAN DIABETES ASSOCIATION. Role of cardiovascular risk factors in prevention and treatment of macrovascular disease in diabetes. *Diabetes Care* 12: 573–579, 1989, Consensus S.
2. ANDERSON, S., and BRENNER, B. Pathogenesis of diabetic nephropathy: hemodynamic considerations. *Diabetes/Metab. Rev.* 4: 163–177, 1988.
3. BEYER-MEARS, A., CRUZ, E., EDELIST, T., and VARAGLANNIS, F. Diminished proteinuria in diabetes mellitus by sorbinil, an aldose reductase inhibitor. *Pharmacology* 32: 52–60, 1986.
4. BILOUS, R. W., STEFFES, M. W., GOETZ, F. C., SUTHERLAND, D. M., and MAUER S. M. Pancreas transplantation for more than two years ameliorates glomerular pathology in insulin-dependent diabetic patients. *N. Engl. J. Med.* 321: 8580–8585, 1989.
5. BROWNLEE, M., CERAMI, A., and VLASSARA, H. Advanced glycosylation end products in tissue and the biochemical basis of diabetic complications. *N. Engl. J. Med.* 318: 1315–1321, 1988.
6. BROWNLEE, M., CERAMI, A., and VLASSARA, H. Advanced products of nonenzymatic glycosylation and the pathogenesis of diabetic vascular disease. *Diabetes/Metab. Rev.* 4: 437–451.
7. BUCALA, R., TRACEY, K. J., and CERAMI, A. Advanced glycosylation products quench nitric oxide and mediate defective endothelium-dependent vasodilatation in experimental diabetes. *J. Clin. Invest.* 87: 432–438, 1991.
8. CERAMI, A., VLASSARA, H., and BROWNLEE, M. Role of advanced glycosylation products in complications of diabetes. *Diabetes Care* 11 (Suppl. 1): 3–79, 1988.
9. CHOBANIAN, A. V., ARGUILLA, E. R., CLARKSON, T. B., EDER, H. A., HOWARD, C. F., REGAN, T. J., and WILLIAMSON, J. R. Proceedings on a task force on animals appropriate for studying diabetes mellitus and its complications. *Diabetes* 31(Suppl 1): 54–64, 1982.
10. CHRISTIANSEN, J. S., GAMMELGAARD, J., TRONIER, B., SVENDSEN, P. A., and PARVING, H. H. Kidney function and size in diabetes before and during initial insulin treatment. *Kidney Int.* 21: 683–688, 1982.
11. CRAVEN, P. A., and DERUBERTIS, F. R. Sorbinil suppresses glomerular prostaglandin production in the streptozotocin diabetic rat. *Metabolism* 38: 649–654, 1989.
12. CRAVEN, P. A., DAVIDSON, C. M., and DERUBERTIS, F. R. Increase in deacylglycerol mass in isolated glomeruli by glucose from de novo synthesis of glycerolipids. *Diabetes* 39: 667–674, 1990.
13. COHEN, M. D. Aldose reductase glomerular metabolism and diabetic nephropathy *Metabolism* 35(Suppl 1): 55–59, 1986.
14. DAVIS, M. D. Diabetic retinopathy: a clinical overview. *Diabetes/Metab. Rev.* 4: 291–321, 1988.
15. DCCT RESEARCH GROUP. Diabetes Control and Complications Trial (DCCT): update *Diabetes Care* 13: 427–433, 1990.

16. DCCT RESEARCH GROUP. Diabetes Control and Complications Trial (DCCT): results of feasibility study. *Diabetes Care* 10: 1–19, 1987.

17. DONAHUE, R. R., ABBOTT, R. D., REED, D. M., and YANO, K. Postchallenge glucose concentration and coronary heart disease in men of Japanese ancestry. Honolulu Heart Program. *Diabetes* 36: 689–692, 1985.

18. DRURY, P. L. Diabetes and arterial hypertension. *Diabetologia* 24: 1–9, 1983.

19. ENGERMAN, R. L., and KERN, T. S. Progression of diabetic retinopathy during good glycemic control. *Diabetes* 36: 808–812, 1987.

20. ENGERMAN, R. L., and KERN, T. S. Hyperglycemia and the development of glomerular pathology: diabetes compared with galactosemia. *Kidney Int.* 36: 41–45, 1988.

21. ENGERMAN, R. L., BLOODWORTH, J. M. B., and NELSON, S. Relationship of microvascular disease to metabolic control. *Diabetes* 26: 760–769, 1977.

22. ENGERMAN, R. L., and KERN, T. S. Experimental galactosemia produces diabetic-like retinopathy. *Diabetes* 33: 97–100, 1984.

23. FEINGOLD, K. R., LEE, T. H., CHUNG, M. U., and SIPERSTEIN, M. D. Muscle capillary basement membrane width in patients with vacor-induced diabetes. *J. Clin. Invest.* 78: 102–107, 1986.

24. FRIEDMAN, E. Diabetic renal disease. In: *Ellenberg and Rifkins Diabetes Mellitus, Theory and Practice,* 4 Ed., edited by H. Rifkin and D. Porte. New York: Elsevier, 1990, pp. 684–709.

25. GOLDFARB, S., SIMMONS, D. A., and KERN, E. F. O. Amelioration of glomerular hyperfiltration in acute experimental diabetes mellitus by dietary *myo*-inositol supplementation and aldose reductase inhibition. *Trans. Assoc. Am. Physicians* 99: 67–72, 1986.

26. GONZALEZ, A.-M., SOCHOR, M., HOTERSALL, J. S., and MCLEAN, P. Effect of aldose reductase inhibitor (sorbinil) on integration of polyol pathway, pentose phosphate pathway and glycolytic route in diabetic lens. *Diabetes* 35: 1200–1205, 1986.

27. GREENE, D. A., LATTIMER, S. A., and SIMAN, A. A. F. Sorbitol, phosphoinositides and sodium-potassium-ATPase in the pathogenesis of diabetic complications. *N. Engl. J. Med.* 316: 599–606, 1987.

28. GRYGLEWSKI, R., BOTTING, R. M., and VANE, J. R. Mediators produced by the endothelial cell. *Hypertension* 62: 185–190, 1988.

29. GUPTA, S., COHEN, R., and SUSSMAN, I. Endothelium-dependent inhibition of vascular NaK ATPase activity by high glucose. *Diabetes* 39: 31A, 1990.

30. HARRIS, K. H., and MACLEOD, K. M. Influence of the endothelium on contractile responses of arteries from diabetic rats. *Eur. J. Pharmacol.* 153: 55–64, 1988.

31. HERMAN, W. H., and TEUTSCH, S. M. Kidney diseases associated with diabetes. In: *Diabetes in America, Diabetes Data Compiled 1984,* edited by National Diabetes Data Group. Washington, DC: U.S. Government Printing Office, NIH Publication 85-1468, 1985, Chapter XIV, pp. 1–31.

32. HORAN, M. J. Diabetes and hypertension. In: *Diabetes in America, Diabetes Data Compiled 1984,* edited by National Diabetes Data Group. Washington, DC: U.S. Government Printing Office, NIH Publication 85-1468, Chapter XVII, pp. 1–22.

33. IRELAND, J. T., VIBERTI, G. C., and WATKINS, P. J. The kidney and renal tract. In: *Complications of Diabetes,* 2 Ed., edited by H. Keen and J. Jarrett. London: E. J. Arnold, 1982, pp. 137–178.

34. IWAL, M., YOSHINO, G., MATSUSHITA, M., MORITA, M., MATSUBA, K., KAZUMI, T., and BABA, S. Abnormal lipoprotein composition in normolipidemic diabetic patients. *Diabetes Care* 13: 792–796, 1990.

35. JARRETT, R. J. Cardiovascular disease and hypertension in diabetes mellitus. *Diabetes/Metab. Rev.* 5: 547–557, 1989.

36. JARRETT, R. J., MCCARTNEY, P., and KEEN, H. The Bedford survey: Ten year mortality rates in newly diagnosed diabetics, borderline diabetics and normoglycemic controls and risk indices for coronary heart disease in borderline diabetics. *Diabetologia* 22: 79–84, 1982.

37. JENSEN, T., BORCH-JOHNSON, K., KOFOED-ENEVOLDSEN, A., and DECKERT, T. Coronary heart disease in young type I (insulin-dependent) diabetic patients with and without diabetic nephropathy: incidence and risk factors. *Diabetologia* 30: 144–148, 1987.

38. KANNEL, W. B., and MCGEE, D. L. Diabetes and cardiovascular disease: the Framingham Study. *JAMA* 241: 2035–2038, 1979.

39. KAMATA, K., MIYATA, N., and KASUYA, Y. Impairment of endothelium-dependent relaxation and changes in levels of cGMP in aorta from streptozotocin-induced diabetic rats. *Br. J. Pharmacol.* 97: 614–618, 1989.

40. KERN, T. S., and ENGERMAN, R. L. Arrest of glomerulopathy in diabetic dogs by improved glycemic control. *Diabetes* 39(Suppl. 1): 34A, 1990.

41. KINOSHITA, J. H., DATILES, M. B., KADOR, P. F., and ROBISON, W. G. Aldose reductase and diabetic eye complications. In: *Ellenberg and Rifkins Diabetes Mellitus, Theory and Practice,* 4 Ed., edited by H. Rifkin and D. Porte. New York: Elsevier, 1990, pp. 264–278.

42. KLEIN, R., and KLEIN, B. E. K. Vision disorders in diabetes. In: *Diabetes in America, Diabetes Data Compiled 1984,* edited by National Diabetes Data Group. Washington, DC: U.S. Government Printing Office, NIH Publication 85-1468, 1985, Chapter XIII, pp. 1–36.

43. KLEIN, R., KLEIN, B. E. K., and MOSS, S. E. The Wisconsin Epidemiological Study of Diabetic Retinopathy. *Diabetes/Metab. Rev.* 5: 559–570, 1989.

44. KNOWLES, H. C. JR. The problem of the relationship of the control of diabetes to the development of vascular disease. *Trans. Am. Clin. Climatol. Assn.* 76: 142–147, 1964.

45. KNUIMAN, M. W., WELBORN, T. A., MCCANN, U. S., STANTON, K. D., and CONSTABLE, I. J. Prevalence of diabetic complications in relation to risk factors. *Diabetes* 35: 1332–1339, 1986.

46. KOHNER, E. M., MCLEOD, D., and MARSHALL, J. Diabetic eye disease. In: *Complications of Diabetes,* edited by H. Keen and J. Jarrett. London: E. J. Arnold, 1982, pp. 19–108.

47. KROLEWSKI, A. S., CANESSA, M., WARRAM, J. H., LAFFEL, L. M. B., CHRISTLIEB, A. R., KNOWLER, W. C., and RAND, L. I. Predisposition to hypertension and susceptibility to renal disease in insulin-dependent diabetes mellitus. *N. Engl. J. Med.* 318: 140–145, 1988.

48. KROLEWSKI, A. S., KOSINSKI, E. J., WARRAM, J. H., LETAND, O. S., BUSICK, E., ASMAL, A. C., RAND, L. I., CHRISTLIEB, A. R., BRADLEY, R. F., and KAHN, C. R. Magnitude and determinants of coronary artery disease in juvenile-onset, insulin-dependent diabetes mellitus. *Am. J. Cardiol.* 59: 750–755, 1987.

49. KROLEWSKI, A. S., WARRAM, J. H., RAND, L. I., and KAHN, C. R. Epidemiological approach to the etiology of type I diabetes and its complications. *N. Engl. J. Med.* 317: 1390–1398, 1987.

50. LEE, T. S., MACGREGOR, L. C., FLUHARTY, S. J., and KING, G. L. Differential regulation of protein kinase C and (Na,K) adenosine triphosphatase activities by elevated glucose levels in retinal capillary endothelial cells. *J. Clin. Invest.* 83: 90–94, 1989.

51. LEE, T. S., SALTSMAN, K. A., ONASHI, H., and KING, G. L. Activation of protein kinase C by elevation of glucose concentration. Proposal for a mechanism in the development of diabetic vascular complications. *Proc. Natl. Acad. Sci. U.S.A.* 86: 5141–5145, 1989.

52. L'ESPERANCE, F. A., JAMES, W. A., and JUDSON, P. H. The eye and diabetes mellitus. In: *Ellenberg and Rifkins, Diabetes Mellitus, Theory and Practice,* 4th Ed. Edited by H. Rifkin and D. Porte. New York: Elsevier, 1990, pp. 661–683.

53. MANGILI, R., BENDING, J. J., SCOTT, G., LI, L. K., GUPTA, A., and VIBERTI, G. C. Increased sodium-lithium countertransport activity in red cells of patients with insulin-dependent diabetes and nephropathy. *N. Engl. J. Med.* 318: 146–150, 1988.

54. MAUER, S. M., STEFFES, M. W., SUTHERLAND, D. E. R., NAJARIAN, J. S., MICHAEL, A. F., and BROWN, D. M. Studies of the rate of regression of the glomerular lesions in diabetic rats treated with pancreatic islet transplantation. *Diabetes* 24: 280–285, 1975.

55. MOGENSEN, C. E., and ANDERSON, M. J. F. Increased kidney size and glomerular filtration rate in untreated juvenile diabetes: normalization by insulin treatment. *Diabetologia* 11: 221–224, 1975.

56. MOGENSEN, C. E., SCHMITZ, A., and CHRISTENSEN, C. R. Comparative renal pathophysiology relevant to IDDM and NIDDM patients. *Diabetes/Metab. Rev.* 4: 453–483, 1988.

57. MORAN, A., BROWN, D. M., KIM, Y., and KLEIN, D. J. The effects of IGF-I and hyperglycemia on protein and proteoglycan synthesis in human fetal mesangial cells. *Diabetes* 39(Suppl 11): 70A, 1990.

58. MYKKANEN, L., VUSITUPA, M., and PYORALA, K. Asymptomatic hyperglycemia is associated with an increased prevalence of coronary heart disease in the elderly. *Diabetes* 39(Suppl. 11): 38A, 1990.

59. NATHAN, D. M., SINGER, D. E., and HURXTHAL, K. The clinical information value of the glycosylated hemoglobin assay. *N. Engl. J. Med.* 310: 341–346, 1984.

60. NISHIZUKA, Y. The role of protein kinase C in cell surface signal transduction and tumour promotion. *Nature* 308: 693–697, 1984.

61. OSTERBY, R. Basement membrane morphology in diabetes mellitus. In: *Ellenberg and Rifkins, Diabetes Mellitus, Theory and Practice,* 4 Ed., edited by H. Rifkin and D. Porte. New York: Elsevier, 1990, pp. 220–233.

62. PANZA, J. A., QUYYUMI, A. A., BRUSH, J. E. JR., and EPSTEIN, S. E. Abnormal endothelium dependent vascular relaxation in patients with essential hypertension. *N. Engl. J. Med.* 233: 22–27, 1990.

63. PARVING, H. H., VIBERTI, G. C., KAN, H., CHRISTIANSEN, J. S., and LASSEN, N. A. Hemody-

namic factors in the genetics of diabetic microangiopathy. *Metabolism* 32: 943–949, 1983.

64. PERLMUTTER, J., JACOBS, J., ZIYADEG, F., SENESKY, D., SIMMONS, D. A., KERN, E. F. D., and GOLDFARB, S. Reduced renal vasoconstrictive response to adenosine and reversal by aldose reductase inhibition in acute experimental diabetes. *Clin. Res.* 37: 583A, 1989.

65. PIRART, J. Diabetes mellitus and its degenerative complications. A prospective study of 4400 patients observed between 1947 and 1973. *Diabetes Care* 1: 168–188, 252–263, 1978.

66. RAMSAY, R. C., GOETZ, F. C., SUTHERLAND, D. E. R., MAUER, S. M., ROBINSON, L. L., CANTRILL, H. L., KNOWBLACH, W. H., and NAJARIAN, J. S. Progression of diabetic retinopathy after pancreas transplantation for insulin-dependent diabetes mellitus. *N. Engl. J. Med.* 318: 208–214, 1988.

67. RASCH, R. Studies on the prevention of glomerulopathy in diabetic rats. *Acta Endocrinol.* (Suppl. 242): 43–44, 1981.

68. ROBERTSON, W. B., and STRONG, J. P. Atherosclerosis in persons with hypertension and diabetes mellitus. *Lab. Invest.* 18: 538–551, 1968.

69. ROBISON, W. G., JR., NAGATA, M., LAVER, N., HOHMAN, T. C., and KONSHITA, J. H. Diabetic-like retinopathy in rats prevented with an aldose reductase inhibitor. *Invest. Ophthalmol. Vis. Sci.* 30: 2285–2292, 1989.

70. ROSENSTOCK, J., and RASKIN, P. Diabetes and its complications: blood glucose control vs. genetic susceptibility. *Diabetes/Metab. Rev.* 4: 417–436, 1988.

71. ROY, S., SALA, R., CAGLIERO, E., and LORENZI, M. Overexpression of fibronectin induced by diabetes or high glucose: phenomenon with a memory. *Proc. Natl. Acad. Sci. U.S.A.* 87: 404–408, 1990.

72. RUDERMAN, N. B., and HAUDENSCHILD, C. Diabetes as an atherogenic factor. *Prog. Cardiovasc. Dis.* 26: 373–412, 1984.

73. SEAQUIST, E. R., GOETZ, F. C., RICH, S., and BARBOSA, J. Familial clustering of diabetic kidney disease. Evidence for genetic susceptibility to diabetic nephropathy. *N. Engl. J. Med.* 320: 1161–1165, 1989.

74. SAENZ DE TEJADA, I., GOLDSTEIN, I., ASADZO, I. K., KRANE, R. J., and COHEN, R. A. Impaired neurogenic and endothelium mediated relaxation of penile smooth muscle from diabetic men with impotence. *N. Engl. J. Med.* 320: 1025–1030, 1989.

75. SIMMONS, D. A., KERN, E. F. O., WINEGRAD, A. I., and MARTIN, D. B. Basal phosphatidylinositol turnover controls aortic (Na^+/K^+) ATPase activity. *J. Clin. Invest.* 77: 503–513, 1986.

76. SIMMONS, D. A., and WINEGRAD, A. I. Mechanism of glucose induced (Na^+/K^+) ATPase inhibition in aortic wall of rabbits. *Diabetologia* 22: 402–408, 1989.

77. SKYLER, J. S. Relations of metabolic control of diabetes mellitus to chronic complications. In: *Ellenberg and Rifkins, Diabetes Mellitus, Theory and Practice,* 4 Ed., edited by H. Rifkin and D. Porte. New York: Elsevier, 1990, pp. 856–868.

78. STAMLER, J. Epidemiology: established major risk factors and the primary prevention of coronary heart diseases. In: *Cardiology,* edited by W. Parmley and K. Chatterjee. Philadelphia: Lippincott, 1987, pp. 1–41.

79. STOUT, R. W. Blood glucose and atherosclerosis. *Atherosclerosis* 1: 227–234, 1981.

80. TILTON, R. G., CHANG, K., PUGLIESE, G., EADES, D. M., PROVINCE, M. A., SHERMAN, W. R., KILO, C., and WILLIAMSON, J. R. Prevention of hemodynamic and vascular albumin filtration changes in diabetic rats by aldose reductase inhibitors. *Diabetes* 37: 1258–1270, 1989.

81. VANE, J. R., ANGGARD, E. E., and BLOTTING, R. M. Regulatory functions of the vascular endothelium. *N. Engl. J. Med.* 323: 27–36, 1990.

82. VIBERTI, G. C., and WALKER, J. D. Diabetic nephropathy: etiology and prevention. *Diabetes/Metab. Rev.* 4: 147–162, 1988.

83. WILLIAMS, C. L., HEATH, W., and STRAMM, L. Retinal pericyte proteoglycan metabolism: modulation by protein kinase C. *Diabetes* 39 (Suppl. 11): 32A, 1990.

84. WILLIAMSON, J. R., TILTON, R. G., CHANG, K., and KILO, C. Basement membrane abnormalities in diabetes mellitus: relationship to clinical microangiopathy. *Diabetes/Metab. Rev.* 4: 339–369, 1988.

85. WINEGRAD, A. I. Does a common mechanism induce the diverse complications of diabetes? *Diabetes* 36: 396–406, 1987.

86. WISEMAN, M. J., SAUNDERS, A. J., KEEN, H., and VIBERTI, G. C. Effect of blood glucose control on increased glomerular filtration rate and kidney size in insulin-dependent diabetes. *N. Engl. J. Med.* 312: 617–621, 1988.

87. WOLF, B. A., WILLIAMSON, J. R., EASOM, R. A., CHANG, K., SHERMAN, W. R., and TURK, J.

Diacylglycerol accumulation and microvascular abnormalities induced by elevated glucose levels. *J. Clin. Invest.* 85: 482–490, 1990.

88. WITZTUM, J. L., STEINBRECHER, U. P., KESANIEMI, Y. A., and FISHER, M. Autoantibodies to glucosylated proteins in the plasma of patients with diabetes mellitus. *Proc. Natl. Acad. Sci, USA* 81: 3204–3208, 1984.

89. WOODGETT, J. R., HUNTER, T., and GOULD, K. Protein kinase C and its role in cell growth. In: *Cell Membranes: Methods and Reviews,* edited by E. Elson. New York: Plenum Press, pp. 215–340, 1987.

90. WORLD HEALTH ORGANIZATION MULTINATIONAL STUDY OF VASCULAR DISEASE IN DIABETES. Prevalence of small vessel and large vessel disease in diabetic patients from 14 centers. *Diabetologia* 28: 615–640, 1985.

2

Epidemiology of Hyperglycemia and Atherosclerosis

PETER W. F. WILSON AND WILLIAM B. KANNEL

For three decades in the United States there has been a major decline in atherosclerotic cardiovascular mortality. It is clear, however, that control or prevention of diabetes has not contributed significantly to this decline since the National Health and Nutrition Examination Survey (NHANES) indicates a continued high prevalence of diabetes, largely undetected, among the general population (2). Despite improved diagnostic methods and better treatment, physicians continue to encounter a high rate of atherosclerotic cardiovascular sequelae in their diabetic patients.

This chapter examines the occurrence of diabetes, its precursors, associated cardiovascular risk factors, and the net and joint contribution of impaired glucose tolerance to the development of atherosclerotic cardiovascular disease. It is based on 30 years of follow-up of the Framingham study, a cohort of 5,209 men and women who were examined biennially for new development of cardiovascular disease in relation to antecedent risk factor levels.

METHODS

The Framingham Heart Study was initiated in 1948 and included 5,209 men and women 30–62 years of age who were followed for the occurrence of cardiovascular disease. Participants were seen in the clinic every two years. At each visit a history was obtained and a physical examination was performed (8).

Blood was drawn for glucose at all biennial clinic visits (except visits 5, 7, and 11), and the Somogyi-Nelson method was used for determination of glucose in whole blood (10). Participants were classified as diabetic at a given visit if any of the following criteria were met: (1) if casual blood glucose levels exceeded 150 mg/dl on two clinic visits, (2) if a positive glucose tolerance test (100 gm oral glucose load after 12 h fast with glucose $\geqslant$ 160 mg/dl or more at 1 h, $\geqslant$ 140 at 2 h, and at a level still higher at 3 h than when the test began) had been obtained by a local physician, or (3) if insulin or oral hypoglycemic agents had been prescribed (8).

Glucose intolerance was diagnosed if blood sugar levels at the clinic visits were above 120 mg/dl but less than 150 mg/dl on two separate occasions. Glycosuria was diagnosed in the clinic with Clinitest tablets during the first ten biennial exams and with Ames Combustix thereafter (8).

Cholesterol was determined in the serum at biennial exams beginning early in the study. At exam 11, a full fasting lipid profile was performed, with measurement of plasma cholesterol, high-density lipoprotein (HDL)-cholesterol after heparin-manganese precipitation (9), ultracentrifugation of specimens with measurement of bottom fraction cholesterol, and calculation of low-density lipoprotein (LDL)-cholesterol and very low-density lipoprotein (VLDL)-cholesterol by subtraction (9). Fibrinogen was measured at exam 10 after a modification of the Ratnoff method (12).

RESULTS

A comparison of the levels of risk factors in diabetics versus nondiabetics attending the eleventh biennial exam in 1972 is given in Table 2.1 for men and women. Casual glucose levels, systolic blood pressure, body mass index (BMI), and prevalence of left ventricular hypertrophy are all greater in diabetic men and women ($p < 0.001$ in all instances after age adjustment). There was no difference in the prevalence of cigarette smoking between diabetics and nondiabetics.

Mean age-adjusted lipid levels for the same group of men and women examined in 1972 are given in Table 2.2. While there is no difference in level of plasma cholesterol, HDL-cholesterol levels are lower in diabetics of each sex ($p < 0.001$), and VLDL-cholesterol levels are higher among diabetics ($p < 0.001$). Lipid patterns can be examined in more detail by comparing the prevalence of lipid extremes in normal and diabetic individuals of the same sex, as seen in Figure 2.1 for men and Figure 2.2 for women (14). For this figure individuals are classified as having an extreme lipid value if their levels exceeded the 90th percentile (or were lower than the 10th percentile for HDL-

TABLE 2.1. Comparison of risk factor levels, diabetics vs nondiabetics, Framingham cohort 1972 — age-adjusted means

	Men		Women	
Risk factor	Diabetes present (N = 318)	Diabetes absent (N = 1,495)	Diabetes present (N = 328)	Diabetes absent (N = 2,178)
Glucose (mg/dl)	147***	87	134***	86
Systolic BP (mm Hg)	145***	137	149***	140
BMI (kg/m²)	27.4***	26.0	28.0***	25.4
Hematocrit (%)	48.8***	46.2	43.9	41.9
Uric Acid (mg/dl)	5.3***	4.9	4.4***	3.9
LVH (%)	14.5**	7.1	12.4***	5.8
Cigarettes (%)	35.8	43.0	32.3	33.6

Significantly different from the comparable non-diabetic group. *p<0.05, **p<0.01, and ***p<0.001.

TABLE 2.2. Comparison of risk factor levels, diabetics vs nondiabetics, Framingham cohort 1972 — age-adjusted means

Lipids (mg/dl)	Men		Women	
	Diabetes present	Diabetes absent	Diabetes present	Diabetes absent
Cholesterol	223.1	223.4	248.2	248.0
HDL-cholesterol	42.1***	46.1	53.0***	57.6
LDL-cholesterol	138.2	143.1	155.9	156.0
VLDL-cholesterol	37.3***	30.1	33.1***	27.9

***$p < 0.001$.

cholesterol) for their respective age and sex, according to the Lipid Research Clinic Program data, which were obtained using similar methodology (9). As with the data for means, there was a trend toward extremely high triglycerides ($p < 0.01$ both sexes) and VLDL-cholesterol ($p < 0.05$ in men), accompanied by low HDL-cholesterols ($p < 0.001$ both sexes).

Similar comparisons for systolic and diastolic blood pressure elevations among normal and diabetic adults at the twelfth examination of the Framingham cohort show that the prevalence of systolic pressures greater than 160 mm Hg and diastolic pressures exceeding 95 mm Hg were more common in diabetics (both sexes combined—no statistical test done) age 50–79 (Figure 2.3).

Fibrinogen was determined in the Framingham cohort at the tenth examination, and published reports show associations with risk factors such as diabetes, obesity, cigarette smoking, hypertension, hematocrit, and serum cholesterol. When compared to casually obtained blood glucose levels at the tenth examination, it is even possible to show a linear association between glucose

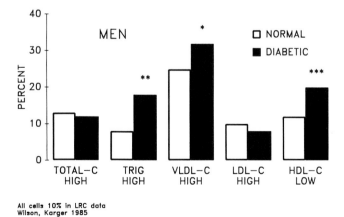

FIGURE 2.1. Frequency of lipid extremes in men 50–80 years of age, according to diabetic status. Key *$p < 0.05$; **$0.01 < p < 0.05$; ***$0.001 < p < 0.01$.

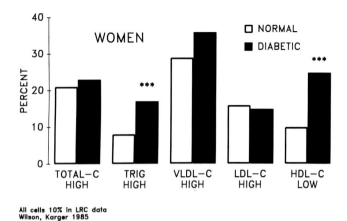

FIGURE 2.2. Frequency of lipid extremes in women 50–80 years of age, according to diabetic status. Key *p<0.05; **0.01<p<0.05; ***0.001<p<0.01.

level and fibrinogen level for both sexes ($p < 0.05$ for men; $p < 0.05$ for women) [(6); Fig. 2.4].

As shown above, diabetes is highly associated with many cardiovascular risk factors. The actual 30-year risk of vascular disease and its components is likewise increased in Framingham diabetic men and women, as shown in Figure 2.5 (age 35–64 yr) and Figure 2.6 (age 65–94 yr). The heights of the bars in each of these figures represent the risk of a diabetic for a given event relative to the risk of a nondiabetic. The numbers above each bar represent the actual age-adjusted risk for diabetics. For example, among men 35–64, the coronary heart disease (CHD) rate is 20/1,000/yr among diabetic men and 19/1,000/yr among diabetic women. The relative risk of CHD among these dia-

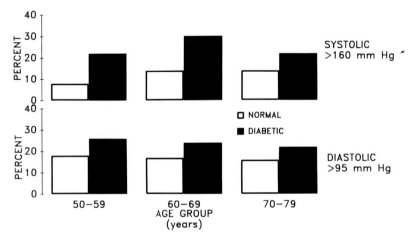

FIGURE 2.3. Prevalence of elevated systolic and diastolic pressures in Framingham cohort participants according to age group and diabetic status.

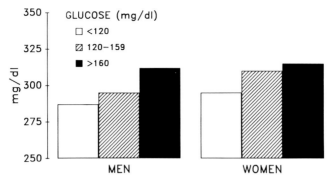

FIGURE 2.4. Age-adjusted mean fibrinogen levels in men and women 45–74 years of age according to casually obtained blood glucose, which was measured simultaneously.

betics is approximately 2 in men ($p < 0.001$) and 3.8 in women ($p < 0.001$) (7).

As seen in the 35–64 yr age group (Fig. 2.5), the relative risk for the various vascular events in diabetics versus nondiabetics is generally twofold in men and threefold in women. In the case of claudication and cardiac failure, however, the relative risk is quite high in women and exceeds 8. Similar trends are seen in the 65–94 yr age group (Fig. 2.6), but there is no extremely accentuated risk for any of the cardiovascular events among people of either sex.

The net effect of diabetes on cardiovascular disease, abstracted from logistic regression analyses is given in Table 2.3. The first two rows represent the relative odds of cardiovascular disease among diabetics without (univariate line) and with age adjustment (age-adjusted line). For example, among men aged 35–64 yr the risk of CVD is 2.4 times that of nondiabetics ($p < 0.001$), and the univariate estimate does not change after age adjustment ($p < 0.001$).

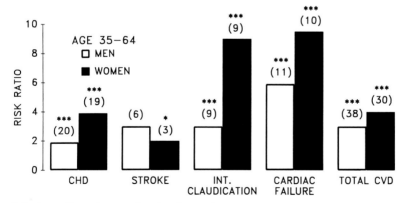

FIGURE 2.5. Age-adjusted annual risk of vascular disease end points over 30 yr follow-up in Framingham men and women 35–64 years of age. Heights of bars represent risk ratios, and numbers above bars show age-adjusted annual rates. Key *p<0.05; **0.01<p<0.05; ***0.001<p<0.01.

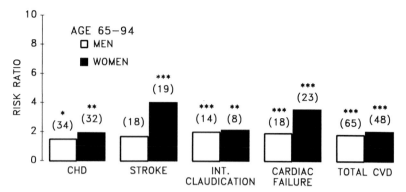

FIGURE 2.6. Age-adjusted annual risk of vascular disease end points over 30 yr follow-up in Framingham men and women 65–94 years of age. Heights of bars represent risk ratios, and numbers above bars show age-adjusted annual rates. Key *p<0.05; **0.01<p<0.05; ***0.001<p<0.01.

When multivariate logistic regression is undertaken, and the diabetes risk is calculated when age, cholesterol level, systolic blood pressure, cigarette smoking, and left ventricular hypertrophy are factored into the model, the risk of CVD among diabetics falls to 2.0 ($p < 0.001$). In general, the excess risk of vascular disease in diabetics holds for both the young (35–64 yr) and the old participants (65–94 yr) in Framingham. It is of interest that the risk for CVD among all diabetics drops from 3.8 in the age-adjusted model to 2.3 in the multivariate model, but for men alone, the risk falls from only 2.4 to 2.0 in the same model. This finding suggests that a considerable portion of the excess risk of CVD among young women is due to the common risk factors. Such is not the case for young men or for older people of either sex.

Overall mortality risk is elevated in diabetics ($p < 0.001$ for men and women, 35–64 and 65–94 yr), and the relative risk estimates are greatest for coronary mortality among individuals 35–64 ($p < 0.01$ for men; $p < 0.05$ for women) (Table 2.4).

DISCUSSION

Three decades of epidemiologic research from the Framingham study indicate that diabetes is a powerful predisposing factor for atherosclerotic disease, particularly coronary heart disease (4,5). For all age groups and both sexes, the

TABLE 2.3. Net effect of diabetes on CVD, Framingham cohort — 30-year follow-up

	35–64 years		65–94 years	
Diabetes effect	Men	Women	Men	Women
Univariate	2.4***	3.9***	1.9***	2.1***
Age-adjusted	2.4***	3.8***	1.9***	2.0***
Risk factor adjusted*	2.0***	2.3***	1.9***	1.7***

*Adjusted for age, cholesterol, systolic blood pressure, cigarettes, LVH. ***Value significantly different from that of a comparable individual without diabetes, p<0.001.

TABLE 2.4. Mortality risk in diabetics, Framingham cohort 30-year follow-up

Mortality type	35–64 years		65–94 years	
	Men	Women	Men	Women
Overall	2.1***	2.2***	1.5***	3.6***
Cardiovascular	2.2**	6.0***	1.9***	3.1***
Coronary	2.3**	9.0*	1.8***	4.0***
Stroke	—	—	2.0*	2.0 ns

Values significantly different from that of individuals without diabetes. *p<0.05, **p<0.01, and ***p<0.001, ns = not significant.

incidence of cardiovascular disease is higher among diabetics: an average two-fold for men and threefold for women. This impact diminishes somewhat with advancing age in women, suggesting that late-onset diabetes may be less atherogenic. At all ages the impact of diabetes is substantially greater for women, which eliminates their advantage over men. The relative impact (risk ratio) is greatest for peripheral arterial disease, but coronary heart disease is the most common and most lethal sequela of diabetes. In women diabetes also has a significant effect on stroke and cardiac failure incidence.

Impaired glucose tolerance is predictive of cardiovascular events, whether the impairment is manifested by a diagnosis of diabetes, hyperglycemia (> 130 mg/dl), glycosuria, or abnormal glucose tolerance. Blood glucose levels are an independent risk factor for cardiovascular disease in women, even within relatively normal blood sugar ranges. Diabetics had higher levels of atherogenic risk factors than nondiabetics for blood pressure, blood sugar, total/HDL-cholesterol ratio, triglyceride, VLDL-cholesterol, uric acid, left ventricular hypertrophy (LVH), hematocrit, and blood fibrinogen. The impact of diabetes on atherosclerotic cardiovascular disease is not entirely attributable to associated higher levels of cardiovascular risk, which indicates that there is some unique effect of diabetes that heightens risk of CVD. In addition, cardiovascular risk factors do not appear to operate with greater potency in diabetics than nondiabetics. However, cardiovascular risk in diabetics is not uniform and varies widely, depending on the level of associated cardiovascular risk factors. Diabetes also worsens the prognosis once myocardial infarction has occurred, as subsequent heart failure and LVH are more common, particularly among women.

Because the influence of diabetes is independent of the atherogenic risk factors that often accompany it, a unique effect on thrombogenesis is suggested. Elevated fibrinogen levels have been demonstrated to increase coronary and cardiovascular risk, and elevated values are more common among diabetics. The excess risk of cardiovascular disease in the diabetic persists after adjustment for fibrinogen level, but the coronary heart disease risk in diabetics seems to be predominantly in those with high fibrinogen values.

Late-onset non-insulin-dependent diabetes mellitus (NIDDM) is common. In the Framingham study, 7.8% of men and 6.2% of women developed diabetes, and the incidence increased sharply with age. A positive family history and obesity (especially abdominal obesity) were the strongest predisposing factors. Diabetes tended to arise from those in the high end of the normal distribution of blood sugars. Blood sugar tended to increase with age in both sexes. Examination of secular trends in the prevalence of diabetes indicates an increasing occurrence in Framingham. Thus, we need more efforts at primary prevention such as weight control and exercise. Also, as elevated triglyceride and VLDL-cholesterol levels often precede diabetes, control of lipids may be of value.

In persons who have already developed diabetes, optimization of risk appears to require a multifactorial approach. Since the high risk of coronary heart disease in diabetics is concentrated in those with one or more associated risk factors, prevention requires more than normalization of the blood sugar. Rational preventive measures include weight reduction, exercise, a fat-modified diet, quitting cigarette smoking, lowering blood pressure, raising HDL-cholesterol, and lowering LDL-cholesterol. These measures can be expected to be associated with a concomitant decrease in fibrinogen and overall decreased risk of vascular disease.

Evidence from the Framingham study and elsewhere indicates a rising prevalence of diabetes in the population, not only because of an aging population of increased size, but age-specifically as well. Up to now treatment directed at impaired glucose tolerance has proved disappointing in reducing cardiovascular sequelae (1,3,11). Perhaps measures taken to improve the entire cardiovascular risk profile of the diabetic will prove more successful. Such a favorable change has not been demonstrated, but a test of this hypothesis would seem long overdue. Most diabetics detected in health maintenance or screening programs are adult-onset, obesity-related, hyperinsulinemic, and keto-resistant. The major sequela of this disease is accelerated atherogenesis and not acute metabolic ketoacidosis and coma. Diabetics have more cardiovascular risk factors such as hypertension, low HDL-cholesterol, high VLDL-cholesterol, and obesity. Hence they require evaluation of cardiovascular risk, since this risk varies considerably in the diabetic, depending on the level of the coexistent risk factors (Table 2.5). Since these risk factors operate similarly to promote atherosclerosis in the diabetic and in the nondiabetic, there is a distinct possibility that diabetics can reduce their cardiovascular risk by controlling their other risk factors.

TABLE 2.5. 8-year probability of cardiovascular events in diabetics aged 50 years, according to associated risk factors[a]

Risk factors	Rate per 1,000	
	Women	Men
None	50	54
Hypertension (165 mm Hg)	117	139
HBP + CHOL. (>260 mg/dl)	159	213
HBP + CHOL. + CIG's.	193	326
HBP + CHOL. + CIG's. + ECG-LVH[b]	323	622

[a]26-year follow up. Framingham study.
[b]Electrocardiographic evidence of left ventricular hypertrophy.

Diabetes screening would seem worthwhile for vulnerable subgroups of the population who are obese, hypertriglyceridemic, or diabetes-prone because of a family history. Such general population screening is indicated if it is undertaken with caution not to mislabel persons as "diabetic" and if it is done as part of a cardiovascular health program in conjunction with hypertension and cholesterol detection and control.

REFERENCES

1. FULLER, J. H., SHIPLEY, M. J., ROSE, G., JARRETT, R. J., and KEEN, H.: Coronary heart disease risk and impaired glucose tolerance: the Whitehall Study. *Lancet* 1: 1373–1376, 1980.
2. HARRIS, M. I., HADDEN, W. C., KNOWLER, W. C., and BENNETT, P. H.: Prevalence of diabetes and impaired glucose tolerance and plasma glucose levels in U.S. population aged 20–74 yr. *Diabetes* 36: 523–534, 1987.
3. KEEN, H., JARRETT, R. J., FULLER, J. H., and MCCARTNEY, P.: Hyperglycemia and arterial disease. *Diabetes* 30(Suppl 2): 49–53, 1981.
4. KANNEL, W. B., and MCGEE, D. L.: Diabetes and cardiovascular risk factors: the Framingham Study. *Circulation* 59: 8–13, 1979.
5. KANNEL, W. B., and MCGEE, D. L.: Diabetes and cardiovascular disease: the Framingham study. *JAMA* 241: 2035, 1979.
6. KANNEL, W. B., WOLF, P. A., CASTELLI, W. P., and D'AGOSTINO, R. B.: Fibrinogen and risk of cardiovascular disease. *JAMA* 258: 1183–1186, 1987.
7. KANNEL, W. B., WOLF, P. A., and GARRISON, R. J.: The Framingham Study: an epidemiological investigation of cardiovascular disease, Section 34. Some risk factors related to the annual incidence of cardiovascular disease and death using pooled repeated biennial measurements. *Framingham Heart Study, 30-Year Follow-Up.* Washington, DC: U.S. Dept. Commerce 1988. PB 87-1777499.
8. KANNEL, W. B., WOLF, P. A., and GARRISON, R. J.: The Framingham Study, Section 35: Survival following initial cardiovascular events. *Framingham Heart Study, 30-Year Follow-Up.* Washington, DC: U.S. Dept. Commerce 1988. PB 88-204029.
9. LIPID RESEARCH CLINICS PROGRAM. *Manual of Laboratory Operations,* vol 1: *Lipid and Lipoprotein Analysis.* Washington, DC: DHEW publ. (NIH) 75-628. Bethesda, MD, National Institutes of Health, 1974.
10. NELSON, N.: A photometric adaptation of the Somogyi method for the determination of glucose. *J. Biol. Chem.* 153: 375–380, 1944.
11. RUDERMAN, N. B., and HAUDENSHILD, C.: Diabetes as an atherogenic factor. *Prog. Cardiovasc. Dis.* 26: 373–412, 1984.
12. SWAIN, W. R., and FEDERS, M. B.: Fibrinogen assay. *Clin. Chem.* 13: 1026–1028, 1967.
13. WILSON, P. W. F., ANDERSON, K. M., and KANNEL, W. B.: Epidemiology of diabetes mellitus in the elderly: the Framingham Study. 80 (suppl 5A): 3–9, 1986.
14. WILSON, P. W. F., KANNEL, W. B., and ANDERSON, K. M.: Lipids, glucose intolerance and vascular disease: the Framingham Study. *Monographs in Atherosclerosis.* New York, Basel: Karger 13:1–11, 1985.

3

Altered Platelet Function in Diabetes Mellitus: Effect of Glycemic Regulation and Antiplatelet Agents

JOHN A. COLWELL, CHRISTOPH GISINGER, AND RICHARD KLEIN

Accelerated atherosclerosis is characteristic of diabetes mellitus. People with diabetes have a risk of dying from cardiovascular disease that is about fourfold greater than the risk for age and sex-matched nondiabetic individuals. This increased risk is not explained by the coexistence of diabetes with the classical major vascular risk factors of hypertension, hypercholesterolemia, and cigarette smoking (26). It appears that there is something else about diabetes that makes this disease a major cardiovascular risk factor, and studies of the pathogenesis of atherosclerosis in diabetes have provided insight into this issue.

The process of atherosclerosis is complicated, with many factors interrelating in its pathogenesis (95–97). The response to injury hypothesis views endothelial damage as an early lesion, with adherence of monocyte-derived macrophages to the area of injury. Macrophage accumulation of cholesterol may occur, and a fatty streak develops. Platelets may adhere to the site of injury and, unless counter-regulation occurs, may aggregate and release intraplatelet materials. Among these is the arachidonic acid–derived metabolite, thromboxane, a potent vasoconstrictor and platelet aggregant. Lipoproteins may accumulate at the site of injury and infiltrate the vascular wall, interact with macrophages to form foam cells, and/or interact with platelets to promote aggregation and thromboxane generation. Platelet–macrophage interaction may lead to foam cell production. Growth factors released by platelets, monocytes, and endothelial cells may contribute to proliferation of smooth muscle cells and other cells in the area of injury. Finally, if these processes are not arrested, thrombosis and vascular occlusion may occur.

There is evidence that many of these steps are altered in experimental and clinical diabetes mellitus. Review articles have considered this in depth (24–28). In particular, altered platelet function is frequently found in diabetes and may parallel metabolic regulation. In diabetes, platelets are more adhesive than normal, often have increased sensitivity to aggregating agents, may release increased amounts of thromboxane on stimulation, and undergo platelet–plasma interactions with such circulating proteins as von Willebrand factor (vWF) immune complexes, fibrinogen, and lipoproteins.

A vicious circle may be operative in diabetes to contribute to accelerated atherosclerosis via altered platelet behavior as a result of platelet–plasma in-

30

teractions. Thus, plasma levels of vWF, immune complexes, and fibrinogen may be elevated in diabetes and may interact with platelets to promote agonist-induced aggregation and thromboxane release. Both qualitative and quantitative changes in lipoproteins may promote these platelet responses. Elevated plasma low-density lipoprotein (LDL) levels may lead to platelet hypersensitivity and release, and there is some evidence that triglyceride-laden very low-density lipoprotein may do the same. Glycated LDL and/or glycated VLDL will accentuate platelet aggregation in vitro. Recently, increased oxidation of lipoproteins has been described in diabetes. Autooxidation of glycated lipoproteins may occur, and interaction of these altered lipoproteins with platelets is under study.

While many factors may contribute to the accelerated atherosclerosis that characterizes the diabetic state, altered platelet function and platelet–plasma interactions are likely to be significant factors. In this chapter, we review some of the evidence that forms the basis for these views.

ALTERED PLATELET FUNCTION IN DIABETES

Platelet Aggregation

Platelet aggregation and release may be studied in vitro with relative ease. Careful instructions to volunteers to avoid ingestion of salicylates, nonsteroidal inflammatory agents, and other drugs that have potent effects on platelet function are necessary to achieve reproducible in vitro results. Many investigators have recognized this fact, and an extensive literature on in vitro platelet function in diabetes and in normal controls has emerged (24–28).

Generally, when studied in platelet-rich citrated plasma in the fasted state, platelets from individuals with diabetes show increased sensitivity to aggregation induced by ADP, epinephrine, collagen, arachidonic acid, and thrombin. The major result is demonstration of the platelet-release phenomenon at lower concentrations of an aggregating agent than occurs in age- and sex-matched controls. This can be found in diabetic patients with or without apparent vascular complications, in type I as well as type II patients, and in animal models of diabetes. An important mechanism appears to be increased synthesis of thromboxane by platelets from diabetic subjects.

Platelet Prostanoid Metabolism

The possibility that prostanoids could cause platelets to aggregate together was suggested by the experiments of Silver et al. (104), who found that arachidonic acid, but no other unsaturated fatty acid, caused rapid and irreversible platelet aggregation when added to human platelet-rich plasma (PRP). Addition of thrombin also caused platelet aggregation and resulted in the release of the prostanoids $PGF_{2\alpha}$ and PGE_2. Pretreatment of platelets with aspirin to block cyclooxygenase inhibited thrombin-induced platelet aggregation and abolished the formation of both prostaglandins. This led to the proposal that the release of a prostaglandin by platelets caused the platelets to aggregate. Since neither PGE_2 nor $PGF_{2\alpha}$ directly affects platelet function (74), another product of arachidonic acid had to be responsible. Willis et al. (120,121) described an unstable arachidonic acid product with powerful platelet aggregatory activity, which was named *labile aggregation stimulatory substance* (LASS). It is now clear that LASS is a mixture of PGD_2, PGH_2, and thromboxane A_2 (TxA_2). It is mainly TxA_2 which is responsible for arachidonic acid–induced platelet aggregation.

In contrast, prostacyclin (PGI_2), PGE_1, PGD_2, and 6-oxo-PGE_1 are potent inhibitors of human platelet aggregation, with PGI_2 having the highest potency in humans. This has been shown in vitro (36) and in vivo (43). Antagonism between TXA_2 and PGI_2 led to the concept proposed by Moncada and Vane (88) that the balanced synthesis and action of proaggregatory, vasoconstrictor TXA_2 by platelets and antiaggregatory, vasoilator PGI_2 by vascular tissue was of physiological importance.

Soon after their early discovery of platelet activation in diabetes (98), Colwell et al. (22) described an increased release of LASS. In subsequent studies, this activity was first thought to be PGE_2 (52), but was later identified as TxA_2 (53). In addition, decreased endothelial PGI_2 synthesis (47), and reduced platelet sensitivity to the anti-aggregatory effect of PGI_2 (64,99) have also been reported in patients with diabetes mellitus, so that it is now generally accepted that platelet activation in diabetes is associated with an imbalance in the TxA_2:PGI_2 system. Several studies attempted to clarify the cause of impaired platelet and/or endothelial cell prostanoid synthesis in diabetes. There is evidence that an altered membrane fatty acid composition, an increased arachidonic acid release from membrane phospholipids, and/or increased phospholipase activity may be involved (24–28,113).

Several studies indicate that insulin treatment to produce near normoglycemia in patients with insulin-dependent diabetes mellitus (IDDM) prevents certain platelet abnormalities in diabetes (58,67,84,86). Normoglycemia induced by ultralente insulin or by sulfonylurea therapy has been shown to reduce platelet sensitivity to agonist stimulation in subjects with non-insulin-dependent diabetes mellitus (NIDDM) (41). Insulin-induced reduction of platelet aggregation can be shown in vitro, and is a dose-dependent phenomenon (115). The phenomenon can be shown in vivo at physiological plasma insulin concentrations (115).

Other studies suggest a critical role of free fatty acids (87), or of glycated lipoproteins (119). Since these metabolic factors may be interrelated, it is important to emphasize the clinical significance of optimized diabetes treatment, both in the prevention of platelet abnormalities and in the normalization of lipid metabolism (79). Unfortunately, complete metabolic long-term normalization cannot always be achieved, and platelet prostanoid abnormalities (49) or altered platelet aggregation (84) may be found in fairly well-controlled patients. Therefore, adjunctive approaches to alter platelet function in diabetes have been widely considered (see below).

Platelet–Plasma Interactions

Platelets are normally operative in circulating blood and at tissue interfaces. They are exposed to, and interact with, many plasma proteins. As a result of this interaction, platelet function is affected, as is platelet adherence to sites of exposure. There are four major platelet–plasma interactions that may have significance in diabetes mellitus: platelet interaction with von Willebrand factor, immune complexes, fibrinogen, and lipoproteins.

von Willebrand Factor

Von Willebrand factor (vWF) factor is synthesized by endothelial cells and by megakarocytes, and it can also be isolated from platelets. Physiologically, it is thought to promote interactions of platelets with vascular endothelium. An elevated plasma level of plasma vWF is often seen in diabetes mellitus, and it probably reflects endothelial damage (24–28). This finding is present shortly after the induction of diabetes by streptozotocin, and is partially reversed by insulin therapy. A role in atherosclerosis is supported by studies in which pigs with von Willebrand disease appear to be protected against the development of atherosclerosis (46). Thus, as an endothelial marker and as a platelet-active protein, vWF may well play a role in macrovascular disease in diabetes mellitus.

A link between altered glucose metabolism and endothelial release of vWF has been reported (89). In studies of endothelial cells in vitro, incubation with high glucose concentrations led to an increase in vWF content. This suggests that hyperglycemia in diabetes may increase vWF production or release. Thus, a case may be made that elevated vWF levels in diabetes reflect the effects of hyperglycemia on the endothelium and that platelet–vWF interactions could occur, which would help explain accelerated atherosclerosis in diabetes.

Immune Complexes

A number of studies have demonstrated the existence of circulating immune complexes in the sera of diabetic patients (61) and a correlation with microvascular disease (71,72,118). Immune complexes isolated from diabetic patients induce aggregation of human platelets (13,116,71). Glycosylation renders a variety of proteins immunogenic leading to the formation of lipoprotein immune complexes (125,126). Lipoproteins may be rendered antigenic by the addition of sugar residues (125).

Fibrinogen

Interest in fibrinogen as a contributor to accelerated atherosclerosis in diabetes has increased since the recognition in three separate epidemiologic studies that the plasma fibrinogen level is an independent risk factor for the development of thrombotic vascular disease of the heart or brain (68,110,122). Fibrinogen has been postulated to play a role in the increased sensitivity of platelets to aggregating agents. Fibrinogen binds to platelet receptors and may be critical for in vitro platelet aggregation. Increased binding of fibrinogen to platelets from diabetic subjects after agonist stimulation has been reported (37). Plasma fibrinogen levels may be raised in people with diabetes, and these levels bear a direct relation to the degree of glycemic regulation. Thus, it is reasonable to postulate that fibrinogen–platelet interactions may occur in diabetes, may contribute to the sensitivity of platelets to agonist stimulation, and may play a role in the accelerated atherosclerosis of diabetes mellitus.

Lipoproteins: Nondiabetic Individuals

The degree of involvement of platelets in atherogenesis is presumably dependent on their level of activation, that is, their level of sensitivity to aggregating agents. Evidence for the importance of platelet–lipoprotein interactions in contributing to platelet activation can be found from observations made in vivo and in vitro (4–12,17–19,21–31,119). The dyslipoproteinemias provide ample evidence in vivo for the contribution of platelet–lipoprotein interactions to platelet activation. Patients with hypercholesterolemia have elevated levels of low-density lipoproteins (LDL) and reduced plasma concentrations of high-density lipoproteins (HDL). These patients have been found to have increased platelet adhesion, aggregation, and serotonin release. Circulating levels of platelet factor four and β-thromboglobulin are enhanced, as is the availability of platelet factor three. Platelet life-span is reduced and platelet turnover increased. Circulating levels of malondialdehyde (MDA) and TxA_2, as well as decreased platelet sensitivity to prostacyclin have been described (5,19,21, 29,54,66,80,111). These changes in platelet activity are paralleled by increased levels of cholesterol and phospholipids in the platelets (100).

The involvement of lipid with enhanced platelet activity has also been demonstrated as a result of experiments designed to alter lipid levels and determine platelet activity. Cholesterol feeding in both animals and man has resulted in enhanced platelet sensitivity (66,94). Therapeutic reductions in cholesterol levels by diet or medication have resulted in a parallel depression of platelet function (17,19). Increased concentrations of plasma triglycerides associated with increased plasma VLDL concentrations (type IV hyperlipoproteinemia), but not with chylomicronemia, are associated with increased platelet activity and an increase in platelet cholesterol and phospholipid contents (19,65,100,128). When type IV hyperlipoproteinemic patients are treated with diet or medication, the decrease in plasma triglyceride concentrations is associated with a decrease in platelet activity (106). Thus, the role of platelet–lipoprotein interactions in platelet sensitivity appears to be critical.

Recent studies in vitro have established that the changes in platelet responsiveness could be effected through interaction with lipoprotein. Platelets are particles without a nucleus and, thus, they are unable to synthesize cholesterol (33); therefore, the source of this cholesterol must be either the parent megakaryocyte or the plasma through interaction with the lipoproteins that transport cholesterol. Platelets have indeed been shown to possess specific LDL receptors (4,6,31,34,76,85). Very low-density lipoprotein (VLDL) has also been reported to bind to platelet membranes in a nonspecific, nonsaturable way (76). Recently, two major lipoprotein-binding membrane glycoproteins were purified to apparent homogeneity and appear to be identical with the components of the GPIIb-IIIa complex from human platelet membranes (77).

A direct effect of lipoproteins on platelet activation is determined by incubating physiological concentrations of isolated lipoproteins with preparations of isolated platelets suspended in buffer. Both LDL and VLDL result in enhanced platelet sensitivity to agonists (6–9,55). In contrast, HDL decreases platelet sensitivity (6–9,55) but HDL_3 is ineffective compared to HDL_2 (1). Further fractionation of HDL_2 by heparin–Sepharose chromatography identified the particles rich in apolipoprotein E as the major antiaggregatory subclass of HDL_2 lipoprotein (34). Incubation of platelets with LDL also results in increased TxA_2 and MDA synthesis rates (10) and the release of platelet granules (117). Recent studies suggest that not only lipoprotein type and concentration but also lipoprotein composition may affect platelet sensitivity (117).

Knowledge of mechanisms underlying the observed effects of lipoproteins on platelet sensitivity is limited; recent studies have shown that LDL elicits some of the mechanisms of stimulus/response coupling in platelets in a manner similar to those of other agonists (1,15,75). One of the first physiological responses to stimulation of platelets in suspension is platelet shape change. The addition of LDL to platelets leads to a dose-dependent shape change reaction within 30 s (123). Platelet shape change is associated with the hydrolysis of inositol phospholipid. Low-density lipoprotein enhances the breakdown of phosphatidylinositol-4-monophosphate and phosphatidylinositol-4,5-*bis*-phosphate, which lead to the elevation of platelet diacylglycerol. These changes are counteracted by HDL_3 and albumin (15). Patients with type II hypercholesterolemia, which has been shown to be associated with platelet hypersensitivity, have elevated levels of platelet membrane phosphatidylinositol (91). Phospholipase C in platelets hydrolyzes specifically the inositol-containing phospholipids, and phospholipase C is present in platelet membranes (103). Similarly, high LDL concentrations stimulate arachidonic acid metabolism and TxB_2 secretion (1). At lower LDL concentrations, no mobilization of platelet arachidonic acid occurs. Arachidonate is released predominantly by phospholipase A_2 acting on platelet phosphatidylcholine and phosphatidylethanolamine. Recently, the transfer of phosphatidylcholine from lipoproteins to platelet plasma membranes has been demonstrated (83). This phospholipid is subsequently incorporated into platelet metabolic pathways. The effect of lipoprotein phospholipids in the platelet membranes on subsequent platelet sensitivity remains to be determined.

Lipoproteins: Diabetes Mellitus

In diabetic individuals, the increased sensitivity of platelets to aggregating agents and increased production of thromboxane and MDA have been extensively documented (24–28,123). Intensive insulin therapy in diabetic patients corrects some aspects of the hypersensitivity of platelets from these individuals (58,67,84,86); however, in those subjects in which insulin treatment did correct increased platelet responsiveness, it is difficult to know if this occurred through an effect on the elevated plasma glucose concentrations or an effect on plasma lipids and lipoproteins. Insulin treatment can have effects on both of these metabolic changes that may occur in the diabetic state. We have shown previously that the plasma level of LDL cholesterol in type I diabetic patients is significantly correlated with the sensitivity of the platelets to arachidonic acid (84). This prompted us to examine the effects of low-density lipoproteins isolated from diabetic patients on platelet function.

LDL Glycation

We isolated the LDL fraction from patients with IDDM (119). We demonstrated that LDL isolated from patients with IDDM enhanced platelet aggregation and TxB_2 production to a greater extent that LDL isolated from normal controls.

The enhancement in platelet aggregation and TxB_2 production was due to an increased binding of LDL from diabetic patients to the platelets. The increase in binding appeared to be due to nonenzymatic glycosylation of LDL. Supporting this hypothesis was the positive correlation between the degree of LDL glycosylation and the reactivity of the platelets to thrombin found in platelets incubated with LDL from diabetic patients. We found that increased glycosylation of LDL occurs in IDDM in vivo, and correlates with indexes of metabolic control (81).

Experiments using LDL glycosylated in vitro confirmed that incubation of glycosylated LDL with platelets enhanced both their aggregation and TxB_2 production. When binding of LDL glycosylated in vitro to platelets was compared with that of normal LDL, it was found to be approximately twofold increased. Thus, it appears that LDL may contribute to the hyperaggregability of platelets in diabetes mellitus not only by enhancing the reactivity of platelets to proaggregatory agents but also by increasing the production of TxB_2, a well-known proaggregatory substance.

It has been shown recently that a glycosylated (G-LDL) and a nonglycosylated (N-LDL) subfraction of LDL can be separated from the total LDL fraction obtained from diabetic patients (63). We have employed this procedure to isolate N-LDL and G-LDL from insulin-dependent diabetic patients. To determine if the increased reactivity of platelets observed previously was induced by the G-LDL subfraction of total LDL, we measured the aggregation rate of washed human platelets preincubated with G-LDL or N-LDL. Glycosylated LDL enhanced both ADP and thrombin-induced platelet aggregation (73). In agreement with our previous studies of platelet aggregation enhanced by glycosylated LDL (119), the extent of glycosylation of G-LDL was significantly greater than that of N-LDL. However, the lipid composition of N-LDL and G-LDL differed significantly. Glycosylated LDL, compared to N-LDL was significantly enriched in triglycerides and phospholipids. The influence of altered lipid composition of G-LDL on platelet activation remains to be determined. However, since lipoprotein phospholipids can exchange with platelet membrane phospholipids (83), the abnormal phospholipid content of G-LDL in insulin-dependent diabetic patients may influence platelet membrane fluidity by altering the platelet membrane phospholipid to cholesterol ratio. Reduced platelet membrane fluidity has been associated with enhanced platelet responsiveness to agonists in vitro (101,102,114). Furthermore, the membrane fluidity of platelets isolated from diabetic patients has been shown to be reduced (124).

It is becoming clear that multiple pathways may be involved in the activation of platelets in diabetes (24–28,123). Since several mechanisms may be involved in the hypersensitivity of platelets in diabetes, an inhibitor of one of these mechanisms may not inhibit hypersensitivity of platelets from diabetic subjects to all agonists. More than one agonist is likely to be present at sites of vessel injury where platelet activation would occur and agonists are known to act synergistically when present together. Clearly, more studies are needed to understand the mechanisms of hypersensitivity of platelets in diabetes mellitus and the role of platelet–lipoprotein interaction in the increased atherosclerosis seen in diabetes.

Low-Density Lipoprotein Oxidation

Low-density lipoprotein oxidation has been the subject of a recent and thorough review by Steinberg et al. (108). It is well established that both the lipid and apoprotein moieties of the LDL particle may be damaged in reactions with free radicals (51). Unsaturated fatty acids are particularly susceptible to attack because they have easily abstracted hydrogen atoms on methylene groups adjacent to C=C double bonds. A chain reaction may follow, cleaving the fatty acid chain and releasing reactive fragments such as MDA (45). MDA may in turn initiate further damage to other macromolecules. Oxidative damage to the apoprotein (apo B-100) component of LDL may cause either fragmentation of the apoprotein (14,44), or the formation of higher molecular weight forms.

Oxidation of LDL occurs readily in vitro in the presence of trace quantities of ferrous or cuprous ions (56). This fact must be borne in mind when isolating LDL for subsequent metabolic studies. Such oxidation can be prevented by removing metallic ions with chelating agents (e.g. EDTA) or by adding antioxidants (e.g. butylated hydroxytoluene) (42). Oxidation of LDL also occurs when the lipoprotein is incubated with cultured endothelial cells, smooth muscle cells, and monocyte-macrophages (20,51,57,90)—the three main types of cell found in the arterial intima. The presence of plasma, however, inhibits the oxidation, suggesting that in vivo, LDL oxidation may only take place in the vessel wall and not in the circulation. Again, antioxidants such as butylated hydroxytoluene can inhibit cell-stimulated oxidation of LDL.

Oxidized LDL (Ox-LDL) is cytotoxic to cultured endothelial cells, smooth muscle cells, and fibroblasts (57,90). The identity of the toxic component(s) of the lipoprotein is unknown, but it can be extracted with chloroform and therefore is thought to reside in the lipid moiety of the particle. Ox-LDL is avidly taken up by macrophages, either by the scavenger receptor or another more specific high-affinity receptor for Ox-LDL (3,105), inducing foam cell formation. Ox-LDL has been isolated from atherosclerotic plaques in rabbits (92) and in humans (127).

The interaction of oxidized LDL and other modified LDL particles with platelets was the subject of a recent study (12). Platelet aggregation in response to collagen and ADP, and platelet composition were studied after exposure to LDL, which was modified by phospholipase C, hepatic lipase, acetylation, or oxidation. Ox-LDL was unique in reducing platelet cholesteryl ester content, and it also caused a reduction, by 25%, in collagen- or ADP-induced platelet aggregation. Enzyme-modified LDL, in contrast, increased the cholesteryl ester:phospholipid ratio in platelets (by decreasing phospholipid) and stimulated aggregation. Low-density lipoprotein–induced changes in platelet membrane fluidity, which were mediated by changes in the cholesteryl ester:phospholipid ratio, were thought to underlie the effects on aggregation. Thus, in this case, oxidation of LDL, in contrast to other lipoprotein modifications was found to inhibit a potentially atherosclerotic process.

In conclusion, it is clear that both oxidation and glycation of lipoproteins have effects on lipoprotein–platelet interactions.

ANTIPLATELET AGENTS AND DIABETIC VASCULAR DISEASE

This subject has been recently reviewed, and should be consulted for details (28). A summary of key primary and secondary prevention trials is given in Tables 3.1 and 3.2. Two primary prevention trials, primarily in nondiabetic individuals who were male physicians, have been reported. One study (93) showed no significant effect of aspirin therapy on vascular events. A second study (107) showed a decrease in the risk of myocardial infarction of 44% (239 in placebo group and 139 in aspirin group) after 5 yr of alternate day therapy with 325 mg of aspirin. A subgroup of 275 individuals with diabetes was randomized to aspirin therapy, and there were eleven myocardial infarctions in this group (4.0%). In contrast, there were 26 myocardial infarctions in the 258 diabetic individuals randomized to the placebo group (10.1%). These data suggest that aspirin may be a good strategy as a primary preventive agent in diabetes, but larger studies are needed to firmly establish this point.

There is one large-scale collaborative trial, the ETDRS (38–40) in which diabetic subjects with retinopathy were randomized to aspirin (650 mg/day) or to placebo therapy and followed for up to 10 yr. Major vascular events have been monitored in this study and are under analysis. Results from this trial will give a definitive answer to the issue of safety and efficacy of aspirin therapy as a primary prevention strategy for macrovascular events in diabetes mellitus.

There are many secondary prevention trials in which antiplatelet agents have been used (Table 3.2). These have primarily been done in nondiabetic patients who have had a myocardial infarction or a cerebrovascular accident. Results of from 25 major trials have been pooled and analyzed, using the technique of metaanalysis (2). In all, there were 29,000 patients reviewed, 3,000 of whom had died during the study. Allocation to antiplatelet therapy was associated with a reduction in vascular mortality of 15% and a reduction in nonvascular events of 30%. There were no differences between different types of antiplatelet regimens, and doses of aspirin from 325 to 1,500 mg were equally effective. A daily dose of 325 mg of aspirin was recommended as a secondary prevention strategy.

Subsequently, this large analysis was supported by a study of aspirin's role in evolving myocardial infarction (62). In this study of 17,187 participants, aspirin use was associated with a 49% reduction in nonfatal myocardial infarction and a 23% reduction in cardiovascular death after 5 weeks of therapy.

There are two secondary prevention trials of antiplatelet agents and macrovascular disease in patients with NIDDM. The first, a V.A. Cooperative Study (23), showed no protective effect of aspirin plus dipyridamole in male diabetic patients who had suffered amputation for gangrene, using vascular death and subsequent amputation of the opposite extremity as end points. A protection from strokes and transient ischemic attacks was suggested by subgroup analysis. Similarly, in the AICLA study (16), subgroup analysis suggested a protective effect of antiplatelet therapy for cerebrovascular events in a group of NIDDM patients who had suffered a previous stroke or transient ischemic attack.

There are three antiplatelet studies in diabetic subjects in which microvascular end points were followed. In the DAMAD study (32), aspirin use was

TABLE 3.1. Primary prevention trials — antiplatelet agents

Study	Reference	Diabetes mellitus	Entry group	ASA[a]	DIP[b]	Results Vascular mortality	Non-fatal vascular disease	Myocardial infarction	Total mortality
UK study (MDs)	93	No	Normal males	+	0	0	0	0	0
US study (MDs)	107	No	Normal males	+	0	0	→	→	0
Subgroup	107	Yes	No vascular disease	+	0	0	0		0
ETDRS	38–40	Yes	Early PDR	+	0	——————No data——————			

[a]Aspirin.
[b]Dipyridamole.

TABLE 3.2. Secondary prevention trials — antiplatelet agents

Study	Reference	Diabetes mellitus	Entry group	ASA[a]	DIP[b]	Results			
						Vascular mortality	Non-fatal vascular disease	CVA/TIA[c]	Total mortality
Antiplatelet trialists	2	No	Post CVA or MI[d]	+	±	→	→	0	0
ISIS-2	62	No	Recent MI	+	0	→	→	0	0
VACS #43	23	Yes	Amputation	+	+	0	0	0	0
AICLA (Subgroup)	16	Yes	Post CVA or TIA	+	+	0	0	→	→
						Microan. prog.	High risk ret.		Visual acuity
DAMAD	32	Yes	Background retinopathy	+	±	→	0		0
ETDRS	38–40	Yes	Early proliferative retinopathy	+	0	———— No data ————			
Mayo	35	Yes	Early nephropathy	+	+	25%: Stable renal function			

[a]Aspirin
[b]Dipyridamole
[c]Cerebrovascular accident/transient ischemic attack.
[d]Myocardial infarction.

associated with a diminution in progression of microaneurysm formation. In the ETDRS (38–40), preliminary reports suggest that aspirin use is neither harmful nor beneficial in patients with advanced diabetic retinopathy. Finally, in a nonrandomized study in diabetic patients with nephropathy (35), 25% of patients showed stable renal function while on antiplatelet agents, while 75% showed the expected deterioration. Those who responded had the best renal function on entry. These studies suggest that if antiplatelet therapy is to be successful in microvascular disease, then it must be used early in the course of vascular damage.

Enhancement of prostacyclin synthesis or release is another approach. Decreased PGI_2 production may lead to enhancement of platelet aggregation in diabetes mellitus. Recent studies showed the presence of PGI_2-stimulating activity in sera which was decreased in patients and in animal models of diabetes mellitus (59,60). A short-term change of the TxA_2/PGI_2 balance in diabetes does not appear to be beneficial with respect to retinopathy, since direct administration of PGI_2 in IDDM patients through a 72 h continuous infusion in a double-blind placebo-controlled study did not significantly affect occlusive retinal lesions as assessed by fluorescence angiography (50).

A promising therapeutic possibility is the use of vitamin E, which has been shown to stimulate vascular PGI_2-synthesis (78) and to inhibit platelet aggregation in vitro (109) and in vivo (82,112). Vitamin E deficiency has been demonstrated in platelets obtained from diabetic subjects (69,70). In a double-blind, controlled, cross-over study in 22 type I diabetic patients who received 400 mg DL-α-tocopherol acetate daily for 4 weeks, the thromboxane production by platelets obtained from patients after vitamin E supplementation returned to levels observed in platelets from healthy controls, indicating that those dosages of vitamin E may be appropriate to normalize platelet abnormalities in this fairly well-controlled type I diabetic population without major complications (48).

CONCLUSION

Altered platelet function occurs in diabetes mellitus and is accompanied by increased thromboxane release. It occurs early in the course of IDDM and in animal models, and the hypersensitivity to agonists and thromboxane release may be reversed by insulin therapy. This suggests that hyperglycemia or other metabolic consequences of the diabetic state are contributory. The process is accentuated by platelet–plasma interactions that are characteristic of diabetes under less than ideal metabolic regulation, including interactions with von Willebrand factor, fibrinogen, immune complexes, lipoproteins, and glycated lipoproteins.

These observations suggest that intensive glycemic management would improve platelet function in diabetes and, to the extent that altered platelet function may be involved in vascular complications, favorably alter the course of such complications. However, it would take a large-scale clinical trial to resolve this issue, and such a trial, directed solely at altered platelet function, is unlikely to be carried out.

The emphasis in this chapter has been on the metabolic consequences present in the diabetic state that may lead to altered platelet function. However, it must be recognized that there is a host of data in the diabetic and in the nondiabetic state that altered platelet function may be the result of vascular damage to the endothelium. Thus, it is likely that in diabetes a vicious cycle may be set up in which vascular disease may lead to platelet damage and altered platelet function may contribute to vascular disease.

In any case, whatever the exact sequence of events, it is clear from clinical trial data that a simple approach to altered platelet function in diabetes can be effective. Clinical trials using aspirin therapy have shown efficacy and safety when used as a secondary prevention strategy after major macrovascular events. Promising results are reported in nondiabetic males with aspirin as a primary prevention strategy, and ongoing studies will provide definitive data in diabetic subjects in the near future. There is a suggestion that antiplatelet therapy may also modify the course of microvascular disease, if used before major damage to the microvessels has occurred.

In view of these considerations, it is recommended that diabetic individuals receive one long-acting aspirin preparation (325 mg) each day after they have had a recognized macrovascular event. Use of aspirin as a primary prevention strategy awaits reports from the ETDRS, a large scale randomized controlled trial.

ACKNOWLEDGMENTS

This work was supported by Veterans Administration research funds.

REFERENCES

1. ANDREWS, H. E., AITKEN, J. W., HASSALL, D. G., SKINNER, V. O., and BRUCKDORFER, R. Intracellular mechanisms in the activation of human platelets by low-density lipoproteins. *Biochem. J.* 242: 559–564, 1987.

2. ANTIPLATELET TRIALISTS' COLLABORATION. Secondary prevention of vascular disease by prolonged antiplatelet treatment. *Br. Med. J.* 296: 310–331, 1988.

3. ARI, H., KITA, T., YOKODE, M., NARUMIYA, S., and KAWAI, C. Multiple receptors for modified low density lipoproteins in mouse peritoneal macrophages: different uptake mechanisms for acetylated and oxidized low density lipoproteins. *Biochem. Biophys. Res. Commun.* 159: 1375–1382, 1989.

4. AVIRAM, M., BROOK, J. G., LEES, A. M., et al. Low-density lipoprotein binding to human platelets: role of charge and of specific amino acids. *Biochem. Biophys. Res. Commun.* 99: 308–318, 1981.

5. AVIRAM, M., and BROOK, J. G. The effect of human plasma on platelet function in familial hypercholesterolemia. *Thromb. Res.* 26: 101–109, 1982.

6. AVIRAM, M., and BROOK, J. G. Platelet interaction with high- and low-density lipoproteins. *Atherosclerosis* 46: 259–268, 1983.

7. AVIRAM, M., and BROOK, J. G. Characterization of the effect of plasma lipoprotein on platelet function in vitro. *Haemostasis* 13: 344–350, 1983.

8. AVIRAM, M., and BROOK, J. G. The effect of blood constituents on platelet function: role of blood cells and plasma lipoproteins. *Artery* 11: 297–305, 1983.

9. AVIRAM, M., and BROOK, J. G. Selective release from platelet granules by plasma lipoproteins. *Biochem. Med.* 32: 30–33, 1984.

10. AVIRAM, M., SITORI, C. R., COLLI, S., et al. Plasma lipoproteins affect platelet malondialdehyde and thromboxane B_2 production. *Biochem. Med.* 34: 29–36, 1985.

11. AVIRAM, M., and BROOK, J. G. Platelet activation by plasma lipoproteins. *Prog. Cardiovasc. Dis.* 30: 61–72, 1987.

12. AVIRAM, M. Modified forms of low density lipoprotein affect platelet aggregation in vitro. *Thromb. Res.* 53: 561–567, 1989.

13. BATTERSBY, B., SHERWOOD, T., WINOCOUR, P., and VIRELLA, G. Human platelets aggregate during antigen antibody reactions at different antigen–antibody ratios. *J. Clin. Lab. Immunol.* 15: 57, 1984.

14. BELLAMY, M. F., NEALIS, A. S., AITKEN, J. W., BRUCKDORFER, K. R., and PERKINS, S. J. Structural changes in oxidised low-density lipoproteins and of the effect of the anti-atherosclerotic drug probucol observed by synchrotron X-ray and neutron solution scattering. *Eur. J. Biochem.* 183: 321–329, 1989.

15. BLOCK, L. H., KNORR, M., VOGT, E., et al. Low-density lipoprotein causes general cellular activation with increased phosphatidylinositol turnover and lipoprotein catabolism. *Proc. Natl. Acad. Sci. USA* 85: 885–889, 1988.

16. BOUSSER, M. G., ESCHWEGE, E., HAGUENAU, M., et al. "AICLA" controlled trial of aspirin and dipyridamole in the secondary prevention of athero-thrombotic cerebral ischemia. *Stroke* 14: 5–14, 1983.

17. BROOK, J. G., WINTERSTEIN, G., and AVIRAM, M. Platelet function and lipoprotein levels after plasma exchange in patients with familial hypercholesterolemia. *Clin. Sci.* 64: 637–642, 1983.

18. BROOK, J. G., and AVIRAM, M. Platelet lipoprotein interactions. *Semin. Thromb. Hemostasis* 14: 258–265, 1988.

19. CARVALHO, A. C. A., COLMAN, R. W., and LEES, R. S. Platelet function in hyperlipoproteinemia. *N. Engl. J. Med.* 290: 434–437, 1974.

20. CATHCART, M. K., MOREL, D. W., and CHISOLM, G. M., III. Monocytes and neutrophils oxidize low density lipoprotein making it cytotoxic. *J. Leuk. Biol.* 38: 341–350, 1985.

21. COLMAN, R. W. Platelet function in hyperbetalipoproteinemia. *Thromb. Haemostasis* 39: 284–293, 1978.

22. COLWELL, J. A., CHAMBERS, A., and LAIMINS, M. Inhibition of labile aggregation-stimulating substance (LASS) and platelet aggregation in diabetes mellitus. *Diabetes* 24: 684–687, 1975.

23. COLWELL, J. A., BINGHAM, S. F., ABRAIRA, J. W., ANDERSON, J. P., COMSTOCK, H. C., KWAAN, F., NUTTALL, F. Q., and COOPERATIVE-STUDY GROUP. Veterans Administration Cooperative Study on Antiplatelet Agents in Diabetic Patients after Amputation for Gangrene: II. Effects of aspirin and dipyridamole on atherosclerotic vascular disease rates. *Diabetes Care* 9: 215–224, 1986.

24. COLWELL, J. A., LOPES-VIRELLA, M. L. F., WINOCOUR, P. D., and HALUSHKA, P. V. New concepts about the pathogenesis of atherosclerosis in diabetes mellitus. In: *The Diabetic Foot,* edited by M. L. Levine. St. Louis: C. V. Mosby, 1987, pp. 51–70.

25. COLWELL, J. A., and LOPES-VIRELLA, M. F. A review of the pathogenesis of large vessel disease in diabetes mellitus. *Am. J. Med.* 85: 113–118, 1988.

26. COLWELL, J. A., et al. Consensus Statement: Role of cardiovascular risk factors in prevention and treatment of macrovascular disease in diabetes. *Diabetes Care* 12: 573–579, 1989.

27. COLWELL, J. A., WINOCOUR, P. D., and LOPES-VIRELLA, M. F. Platelet function and platelet–plasma interactions in atherosclerosis and diabetes mellitus. In: *Diabetes Mellitus: Theory and Practice,* edited by H. Rifkin and D. Porte. New York: Elsevier, 1989, pp. 249–256.

28. COLWELL, J. A. Platelet-active drugs in diabetes mellitus. In: *Pharmacology of Diabetes,* edited by E. Standl and C.E. Morgenson. Berlin: DeGruyter, 1990, in press.

29. CORASH, L., ANDERSON, J., POINDEXTER, B. J., et al. Platelet function and survival in patients with severe hypercholesterolemia. *Atherosclerosis* 1: 443–448, 1981.

30. CUCINOTTA, D., TRIFILETTI, A., DiDESARE, E., DiBENEDETTO A., CERUSO, P., and SQUADRITO, G. The effect of strict metabolic control on clotting actors and platelet function in diabetics with vascular disease. *G. Ital. Diabetol.* 5: 311, 1985.

31. CURTISS, L. K., and PLOW, E. F. Interaction of plasma lipoproteins with human platelets. *Blood* 64: 365–374, 1984.

32. THE DAMAD STUDY GROUP. Effect of aspirin alone and aspirin plus dipyridamole in early diabetic retinopathy. A multicenter randomized controlled clinical trial. *Diabetes* 38: 491–498, 1989.

33. DERKSEN, A., and COHEN, P. Extensive incorporation of 2-^{14}C-mevalonic acid into cholesterol precursors by human platelets in vitro. *J. Biol. Chem.* 248: 7396–7403, 1973.

34. DESAI, K., BRUCKDORFER, K. R., HUTTON, R. A., and OWEN, J. S. Binding of apo E–rich high density lipoprotein particles by saturable sites on human blood platelets inhibits agonist-induced platelet aggregation. *J. Lipid Res.* 30: 831–840, 1989.

35. DONADIO, J. V., JR., ILSTRUP, D. M., HOLLEY, K. E., et al. Platelet-inhibitor treatment of diabetic nephropathy: a 10-year prospective study. *Mayo Clin. Proc.* 63: 3–15, 1988.

63. DiMinno, G., Silver, M. J., and deGaetano, G. Prostaglandins as inhibitors of human platelet aggregation. *Br. J. Haematol.* 43: 637–647, 1979.

37. DiMinno, G., Silver, M. J., Cerbone, A. M., et al. Platelet fibrinogen binding in diabetes mellitus. Differences between binding to platelets from nonretinopathic and retinopathic diabetic patients. *Diabetes* 35: 182–185, 1986.

38. Early Treatment Diabetic Retinopathy Study Research Group. Photocoagulation for diabetic macular edema. Early Treatment Diabetic Retinopathy Study Report Number 1. *Arch. Ophthalmol.* 103: 1796–1806, 1985.

39. Scientific Reporting Section, National Institutes of Health. Conclusions of the Early Treatment Diabetic Retinopathy Study, October 1989.

40. Fact Sheet. National Eye Institute, National Institutes of Health. November 1989.

41. Evans, R. J., Lane, J., Holman, R. R., et al. Induced basal normoglycemia and altered platelet aggregation in non-insulin-dependent diabetes. *Diabetes Care* 5: 433–437, 1982.

42. Evensen, S. A., Galdal, K. S., and Nilsen, E. LDL-induced cytotoxicity and its inhibition by anti-oxidant treatment in cultured human endothelial cells and fibroblasts. *Atherosclerosis* 49: 23–30, 1983.

43. Fitzgerald, G. A., Friedman, L. A., Miyamori, I., O'Grady, J., and Lewis, P. J. A double blind placebo-controlled crossover study of prostacyclin in man. *Life Sci.* 25: 665–672, 1979.

44. Fong, L. G., Parthasarathy, S., Witztum, J. L., and Steinberg, D. Nonenzymatic oxidative cleavage of peptide bonds in apoprotein B-100. *J. Lipid Res.* 28: 1466–1477, 1987.

45. Frankel, E. N., and Neff, W. E. Formation of malondialdehyde from lipid oxidation products. *Biochim. Biophys. Acta* 754: 264–270, 1983.

46. Fuster, V., Bowie, E. J. W., Lewis, J. C., et al. Arteriosclerosis in von Willebrand and normal pigs: spontaneous and high-cholesterol diet induced. *J. Clin. Invest.* 61: 722–730, 1978.

47. Gerrard, J. M., Stuart, M. J., Rao, G. H. R., Steffes, M. W., Mauer, S. M., Brown, D. M., and White, J. C. Alterations in the balance of prostaglandins and thromboxane synthesis in diabetic rats. *J. Lab. Clin. Med.* 95: 950–958, 1980.

48. Gisinger, C., Jeremy, J., Speiser, P., Mikhailidis, D., Dandona, P., and Schernthaner, G. Effect of vitamin E supplementation on platelet thromboxane A2 production in type I diabetic patients. *Diabetes* 37: 1260–1264, 1988.

49. Gisinger, C., and Schernthaner, G. Increased platelet malondialdehyde, but normal platelet sensitivity to adenosin-5-diphosphate and prostacyclin in well controlled type I diabetics without vascular complications. *Diabetes Res.* 3: 401–404, 1986.

50. Gottlob, I., Schernthaner, G., Riss, B., Gisinger, C., Klemen, U. M., and Freyler, H. Effect of prostacyclin treatment on diabetic retinopathy in type-I diabetics: a double blind controlled study. In: *Proceedings VIIth Congress European Society of Ophthalmology.* Helsinki, 1985.

51. Halliwell, B., and Gulteridge, J. M. C. Free radicals in biology and medicine. In: Oxford: Clarendon Press, 1985, pp. 146–169.

52. Halushka, P. V., Lurie, D., and Colwell, J. A. Increased synthesis of prostaglandin-E-like material by platelets from patients with diabetes mellitus. *N. Engl. J. Med.* 297: 1306–1310, 1977.

53. Halushka, P. V., Rogers, R. C., Loadholt, C. B., and Colwell, J. A. Increased platelet thromboxane synthesis in diabetes mellitus. *J. Lab. Clin. Med.* 97: 87–96, 1981.

54. Harker, L. A., and Hazzard, W. Platelet kinetic studies in patients with hyperlipoproteinemia: effect of clofibrate therapy. *Circulation* 60: 492–496, 1979.

55. Hassall, D. G., Owen, J. S., and Bruckdorfer, K. R. The aggregation of isolated platelets in the presence of lipoproteins and prostacyclin. *Biochem. J.* 216: 43–49, 1983.

56. Heinecke, J. W. Free radical modification of low-density lipoprotein: mechanisms and biological consequences. *Free Radical Biol. Med.* 3: 65–73, 1987.

57. Hessler, J. R., Morel, D. W., Lewis, L. J., and Chisolm, G. M. Lipoprotein oxidation and lipoprotein-induced cytotoxicity. *Arteriosclerosis* 3: 215–222, 1983.

58. Hiramatsu, K., Nozaki, H., and Arimori, S. Reduction of platelet aggregation induced by euglycaemic insulin clamp. *Diabetologia* 30: 310–313, 1987.

59. Inoguchi, T., Imeda F., Ono, H., Kunisaki, M., Watanabe, J., and Newata, H. Abnormality in prostacyclin-stimulatory activity in sera from diabetics. *Metabolism* 38: 837–842, 1989.

60. Inoguchi, T., Umeda, F., Watanabe, J., and Ibayashi, H. Reduced serum-stimulatory activity on prostacyclin production by cultured aortic endothelial cells in diabetes mellitus. *Haemostasis* 16: 447–452, 1986.

61. Irvine, W. J., Al-Kateeb, S. F., Di Mario, U., Feek, C. M., Gray, R. S., Edmond, B., and

DUNCAN, L. J. P. Soluble immune complexes in the sera of newly diagnosed insulin dependent diabetics and in treated diabetics. *Clin. Exp. Immunol.* 30: 16–21, 1977.

62. ISIS-2 (SECOND INTERNATIONAL STUDY OF INFARCT SURVIVAL) COLLABORATIVE GROUP. Randomized trial of intravenous streptokinase, oral aspirin, both, or neither among 17,187 cases of suspected acute myocardial infarction: ISIS-2. *Lancet* 1: 349–360, 1988.

63. JACK, C. M., SHERIDAN, B., KENNEDY, L., and STOUT, R. W. Non-enzymatic glycosylation of low-density lipoprotein. Results of an affinity chromatography method. *Diabetologia* 31: 126–128, 1988.

64. JOHNSON, M., and HARRISON, H. E. Platelet abnormalities in experimental diabetes. *Thromb. Haemostasis* 42: 333, 1981.

65. JOIST, J. H., BAKER, R, K., and SCHONFELD, G. Increased in vivo and in vitro platelet function in type II and type IV hyperlipoproteinemia. *Thromb. Res.* 15: 95–108, 1974.

66. JOIST, J. H., DOLEZEL, G., KINLOUGH-RATHBONE, F. L., and MUSTARD, J. F. Effect of diet-induced hyperlipidemia on in vitro function of rabbit platelets. *Thromb. Res.* 9: 435–439, 1976.

67. JUHAN, I., BUONOCORE, M., JOUVE, R., VAUGE, P. H., MOULIN, J. P., and VIALETTES, B. Abnormalities of erythrocyte deformability and platelet aggregation in insulin-dependent diabetics corrected by insulin in vivo and in vitro. *Lancet* 1: 535–537, 1982.

68. KANNEL, W. B., WOLF, P. A., CASTELLI, M. D., et al. Fibrinogen and risk of cardiovascular disease. *JAMA* 258: 1183–1186, 1987.

69. KARPEN, C. W., PRITCHARD, K. A., ARNOLD, J. H., CORNWELL, D. G., and PANGANAMALA, R. V. Restoration of prostacyclin/thromboxane A2 balance in the diabetic rat: influence of dietary vitamin E. *Diabetes* 31: 947–951, 1982.

70. KARPEN, C. W., CATALAND, S., O'DORISIO, T. M., and PANGANAMALA, R. V. Interrelation of platelet vitamin E and thromboxane synthesis in type I diabetes mellitus. *Diabetes* 33: 239–243, 1984.

71. KILPATRICK, J. M., and VIRELLA, G. Isolation and characterization of soluble insulin–anti-insulin immune complexes formed in vitro and in vivo in sera from patients with diabetes mellitus. *Clin. Exp. Immunol.* 40: 445, 1980.

72. KILPATRICK, J. M., and VIRELLA, G. Statistical analysis of five immune complex screening assays: patterns of detection in patients with rheumatoid arthritis, systemic lupus erythematosus, infectious endocarditis, and diabetes mellitus. *J. Clin. Lab. Immunol.* 1: 57, 1983.

73. KLEIN, R. L., LOPES-VIRELLA, M. F., and COLWELL, J. A. Enhancement of platelet aggregation by the glycosylated subfraction of low density lipoprotein (LDL) isolated from patients with insulin-dependent diabetes mellitus (IDDM). *Diabetes* 39(Suppl 1): 44a, 1990.

74. KLOEZE, J. Influence of prostaglandins on platelet adhesion and platelet aggregation. In: *Proceedings of the 2nd Nobel Symposium,* edited by S. Bergstrom and B. Samuelsson. New York: Interscience, 1967, pp. 241–252.

75. KNORR, M., LOCHER, R., VOGT, E., VETTER, W., BLOCK, L. H., FERRACIN, F., LEFKOVITS, H., and PLETSCHER, A. Rapid activation of human platelets by low concentrations of low-density lipoprotein via phosphatidylinositol cycle. *Eur. J. Biochem.* 172: 753–759, 1988.

76. KOLLER, E., KOLLER, F., and DOLESCHEL, W. Specific binding sites on human platelets for plasma lipoproteins. *Z. Physiol. Chem.* 363: 395–405, 1982.

77. KOLLER, E., KOLLER, F., and BINDER, B. R. Purification and identification of the lipoprotein-binding proteins from human blood platelet membrane. *J. Biol. Chem.* 264: 12412–12418, 1989.

78. KUNISAKI, M., UMEDA, F., INOGUCHI, T., ONO, H., and SAKO, Y. Effect of vitamin E on prostacyclin production from cultured aortic endothelial cells. In: *Endothelium in Health and Diabetes.* New York: Plenum, 1988, pp. 113–118.

79. LOPES-VIRELLA, M. F., WOHLTMANN, H. J., MAYFIELD, R. K., LOADHOLT, C. B., and COLWELL, J. A. Effect of metabolic control on lipid, lipoprotein and apolipoprotein levels in 55 insulin-dependent diabetic patients. *Diabetes* 32: 2–25, 1983.

80. LOWE, G. O. O., DRUMMOND, M. M., THIRD, J. L. H., et al. Increased plasma fibrinogen and platelet aggregates in type II hyperlipoproteinemia. *Thromb Haemostasis* 42: 1503–1507, 1979.

81. LYONS, T. J., BAYNES, J. W., PATRICK, J. S., COLWELL, J. A., and LOPES-VIRELLA, M. F. Glycosylation of low density lipoprotein in patients with type I diabetes: correlations with other parameters of glycaemic control. *Diabetologia* 29: 685–689, 1985.

82. MACHLIN, L. J., FILIPSKI, R., WILLIS, A. L., KUHN, D. C., and BRIN, M. Influence of vitamin

E on platelet aggregation and thrombocythemia in the rat. *Proc. Soc. Exp. Biol. Med.* 149: 275–277, 1975.

83. MARTIN-NIZARD, F., RICHARD, B., TORPIER, G., NOUVELOT, A., FRUCHART, J. C., DUTHILLEUL, P., and DELBART, C. Analysis of phospholipid transfer during HDL binding to platelets using a fluorescent analog of phosphatidylcholine. *Thromb. Res.* 46: 811–825, 1987.

84. MAYFIELD, R. K., HALUSHKA, P. V., WOLTMANN, H. J., LOPES-VIRELLA, M. F., CHAMBER, J. K., LOADHOLT, C. B., and COLWELL, J. A. Platelet function during continuous insulin infusion treatment in insulin dependent diabetic patients. *Diabetes* 34: 1127–1133, 1985.

85. MAZUROV, A. V., PREOBRAZHENSKY, S. N., LEYTIN, V. L., et al. Study of low-density lipoprotein interaction with platelets by flow cytofluorimetry. *FEBS Lett.* 137: 319–322, 1982.

86. McDONALD, J. W. D., DUPRE, J., RODGER, N. W., CHAMPION, M. C., WEBB, C. D., and ALI, M. Comparison of platelet thromboxane synthesis in diabetic patients on conventional insulin therapy and continuous insulin infusion. *Thromb. Res.* 28: 705–712, 1982.

87. MIKHAILIDIS, D. P., MIKHAILIDIS, A. M., BARRADAS, M. A., and DANDONA, P. Effect of nonsterified fatty acids on the stability of prostacyclin activity. *Metabolism* 32: 717–721, 1983.

88. MONCADA, S., and VANE, J. R. Arachidonic acid metabolites and the interactions between platelets and blood vessel walls. *N. Engl. J. Med.* 300: 1142–1147, 1979.

89. MORDES, D. B., LAZARCHICK, J., COLWELL, J. A., and SENS, D. A. Elevated glucose concentrations increase factor VIIIR:Ag levels in human umbilical vein endothelial cells. *Diabetes* 32: 876–878, 1983.

90. MOREL, D. W., HESSLER, J. R., and CHISOLM, G. M. Low density lipoproteins cytotoxicity induced by free radical peroxidation of lipid. *J. Lipid. Res.* 24: 1070–1076, 1983.

91. MOSCONI, C., COLLI, S., TREMOLI, E., and GALLI, C. Phosphatidylinositol (PI) and PI-associated arachidonate are elevated in platelet total membranes of type IIa hypercholesterolemic subjects. *Atherosclerosis* 72: 129–134, 1988.

92. PALINSKI, W., ROSENFELD, M. E., YLA-HERTTUALA, S., GURTNER, G. C., SOCHER, S. S., BUTLER, S. W., PARTHASARATHY, S., CAREW, T. E., STEINBERG, D., and WITZTUM, J. L. Low density lipoprotein undergoes oxidative modification in vivo. *Proc. Natl. Acad. Sci. USA* 86: 1372–1376, 1989.

93. PETO, R., GRAY, R., COLLINS, R., et al. Randomized trial of prophylactic daily aspirin in British male doctors. *Br. Med. J.* 296: 313–316, 1988.

94. RENAUD, S., DUMONT, E., GODSEY, F., McGREGOR, L., and MORAZAIN, R. Effect of diet on blood clotting and platelet aggregation. In: *Nutrition in the 1980s. Constrains on Our Knowledge,* edited by N. Selvey and P. L. White. New York: Alan R. Liss, 1981, pp. 361–372.

95. ROSS, R., and GLOMSET, J. A. Atherosclerosis and the arterial smooth muscle cell. *Science* 180: 1332–1339, 1973.

96. ROSS, R., and GLOMSET, J. A. The pathogenesis of atherosclerosis. *N. Engl. J. Med.* 295: 369–377, 1976.

97. ROSS, R. The pathogenesis of atherosclerosis: an update. *N. Engl. J. Med.* 488–500, 1986.

98. SAGEL, J., COLWELL, J. A., CROOK, L., and LAIMINS, M. Increased platelet aggregation in early diabetes mellitus. *Ann. Intern. Med.* 82: 733–738, 1975.

99. SCHERNTHANER, G., SINZINGER, H., SILBERBAUER, K., FREYLER, H., MUHLHAUSER, I., and KALIMAN, J. Vascular prostacyclin, platelet sensitivity to prostaglandins, and platelet-specific proteins in diabetes mellitus. *Horm. Metab. Res.* 11: 33–43, 1981.

100. SHASTRI, K, N., CARVALHO, A. C. A., and LEES, R. S. Platelet function and platelet lipid composition in the dyslipoproteinemias. *J. Lipid Res.* 21: 467–472, 1980.

101. SHATTIL, S. J., and COOPER, R. A. Membrane viscosity and human platelet function. *Biochemistry* 15: 4832–4837, 1976.

102. SHATTIL, S. J., and COOPER, R. A. Role of membrane lipid composition, organization, and fluidity in human platelet function. *Prog. Hemostasis Thromb.* 4: 59–86, 1978.

103. SIESS, W. Molecular mechanisms of platelet activation. *Physiol. Rev.* 69: 48–178, 1989.

104. SILVER, M. J., SMITH, J. B., INGERMAN, C. M., and KOCSIS, C. Arachidonic acid induced human platelet aggregation and prostaglandin formation. *Prostaglandins* 4: 863–875, 1973.

105. SPARROW, C. P., PARTHASARATHY, S., and STEINBERG, D. A macrophage receptor that recognizes oxidized low density lipoprotein but not acetylated low density lipoprotein. *J. Biol. Chem.* 264: 2599–2604, 1989.

106. STEELE, P., and RAINWATER, J. Effect of dietary and pharmacologic alteration of serum lipids on platelet survival time. *Circulation* 58: 354–367, 1978.

107. STEERING COMMITTEE OF THE PHYSICIANS' HEALTH STUDY RESEARCH GROUP. Final report on the aspirin component of the ongoing physicians' health study. *N. Engl. J. Med.* 321: 129–135, 1989.

108. STEINBERG, D., PARTHASARATHY, S., CAREW, T. E., KHOO, J. C., and WITZTUM, J. L. Beyond cholesterol. Modifications of low-density lipoprotein that increase its atherogenicity. *N. Engl. J. Med.* 320: 915, 1989.

109. STEINER, M., and ANASTASI, J. Vitamin E: an inhibitor of the platelet release reaction. *J. Clin. Invest.* 57: 732–737, 1976.

110. STONE, M. C., and THORP, J. M. Plasma fibrinogen—a major coronary risk factor. *J. R. Coll. Gen. Pract.* 35: 565–569, 1985.

111. STRANO, A., DAVI, G., AVERNA, M., et al. Platelet sensitivity to prostacyclin and thromboxane production in hyperlipidemic patients. *Thromb. Haemostasis* 48: 18–20, 1982.

112. STUART, M. J., and OSKI, F. A. Vitamin E and platelet function. *Am. J. Pediatr. Hematol. Oncol.* 1: 227–234, 1979.

113. TAKEDA, H., MAEDA, H., FUKUSHIMA, H., NAKAMURA, N., and UZAWA, H. Increased platelet phospholipase activity in diabetic subjects. *Thromb. Res.* 13: 703–714, 1981.

114. TANDON, N., HARMON, J. T., RODBARD, D., and JAMIESON, G. A. Thrombin receptors define responsiveness of cholesterol-modified platelets. *J. Biol. Chem.* 258: 11840–11845, 1983.

115. TROVATI, M., ANFOSSI, G., CAVALOT, F., et al. Insulin directly reduces platelet sensitivity to aggregating agents. *Diabetes* 37: 780–786, 1988.

116. VAN ZILE, J., KILPATRICK, M., LAIMINS, M., SAGEL, J., COLWELL, J., and VIRELLA, G. Platelet aggregation and release of ATP after incubation with soluble immune complexes purified from the serum of diabetic patients. *Diabetes* 30: 575–579, 1981.

117. VIENER, A., BROOK, G., and AVIRAM, M. Abnormal plasma lipoprotein composition in hypercholesterolemic patients induces platelet activation. *Eur. J. Clin. Invest.* 14: 207–213, 1984.

118. VIRELLA, G., WOHLTMANN, H., SAGEL, J., LOPES-VIRELLA, M. F. L., KILPATRICK, M., PHILLIPS, C., and COLWELL, J. Soluble immune complexes in patients with diabetes mellitus: detection and pathological significance. *Diabetologia* 21: 184–191, 1981.

119. WATANABE, J., WOHLTMANN, H. J., KLEIN, R. L., COLWELL, J. A., and LOPES-VIRELLA, M. F. Enhancement of platelet aggregation by low-density lipoproteins from IDDM patients. *Diabetes* 37: 1652–1657, 1988.

120. WILLIS, A. L. An enzymatic mechanism for the antithrombotic and antihemostatic actions of aspirin. *Science* 183: 325–327, 1974.

121. WILLIS, A. L., KUHN, D. C., and WEISS, H. J. Acetylenic analog of arachidonate that acts like aspirin on platelets. *Science* 183: 327–329, 1974.

122. WILHELMSEN, L., SVARDSUDD, K., KORSA-BENGTSEN, K., et al. Fibrinogen as a risk factor for stroke and myocardial infarction. *N. Engl. J. Med.* 311: 501–505.

123. WINOCOUR, P. D. The role of platelets in the pathogenesis of diabetic vascular disease. In: *Molecular and Cellular Biology of Diabetes Mellitus*, Vol. III, edited by B. Draznin, S. Melmed, D. LeRoith. New York: Alan R. Liss, 1989, pp. 37–47.

124. WINOCOUR, P. D., BRYSZEWSKA, M., WATALA, C., et al. Reduced membrane fluidity in platelets from diabetic patients. *Diabetes* 39: 241–244, 1990.

125. WITZTUM, J., STEINBRECHER, U. P., FISHER, M., and KESANIEMI, A. Nonenzymatic glucosylation of homologous low density lipoprotein and albumin renders them immunogenic in the guinea pig. *Proc. Natl. Acad. Sci. USA* 80: 2757–2761, 1983.

126. WITZTUM, J., STEINBRECHER, U., KESANIEMI, Y., and FISHER, M. Autoantibodies to glucosylated proteins in the plasma of patients with diabetes mellitus. *Med. Sci.* 81: 3204–3208, 1984.

127. YLA-HERTTUALA, S., PALINSKI, W., ROSENFELD, M. E., and PARTHASARATHY, S. Evidence for the presence of oxidatively modified low density lipoprotein in atherosclerotic lesions of rabbit and man. *J. Clin. Invest.* 84: 1086–1095, 1989.

128. ZAHAVI, J., BETTERIDGE, J. D., JONES, N. A. G., et al. Enhanced in vivo platelet-release reaction and malondialdehyde formation in patients with hyperlipidemia. *Am. J. Med.* 70: 59–64, 1981.

4

Diabetes Mellitus and the Vascular Endothelium

RICHARD A. COHEN AND BELAY TESFAMARIAM

The endothelium plays an important role in the function of blood vessels. Under normal circumstances substances released from the endothelium, such as endothelium-derived factor(s), prostaglandins, and peptides, modulate the tone of vascular smooth muscle, prevent platelet aggregation and thrombosis in the blood vessel lumen, and may modulate vessel growth. It is well known that vasomotor, thrombotic, and growth control mechanisms are abnormal in blood vessels from humans and animals with atherosclerosis. It is also recognized that the progression and complications of atherosclerosis are increased in patients with diabetes. This chapter will review recent evidence that diabetes and hyperglycemia cause specific abnormalities in the vasomotor function of the endothelium. Because these vasomotor abnormalities result from the abnormal release of substances from the endothelium that may play a role in thrombosis and growth, an understanding of their mechanism of action may provide new insights to the basis of vascular complications in diabetes mellitus.

VASOMOTOR ROLE OF THE ENDOTHELIUM IN DIABETES MELLITUS

In 1980 Robert Furchgott reported that the endothelium is responsible for the vasodilator response to acetylcholine (5). He demonstrated that rings of isolated rabbit aorta contracted with phenylephrine failed to relax upon the addition of acetylcholine when the endothelium had been selectively removed by rubbing the intimal surface of the blood vessel. Subsequently, the relaxation of vascular preparations with intact endothelium in response to acetylcholine and many other vasodilators, including thrombin, bradykinin, substance P, serotonin, ATP, and ADP, have been ascribed to the release from the endothelium of vasodilator(s) termed *endothelium-derived relaxing factor(s)* (EDRF). The primary vasodilator released from the endothelium has been identified as nitric oxide (14), or a related molecule such as S-nitrosocysteine (12), which is formed by the breakdown of arginine (14). The endothelium-derived nitrosylated compound activates guanylate cyclase in the smooth muscle to cause relaxation by a mechanism similar to that by which nitroprusside or nitroglycerin causes relaxation (16). The release of EDRF is initiated by agonists such

48

as acetylcholine, which act by causing increases in endothelial cell calcium (3). They appear to do so both by stimulating receptor activation of phospholipase C, with the consequent formation of inositol triphosphate and release of intracellular calcium stores, and by enhancing the influx of extracellular calcium (15). The release of EDRF may be stimulated without the involvement of endothelial cell receptors when intracellular calcium is increased by the calcium ionophore A23187. The release of EDRF parallels that of prostaglandins caused by cell calcium increases, but the release may depend differently on intracellular calcium than on extracellular calcium (10).

Blood vessels of some animals with diabetes, including the aortas of streptozotocin-treated rats and BB rats demonstrate abnormal endothelium-dependent relaxations (11,13). Likewise, in coronary arteries from the same chronically diabetic dogs in which Engerman et al. have studied the development of retinopathy (4), we found that the endothelium-dependent relaxation caused by thrombin was abnormal (Figure 4.1). Arteries from two diabetic dogs maintained for 5 yr were studied. The coronary artery rings from a dog in which glucose was maintained in the near-normal range with daily injections of insulin showed normal relaxations to thrombin and ADP. In contrast, in the coronary arteries from this dog's littermate whose hyperglycemia was not effectively controlled, the rings showed impaired relaxations to thrombin. Relaxation induced by adenosine diphosphate in the rings from the dog with poor diabetic control was normal, implying that the endothelium was functionally intact, and that the impairment in endothelial cell function was selective for certain agonists.

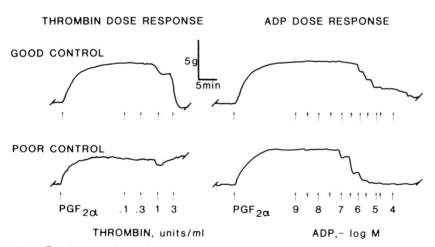

DIABETIC CANINE CORONARY ARTERY

THROMBIN DOSE RESPONSE ADP DOSE RESPONSE

GOOD CONTROL

5g

5min

POOR CONTROL

PGF$_{2\alpha}$ .1 .3 1 3   PGF$_{2\alpha}$ 9 8 7 6 5 4

THROMBIN, units/ml ADP,- log M

FIGURE 4.1. Tension recordings of coronary artery rings from two diabetic dogs contracted with prostaglandin F$_{2\alpha}$ (PGF$_{2\alpha}$). The upper ring is that of a dog in good diabetic control achieved by daily insulin doses. The lower ring is that of a dog in poor diabetic control. The ring from the treated dog relaxes normally in response to thrombin; an endothelium-dependent vasodilator, but the response of the artery from the dog in poor diabetic control is decreased. The rings from both dogs relax normally in response to another endothelium-dependent vasodilator, adenosine diphosphate (ADP).

The only observations reported on human diabetic vascular tissues have been made in biopsies of penile corpora cavernosa from impotent diabetic men which were obtained at the time of implantation of penile prostheses [(17); Fig. 4.2]. Compared to controls, relaxations induced by acetylcholine were decreased or absent in penile tissue from these diabetic individuals, despite a morphologically intact endothelium. Abnormal vasodilation mediated by the endothelium could be an important contributor to impaired erectile function.

To study endothelium-dependent function in a more convenient and accessible diabetic animal model, further studies have been conducted in New Zealand white rabbits made diabetic with alloxan (23). These rabbits had plasma glucose levels averaging 360 mg/dl and were studied after being diabetic for 6 weeks. Figure 4.3 shows an example of the abnormal response to acetylcholine of a ring of the abdominal aorta from a diabetic rabbit. Unlike the normal aorta, in which each concentration of acetylcholine causes relaxation, the diabetic aorta relaxes and then contracts in response to acetylcholine. Furthermore, higher concentrations of this agonist cause contractions in diabetic aorta. This abnormality in endothelium-dependent relaxation in diabetes is selective for receptor-mediated agonists, because relaxations in response to ionophore A23187 are normal (23). Relaxations to nitroprusside, a direct smooth muscle vasodilator, also are normal suggesting an impaired release of EDRF in the diabetic animals following acetylcholine stimulation. Indeed, a decrease in acetylcholine-induced stimulation of cyclic 3',5'-guanosine monophosphate levels in diabetic rabbit aorta is consistent with a decreased release of EDRF from the diabetic rabbit aortic endothelium (1).

However, several lines of evidence indicate that the abnormality in endothelial cell function in diabetes results from the abnormal production of vasoconstrictor prostaglandins by the endothelium of the diabetic rabbit aorta (23). First, treatment of the isolated aortic ring with the cyclooxygenase inhibitor

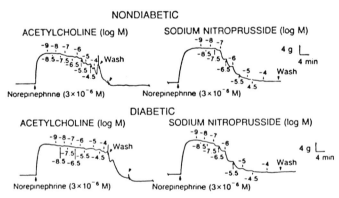

FIGURE 4.2. Tension recordings of biopsies of human corpus cavernosae from nondiabetic (*top*) and diabetic (*bottom*) men. The tissue is contracted with norepinephrine and subsequently exposed to increasing concentrations of acetylcholine (*left*) or sodium nitroprusside (*right*). The tissue from the nondiabetic man relaxes in response to acetylcholine, but that from the diabetic man does not. Both tissues relax normally in response to sodium nitroprusside. [From reference 17 by permission of the *New England Journal of Medicine*.]

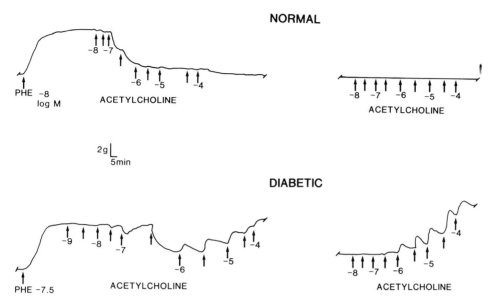

FIGURE 4.3. Recording of acetylcholine-induced relaxations and contractions of normal and diabetic rabbit aortic rings. *Left*: In aorta from diabetic rabbits, rings contracted with phenylephrine (PHE) show decreased relaxations at low concentrations. *Right*: Acetylcholine caused contraction of resting aortic rings from diabetic rabbits, but not from normal rabbits. [From reference 23 by permission of the American Physiological Society.]

indomethacin normalizes the relaxation of the diabetic aorta. Second, the thromboxane (Tx) A_2/prostaglandin (PG) H_2 receptor antagonist SQ29548 also normalizes the relaxation. Third, in separate experiments, radioimmunoassay of incubates of segments of aorta with intact endothelium (3 cm long) showed increased levels of TxA_2 produced by the diabetic aorta (Fig. 4.4). The increased release of the vasoconstrictor prostanoid occurred only in segments with intact endothelium and was stimulated by acetylcholine, suggesting the endothelium was responsible for the increased release, and that the prostanoid could account for the abnormal relaxation. In contrast to TxA_2, the release of PGI_2, which is also primarily derived from endothelial cells, was not significantly changed by diabetes.

INFLUENCE OF GLUCOSE ON THE ENDOTHELIUM

Further studies have been performed in normal rabbit aorta exposed in vitro to elevated concentrations of glucose (20). The studies cited above on diabetic rabbit aorta were done in physiological solution containing 11 mM (200 mg/dl) glucose. When normal aorta is incubated for 6 h at 37°C in glucose (11 mM), there is no time-dependent change in the acetylcholine relaxation. Also, similar relaxations are seen in arteries incubated for 6 h in 5.5 mM (100 mg/dl) glucose. However, when normal aorta is incubated for 6 h in media containing 44 mM (800 mg/dl) glucose, acetylcholine relaxations are abnormal (Fig. 4.5).

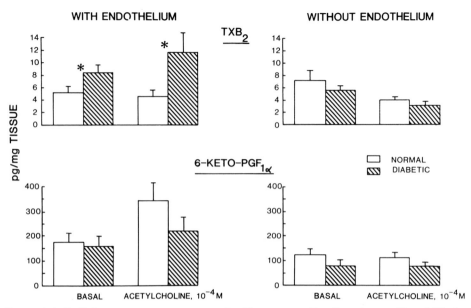

FIGURE 4.4. Radioimmunoassay measurements of immunoreactive thromboxane B_2 and 6-keto-$PGF_{1\alpha}$ as measures of thromboxane A_2 and PGI_2, respectively, in the incubation media of aortic segments from normal and diabetic rabbits. In segments with endothelium (left), basal and acetylcholine-stimulated levels of thromboxane B_2 were significantly higher in aorta from diabetic rabbits (*$p<0.05$). Levels of 6-keto-$PGF_{1\alpha}$ were not significantly different in aortic segments from normal and diabetic rabbits. In segments without endothelium (right), the levels of thromboxane B_2 and 6-keto-$PGF_{1\alpha}$ were significantly lower than in segments with endothelium, indicating that the major source of the prostanoids is the endothelium.

The response after exposure to elevated glucose resembles that observed in diabetic aorta in that acetylcholine causes contractions following relaxation in response to each concentration added. The effect of glucose apparently is not due to the hyperosmolarity associated with the high concentration used, because mannose at the same concentration does not simulate the effect of glucose (Fig. 4.5). For the effect of glucose to be elicited within 6 h, requires concentrations greater than 22 mM. Likewise at least 3 h of incubation is needed to see an effect at 44 mM glucose. The similar effect of incubation in vitro with 44 mM glucose and 6 weeks of diabetes in which the endothelium is exposed to a plasma glucose concentration of 360 mg/dl (20 mM) supports the notion that glucose in the diabetic milieu is the primary etiologic agent causing endothelial cell dysfunction. The similarity between endothelial cell function in aorta exposed to glucose in vitro and in the diabetic rabbit also extends to the involvement of vasoconstrictor prostaglandins. The abnormal relaxations caused by high concentrations of glucose in vitro are prevented by cyclooxygenase inhibitors or by the PGH_2/TxA_2 receptor blocker, SQ29548 (Fig. 4.5). In addition, there are similar increases in the acetylcholine-induced release of immunoassayable TxA_2 and $PGF_{2\alpha}$ in aorta incubated in 44 mM glucose (20). The changes described in endothelium-dependent relaxations of rabbit aorta are not specific for acetylcholine, because endothelium-dependent relaxations

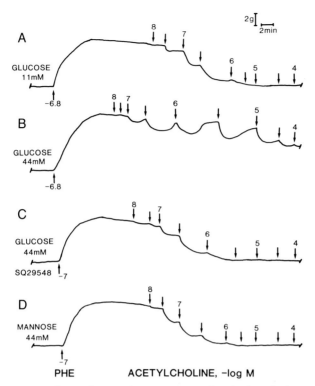

FIGURE 4.5. Tension recordings of rings of aorta contracted with phenylephrine (PHE) and then exposed to acetylcholine. Aortic rings incubated for 6 h in control glucose (11mM) show normal relaxations (A), but those incubated in elevated glucose (44 mM) show decreased relaxations to acetylcholine (B). Treatment with SQ 29548 (3×10^{-6} M) normalized the abnormal responses in aorta incubated in elevated glucose (C). Aorta incubated in mannose (44 mM), to serve as a hyperosmotic control, relaxed to acetylcholine normally (D). [From reference 20 by permission of the *Journal of Clinical Investigation*.]

of the rabbit aorta in response to ADP are also abnormal at high glucose concentrations and are prevented by cyclooxygenase blockade (Fig. 4.6). This is in contrast to the normal ADP relaxations in coronary artery from diabetic dog, which may be due, at least in part, to differences in the species, type of vascular bed, and/or duration of diabetes. Observations of changes in endothelium-dependent responsiveness caused by elevated glucose have not been restricted to the rabbit aorta. For instance, the endothelium-dependent relaxation of pig coronary artery to bradykinin is also abnormal after exposure to elevated concentrations of glucose in vitro (Fig. 4.7).

MECHANISM OF GLUCOSE EFFECT ON ENDOTHELIUM

Studies now underway in our laboratory are aimed at determining the mechanism by which a high concentration of glucose influences the release of endothelium-derived vasoactive substances.

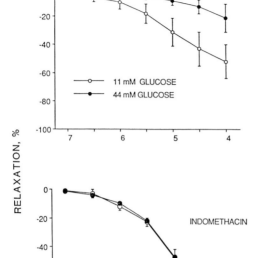

FIGURE 4.6. Comparison of relaxations induced by adenosine diphosphate of aortic rings incubated in control (11 mM) or elevated (44 mM) glucose for 6 h. *Top:* Relaxations were significantly fewer in aortic rings incubated in elevated glucose than in those incubated in control glucose. *Bottom:* In rings treated with indomethacin during the 6 h incubation, the incidence of ADP-induced relaxation of rings incubated in elevated glucose was not significantly different from that of rings incubated in control glucose. Values are means ± SE; n = 4.

Aldose Reductase and Myo-inositol

Greene et al. have suggested that hyperglycemia may contribute to the pathogenesis of many of the complications of diabetes mellitus by increasing flux through the enzyme aldose reductase, which converts glucose to sorbitol. The hypothesis is based on measurements of increased levels of sorbitol in diabetic tissues and the ameliorating effects of aldose reductase inhibitors, such as sorbinil, in diabetic neuropathy. They suggest that high concentrations of glucose and the resultant increased amounts of sorbitol lead to decreases in a cellular pool of myo-inositol, which in turn leads to abnormal cell signaling. With this hypothesis in mind, the effects of sorbinil and *myo*-inositol repletion on endothelial cell function were examined in rabbit aorta exposed to an elevated glucose concentration. When sorbinil (1 mM) or *myo*-inositol (1 mM) were added to the incubation media, aortic rings exposed for 6 h to 44 mM glucose had normal endothelium-dependent relaxations in response to acetylcholine (22). This suggests the importance of altered aldose reductase activity and *myo*-inositol depletion in the abnormal endothelial cell function observed in these studies. It has been suggested that depletion of *myo*-inositol decreases the turnover of a pool of phosphatidylinositol, which is involved in the regulation of Na^+K^+-ATPase (18). High concentrations of glucose decrease Na^+K^+-ATPase activity in rabbit aorta, and this effect is prevented by adding to the medium aldose reductase inhibitors or supplemental *myo*-inositol (19). The in-

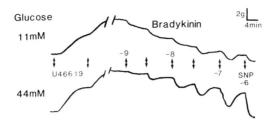

FIGURE 4.7. Tension recording of two rings of pig coronary artery after incubation for 6 h in control (11 mM) or elevated (44 mM) glucose. The rings were contracted with the thromboxane A$_2$-mimetic U46619, and relaxations were elicted with bradykinin. In the ring incubated with elevated glucose, relaxations are fewer and the response to each concentration of bradykinin is followed by a contraction.

hibition of rabbit aortic Na$^+$K$^+$-ATPase activity by glucose is endothelium dependent (8). Thus, reduced Na$^+$K$^+$-ATPase activity secondary to *myo*-inositol depletion may explain the endothelial cell dysfunction caused by elevated glucose.

Endothelial Cell Calcium

As in the aorta of diabetic rabbit, non-receptor-mediated endothelium-dependent relaxations caused by the calcium ionophore A23187 are normal in aorta incubated with 44 mM glucose. Exposure to elevated glucose may therefore interfere with steps in the activation of endothelial cell receptors by acetylcholine or other receptor-mediated vasodilators. In addition, prostaglandin release from endothelial cells, which is also modulated by calcium, is abnormal with acetylcholine but not with ionophore A23187. These possibilities suggest that the formation of inositol triphosphate by phospholipase C in response to endothelial receptor activation may be abnormal in endothelium exposed to elevated glucose. This hypothesis would require direct measurements of phospholipids and calcium.

Role of G Proteins

It has been reported that G$_i$ protein is deficient in the liver of streptozotocin-induced diabetic rats (6). Pertussis toxin, which inactivates G$_i$ protein by ADP ribosylation (24), has been used to examine its role in endothelium-mediated relaxation. Rings of rabbit aorta were incubated with pertussis toxin 100 ng/ml for 2 h in media containing (control 11 mM or elevated 44 mM) glucose. The relaxation caused by acetylcholine, but not ionophore A23187, was inhibited following treatment with pertussis toxin in the aortas incubated in control glucose concentration. In contrast, pertussis toxin did not have any effect on the abnormal response to acetylcholine observed at 44 mM glucose. The abnormal acetylcholine relaxations caused by pertussis toxin were similar to those caused by incubation in elevated glucose, suggesting involvement of the G$_i$ protein in the endothelial cell dysfunction caused by hyperglycemia.

Protein Kinase C

Recent studies by King and colleagues suggest that cultured endothelial cells and other vascular cells exposed to elevated concentrations of glucose have an increase in the de novo synthesis of diacylglycerol and subsequent increase in protein kinase C activity (9). The effects of the protein kinase C activator, phorbol myristate acetate (PMA), and of the protein kinase C inhibitors, H-7 and sphingosine, have been investigated on endothelial cell function in aortic rings (21). In normal rabbit aorta a 10 min exposure to PMA (10^{-8} M), which itself caused no contraction and did not interfere with the contraction caused by phenylephrine, resulted in an abnormal acetylcholine relaxation. The latter resembled the abnormality observed in aorta exposed to 44 mM glucose for 6 h, in that contractions followed relaxation in response to each added concentration of acetylcholine. There was no additive effect of a 10 min exposure to PMA in rings incubated in 44 mM glucose for 6 h, suggesting a common mechanism for the abnormal acetylcholine relaxation. Incubation of segments of rabbit aorta in 11 mM glucose containing PMA resulted in increased acetylcholine-induced release of vasoconstrictor prostaglandins in a pattern nearly identical to that of the diabetic aorta and to normal aorta exposed to 44 mM glucose for 6 h. Furthermore, the inhibitors of protein kinase C prevented both the abnormal acetylcholine relaxations and the increased release of vasoconstrictor prostanoids caused by 6 h exposure to elevated glucose. These studies strongly implicate protein kinase C in the abnormal endothelium-dependent relaxations to acetylcholine and the increased release of vasoconstrictor prostaglandins caused by a high concentration of glucose (Fig. 4.8). Activation of protein kinase C inactivates G_i protein by phosphorylation (25). It is tempting to speculate that this mechanism may be responsible for the impairment of endothelial cell receptor–mediated signal transduction.

IMPLICATIONS FOR DIABETIC VASCULAR DISEASE

These studies demonstrate that elevated concentrations of glucose could directly cause endothelial cell dysfunction in diabetes mellitus. They also raise the possibility that alterations in vascular responsiveness caused by glucose may contribute to abnormal vascular reactivity in diabetes such as that exists in the eye, skin, kidney, brain, and heart. Furthermore, it is important to consider the effects of abnormally produced prostanoids by diabetic blood vessels. Augmented thromboxane A_2 production by the endothelium may contribute to an accelerated rate of platelet aggregation in diabetic blood vessels noted in many clinical studies (2). The platelet proaggregatory action and the vascular smooth muscle growth-promoting activity of TxA$_2$ could increase the rate of atherogenesis in diabetic blood vessels (2). Thus, the increased rate of both thrombotic and atherosclerotic vascular disease could be attributed to an influence of glucose on the endothelium. Whether these results will lead to new treatment modalities or a different use of older approaches for diabetic vascular disease requires further study. These modalities might include cyclooxygenase or TxA$_2$/PGH$_2$ receptor antagonists, aldose reductase inhibitors, and protein kinase C inhibitors.

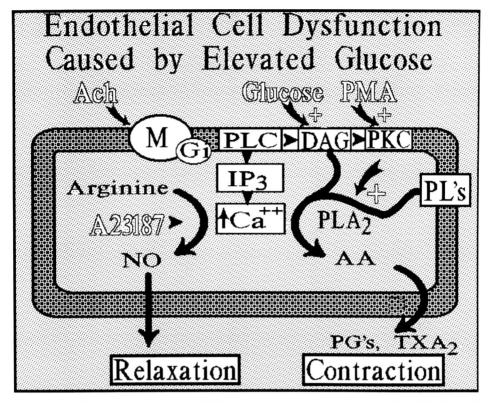

FIGURE 4.8. Hypothetical scheme by which elevated glucose may interfere with endothelial cell signal transduction. Acetylcholine (Ach), by binding to a muscarinic receptor, activates phospholipase C (PLC) to form inositol triphosphate (IP_3), which releases intracellular stores of calcium (Ca^{2+}) and diacylglycerol (DAG), which activates protein kinase C (PKC). Rises in Ca^{2+} lead to release of the arginine-derived vasodilator, nitric oxide (NO), as well as prostaglandins by activation of phospholipase A_2 (PLA_2) which cleaves membrane phospholipids (PLs). Activation of PKC may inactivate the G_i protein by negative feedback inhibition. Increased prostaglandin production could result from free arachidonic acid (AA) derived from DAG by way of diacylglycerol lipase, or PKC may have specific effects on PLA_2 activity. By the activity of cyclooxygenase, prostaglandin H_2 is formed from AA and, together with its prostaglandin (PG) products including thromboxane A_2 (TXA_2), it can cause contraction of underlying smooth muscle cells.

ACKNOWLEDGMENTS

The work was supported by National Institutes of Health grants HL31607 and HL 38731. R. A. Cohen is the recipient of an Established Investigator Award from the American Heart Association. B. Tesfamariam is supported by research grant 190759 from the Juvenile Diabetes Foundation and grant-in-aid 13-551-890 from the American Heart Association, Massachusetts Affiliate, Inc.

REFERENCES

1. ABIRU, T., WATANABE, Y., KAMATA, K., MIYATA, N., and KASUYA, Y. Decrease in endothelium-dependent relaxation and levels of cyclic nucleotides in aorta from rabbits with alloxan-induced diabetes. *Res. Commun. Chem. Pathol. Pharmacol.* 68: 13, 1990.

2. COLWELL, J. A. Platelets, endothelium, and diabetic vascular disease. *Diabetes Metab.* 14: 512, 1988.
3. DANTHULURI, N. R., CYBULSKY, M. I., and BROCK, T. ACh-induced calcium transients in primary cultures of rabbit aortic endothelial cells. *Am. J. Physiol.* 255 (*Heart Physiol.*): H1549, 1988.
4. ERNST, J. T., GOLDSTICK, T. K., and ENGERMAN, R. L. Hyperglycemia impairs retinal oxygen autoregulation in normal and diabetic dogs. *Invest. Opthalmol. Vis. Sci.* 24: 985, 1985.
5. FURCHGOTT, R. F., and ZAWADZKI, J. V. The obligatory role of the endothelial cells in the relaxation of arterial smooth muscle by acetylcholine. *Nature* 288: 373, 1980.
6. GAWLER, D., MILLIGAN, G., SPIEGEL, A. M., UNSON, C. G., and HOUSLEY, M. D. Abolition of the expression of inhibitory guanine nucleotide regulatory protein G_i activity in diabetes. *Nature* 327: 229, 1987.
7. GREENE, D. A., LATTIMER, S. A., and SIMA, A. A. F. Sorbitol, phosphoinositides and sodium-potassium-ATPase in the pathogenesis of diabetic complications. *N. Engl. J. Med.* 316: 599, 1987.
8. GUPTA, S., COHEN, R. A., and SUSSMAN, I. Endothelium-dependent inhibition of vascular Na^+/K^+-ATPase activity by high glucose. *Diabetes* 39(Suppl I): 31A, 1990.
9. LEE, T.-S., MACGREGOR, L. C., FLUHARTY, S. J., and KING, G. L. Differential regulation of protein kinase C and (Na^+/K^+)-adenosine triphosphate activities by elevated glucose levels in retinal capillary endothelial cells. *J. Clin. Invest.* 83: 90, 1989.
10. LUCKHOFF, A., POHL, U., MULSCH, A., and BUSSE, R. Differential role of extra- and intracellular calcium in the release of EDRF and prostacyclin from cultured endothelial cells. *Br. J. Pharmacol.* 95: 189, 1988.
11. MERAJI, S., JAYAKODY, L., SENARATNE, P., THOMSON, A. B. R., and KAPPAGODA, T. Endothelium-dependent relaxation in aorta of BB rats. *Diabetes* 36: 978, 1987.
12. MYERS, P. R., MINOR, R. L., GUERRA, R., BATES, J. N., and HARRISON, D. G. Vasorelaxant properties of the endothelium-derived relaxing factor more closely resemble S-nitrosocysteine than nitric oxide. *Nature* 345: 161, 1990.
13. OYAMA, Y., KAWASAKI, H., HATTORI, Y., and KANNO, M. Attenuation of endothelium-dependent relaxation in aorta from diabetic rats. *Eur. J. Pharmacol.* 131: 75, 1986.
14. PALMER, R. M. J., ASHTON, D. S., and MONCADA, S. Vascular endothelial cells synthesize nitric oxide from L-arginine. *Nature* 333: 664, 1988.
15. PEACH, M. J., SINGER, H. A., IZZO, N. J., and LOEB, A. L. Role of calcium in endothelium-dependent relaxation of arterial smooth muscle. *Am. J. Cardiol.* 59: 35A, 1987.
16. RAPPOPORT, R. M., and MURAD, F. Agonist-induced endothelium-dependent relaxation in rat thoracic aorta may be mediated through cGMP. *Circ. Res.* 52: 352, 1983.
17. SAENZ DE TEJADA, I., GOLDSTEIN, I., AZADZOI, K., KRANE, R., and COHEN, R. Impaired neurogenic and endothelium-dependent relaxation of human penile smooth muscle: the pathophysiological basis for impotence in diabetes mellitus. *N. Engl. J. Med.* 320: 1025, 1989.
18. SIMMONS, D. A., KERN, E. F. D., WINEGRAD, A. I., and MARTIN, D. B. Basal phosphotidylinositol turnover controls aortic Na^+/K^+ ATPase activity. *J. Clin. Invest.* 77: 503, 1986.
19. SIMMONS, D. A., and WINEGRAD, A. I. Mechanism of glucose-induced (Na^+/K^+)-ATPase inhibition in aortic wall of rabbits. *Diabetologia* 322: 402, 1989.
20. TESFAMARIAM, B., BROWN, M. L., DEYKIN, D., and COHEN, R. A. Elevated glucose promotes generation of endothelium-derived vasoconstrictor prostanoids in rabbit aorta. *J. Clin. Invest.* 85: 929, 1990.
21. TESFAMARIAM, B., and COHEN, R. A. Role of protein kinase C in the impairment caused by elevated glucose of receptor-mediated endothelium-dependent relaxation. *Clin. Res.* 38: 413A, 1990.
22. TESFAMARIAM, B., and COHEN, R. A. Role of sorbitol and *myo*-inositol in the endothelial cell dysfunction caused by elevated glucose. *Federation Proc.* 4: A416, 1990.
23. TESFAMARIAM, B., JAKUBOWSKI, J. A., and COHEN, R. A. Contraction of diabetic rabbit aorta due to endothelium-derived PGH_2/TxA_2. *Am. J. Physiol.* 257 (*Heart Physiol.*): H1327, 1989.
24. UI, M. Islet-activating protein, pertussis toxin: a probe for functions of the inhibitory guanine nucleotide regulatory component of adenylate cyclase. *Trends Pharmacol. Sci.* 5: 227, 1984.
25. WATSON, S. P., and LAPETINA, E. G. 1,2-diacylglycerol and phorbol ester inhibit agonist-induced formation of inositol phosphate in human platelets: possible implications for negative feed back regulation of inositol phospholipid hydrolysis. *Proc. Natl. Acad. Sci. USA* 82: 2623, 1985.

5

Cerebral Microvascular Transport and Metabolism: Implications for Diabetes

ANTHONY L. MCCALL

Diabetes mellitus affects many organs of the body. While the eyes, kidneys, cardiovascular system, and peripheral nervous system are most widely recognized to be harmed by diabetes, the impact of diabetes on the central nervous system (CNS) has gained attention only recently (172,213). Altered cerebral microvascular transport and metabolism may be relevant to three clinical areas in diabetes—stroke, hypoglycemia, and chronic cognitive dysfunction. Knowledge of the basic physiology of brain transport of glucose has mushroomed, especially since the cloning of the glucose-transport proteins. As a result, descriptive in vivo studies of physiology can now be extended, and precise molecular mechanisms underlying transport changes can be determined. Recent studies also extend basic knowledge of how diabetes affects microvascular function and metabolism in the brain.

This chapter will cover the effects of diabetes and hypoglycemia on blood–brain transport of metabolic fuels. Evidence will be presented that glucose regulates its own transport into the brain and that diabetes and hypoglycemia alter both the metabolism of glucose and other fuels by cerebral microvessels and their transport across the blood–brain barrier. The importance of glucose to the energy state of isolated microvessels will also be discussed. The last section of the chapter will discuss the potential consequences of such alterations in the microvasculature for clinical diabetes and brain function, particularly in relation to stroke and hypoglycemia.

BLOOD–BRAIN TRANSPORT

Blood–Brain Barrier: Origin of the Concept and Anatomy

In 1913, E. E. Goldmann extended the studies of his mentor Paul Ehrlich on the administration of vital dyes to animals (86,87). He injected trypan blue, an acidic, water-soluble, albumin-bound dye into the venous circulation. Almost all tissues stained intensely except the brain, which remained "snow white." In a crucial companion experiment, he injected trypan blue into the cerebrospinal fluid, strongly staining the brain. He concluded that a blood–brain barrier (*Blut-Gehirn-Schranke* in the original German) must exist. He postulated that the barrier was formed by the astrocytic foot processes adjacent to the endothelial basement membrane in brain capillaries (the glial limiting membrane, or *gliose Grenzmembran* in German). Ehrlich, however, felt that the notion of a barrier between blood and brain seemed to violate rational physiology. If a blood–brain barrier existed, how could the brain acquire essential nutrients? Goldmann surmised that the choroid plexus regulated the entry of nutrients into the brain. Present evidence suggests that the choroid plexus plays a minor role in regulating brain interstitium when compared to brain capillaries. Perhaps calling the interface between blood and brain a "gateway" rather than a barrier would have been a more apt metaphor.

Ultrastructural Anatomic Basis for the Barrier

The anatomic basis of the blood–brain barrier is tight junctions between endothelial cells in brain capillaries. Brightman and Reese and their colleagues first defined the anatomical nature of the blood–brain barrier. In a series of papers (30,31,204), they performed experiments analogous to that of Goldmann and examined the ultrastructural detail of brain capillaries using electron-dense markers and transmission electron microscopy. In 1967 Reese and Karnovsky (204) examined brain capillary endothelium after injection of horseradish peroxidase, an enzyme (MW = 40,000) with a reaction product that has a high affinity for osmium tetroxide. Peroxidase was confined to the capillary lumen; five layered "tight junctions" (zonula occludens) appeared at the overlapping interendothelial cell sites of apposition. This continuous seal occurred between endothelial cells in parenchymal blood vessels, between epithelial cells of the choroid plexus, and between ependymal cells overlying the median eminence and the area postrema. Membranes were not fused but were connected by a series of common fibrillar strands as shown by freeze-fracture studies (30). Effectively, these circumferential tight junctions occlude paracellular movement of water-soluble materials. These studies were later confirmed with smaller molecular weight, electron-dense markers, cytochrome c (MW = 17,000), microperoxidase (MW = 1,800), and lanthanum hydroxide or ionic lanthanum [(31); diameters less than 20 and 10 Å, respectively].

Transport of Metabolic Substrates

Reservations about the initial, unrefined concept of a barrier between blood and brain were realistic. Some compounds, including metabolic substrates, must be able to pass the barrier in a selective manner. Table 5.1 lists the different types of mechanisms of transport, their physiological basis, and some representative substrates (187). One manner of circumventing the blood–brain barrier is penetration of lipid-soluble compounds through the endothelial cell's phospholipid cell membranes via simple diffusion. Anesthetics and drugs of abuse are notoriously lipid soluble; penetration into the brain is predicted by their high oil:water partition coefficient. In contrast, metabolic substrates are weak electrolytes and are sparingly lipid soluble. Thus, fuels for brain energy metabolism (glucose, ketone bodies, and lactate) and precursors to brain neurotransmitters (tryptophan, tyrosine, and choline) are largely transported by

TABLE 5.1. Types of blood–brain barrier transport

Type of transport	Physiologic basis	Representative substrates
Simple diffusion	Lipid solubility	Heroin, ethanol, nicotine
Facilitated diffusion	Protein carrier molecules	Glucose, tyrosine, choline
Active transport	Carrier molecules	Na^+,K^+,-glutamate (efflux)
Endocytosis (receptor-mediated)	Specific receptors	Insulin, peptides, other hormones

carrier systems with enzyme-like specificity. Transport systems currently described for metabolic substrates include those listed in Table 5.2 (12).

Under normal circumstances, the primary fuel for brain energy metabolism is glucose. Christian Crone (48,49) used the indicator diffusion technique to study transport of D-glucose into dog brain. He first demonstrated that the brain had a saturable transport system for glucose. Several attributes characterize this transport process, which is termed facilitated diffusion. They include (1) saturation, (2) competition between substrates if more than one binds to the carrier protein, (3) lack of direct dependence on cellular energy, (4) equilibration-movement of substrates down a concentration gradient, and (5) bidirectional symmetry. In addition, hexose transport possesses a property known as *accelerated exchange diffusion:* the activity of the carrier protein (i.e. glucose transport) increases dramatically shortly after a brief exposure to very high concentrations of hexoses, e.g. 50 mM glucose.

The transport of the acidic class of amino acids (e.g. glutamate and aspartate), like the transport of ions (88), is asymmetrically distributed between the blood (luminal) and brain (abluminal) sides of brain capillaries, unlike most other facilitated diffusion systems (186). Similarly, transport for small, polar amino acids is asymmetric in its distribution in brain capillaries (89), probably due to induction of their transport systems by astrocytes (8,35,52,53) on the abluminal or brain side of cerebral capillaries. Recent evidence suggests that astrocyte products may also induce transport of glucose (159).

Normally, the entry of proteins into the brain is limited by their large size and sparing lipid solubility. Receptor-mediated transendothelial passage may

TABLE 5.2. Transport systems for metabolic substrates at the blood–brain barrier

System	Substrates transported
Hexoses	D-Glucose, 2-deoxy-D-glucose, D-galactose
Monocarboxylic acids	Ketone bodies, L-lactate, L-pyruvate
Large neutral amino acids	L-tyrosine, L-tryptophan, L-leucine
Basic amino acids	L-lysine, L-arginine
Acidic amino acids	L-glutamate, L-aspartate
Amines	Choline
Purine nucleosides	Adenosine
Purine bases	Adenine

represent one mechanism of entry circumventing these restrictions. Insulin may enter into the brain by such a mechanism. Fluid-filled pinocytosis is not a likely mechanism for protein uptake normally, since it is minimal in unperturbed brain vasculature; however, it increases with a variety of insults (25).

Brain microvessels possess Na^+K^+-ATPase activity (88,95), bind ouabain (96), and take up the potassium analog ^{86}Rb. ^{22}Na movement across the blood–brain barrier has also been studied in vivo (142). Another aspect of the barrier or gateway function of brain capillaries is their high content of degradative enzymes, which may minimize the effects of circulating compounds on the brain (58,176), e.g. circulating catecholamines are degraded by monoamine oxidase in brain capillaries.

The kinetics of entry of metabolic substrates into the brain suggests that transport characteristics are not fixed; they are modulated in response to a variety of circumstances. As a result of transport adaptations, brain biochemistry may be affected. Situations in which transport adapts include ischemia (14,16), hypoxia (11,13,63), starvation (84), during development (27,46,214), portocaval anastomosis (122,215), mercury intoxication (185), hypoglycemia (162), and diabetes mellitus (85,165,195). It is to these last adaptations we will turn. However, before discussion of these adaptations, some methods used to study transport will be briefly described.

Methods Used to Study Transport

It is beyond the scope of this chapter to comprehensively discuss the merits or limitations of different methods for studying blood-to-brain transport in live animals or people. Readers are referred to some reviews (21,25,187, 189,203,224) for fuller discussions, particularly since proponents of varying methods have not reached full consensus on which approaches are most appropriate. Some discussion of technical aspects is brought out below, however, so that the reader will understand some of the basis for the disagreement over results in studies of blood–brain barrier permeability, especially in experimental diabetes.

In a recent review, Smith (224) has discussed several types of methods used to study blood–brain barrier transport in vivo. They include (1) intravenous administration techniques (83), (2) the in situ brain perfusion method (233), (3) the indicator diffusion method pioneered by Crone (48,49), (4) the brain uptake index of Oldendorf (181,182), and (5) the single injection–external registration method of Raichle (221). As reviewed by Pardridge (187), methods to study brain transport in vivo involve administration of test compounds by several means, including constant infusion or injection either via an intravenous route or an intraarterial route. Sampling of the brain uptake of compounds may be performed by venous sampling or tissue sampling. (This latter may be determined by liquid scintillation counting of brain tissue samples, autoradiography, or some form of external registration, as with positron emission tomography [PET].)

The intravenous administration method and the in situ brain perfusion methods measure transport over relatively long periods involving several circulatory passages through brain. Smith and colleagues have argued that longer uptake makes them more sensitive and accurate at low rates of solute penetration. This is clearly true; such an approach permits accurate measurement of compounds that penetrate the blood–brain barrier poorly, e.g. sucrose. The greater accuracy of measurement may be especially important when determining transport kinetics, i.e. studying inhibition by unlabeled substrates of labeled substrate transport (e.g. ^{14}C-D-glucose inhibited by unlabeled glucose). However, longer periods of study may prove disadvantageous when metabolism is altered, making transport estimates less accurate and more influenced by altered metabolism of labeled compounds.

The last three methods that Smith discusses measure brain unidirectional extraction of compounds over a single circulatory passage and may thus be more suitable for measurement of permeability coefficients for compounds like glucose, which penetrates the brain at high rates. Furthermore, in diabetes mellitus, there are many abnormalities in brain metabolism, including specific changes in glucose metabolism (67,119,156). These metabolic alterations may cause problems in estimation of brain transport by methods that are of long duration.

Brain Uptake Index
A few comments about the Brain Uptake Index (BUI) are needed, because some of the controversy that has developed about abnormal blood–brain barrier transport in experimental diabetes revolves around its perceived limitations. Oldendorf described this single-pass, intracarotid bolus injection technique, known as the Brain Uptake Index. In essence, the BUI uses injection of a 200 μL "bolus" of buffered saline with a radiolabeled test compound, e.g. ^{14}C-D-glucose, and one or two radiolabeled reference compounds, e.g. ^{3}H$_2$O. The ratio of the test and reference compounds in the brain 5–15 s after intracarotid injection is compared to the same ratio in the injection bolus. It is a rapid, non-steady-state method that has been used to delineate details and adaptations of many of the currently understood blood–brain barrier transport systems (84,122,170,187,188,194,216). It has several advantages, including its simplicity, rapidity, and consequent lack of influence of labeled compound metabolism on measured extraction. In recent years, however, it has come under increasing criticism, primarily on theoretical grounds (21,224,233). Among the concerns raised about the BUI is its limited accuracy for estimating low rates of blood–brain barrier penetration. In particular, in kinetic studies it is necessary to measure accurately the rate of radiolabeled substrate transport when it is inhibited by unlabeled substrate. Thus, at low rates of substrate penetration, the BUI method may not be adequate to estimate the half-saturation constant (or K_m) for transport. Other issues are that both anesthetic use and diabetes depress cerebral blood flow. Low viscosity and high pressure of the bolus after rapid intracarotid injection, and the possible backflux of labeled compounds from the brain into the injected bolus, thereby diluting specific activity, are also of potential concern. Similarly, dilution by mixing with plasma constituents may occur. Despite these criticisms, the BUI has been extremely useful, and its results often agree with those of other methods. Pardridge in particular has used the BUI and other techniques with similar results. He has also successfully addressed many of the concerns raised regarding the BUI (187,193).

Regulation of Blood–Brain Barrier Transport

The notion that transport may be regulated, that carrier proteins, like enzymes, may be modified in number or activity, occurred shortly after demonstration of saturable transport itself. Transport of ketone bodies into the brain can be induced by prolonged starvation (84,184) and probably occurs in other ketotic states, such as fat feeding (28,205), during development (27,46,47,174), and ketotic diabetic mellitus (165,211). The brain adapts to use of nonglucose fuels gradually. As part of that adaptation, it makes great teleologic sense to induce the transport mechanism of the blood–brain barrier for ketone bodies, in addition to increasing their production by the liver to raise their circulating blood concentrations. Indeed, this highly coordinated series of events may be under common physiologic regulatory controls, e.g. low insulin levels, high levels of free fatty acids and glucagon. Plasma levels of metabolic fuels and hormones may affect tissue metabolism in several organs, including brain capillaries. Metabolism in brain capillaries in turn may influence their transport of nutrients into brain. The linkage between tissue metabolism (i.e. in brain microvessels), plasma levels, and transport may be an important pattern of control. Delineation of the precise physiological controls that regulate blood–brain barrier transport, as has been done for other aspects of metabolism, may be useful if transport is ever to be manipulated as a form of therapy. As an example, it would be potentially very useful to increase the transport of organic acids such as lactate out of the brain in certain situations.

Transport adaptations thus far identified have been described for most of the known blood–brain barrier transport systems, using one or several transport methods. Transport typically adapts to changing levels of hormones or metabolic levels; the specific regulatory and molecular mechanisms, however, remain elusive or controversial. Some clinically relevant situations in which blood–brain barrier transport adaptations occur in experimental animals include ketosis (84), starvation (184,226), portocaval anastomosis (36,105, 122,123,153–155,216), development (46,47), malnutrition (51,79), after drug administration (185,191,192), and as a result of diabetes (173) or hypoglycemia (162).

Recent Advances in Study of Glucose-Transport Proteins

Investigation of glucose transport, including studies of brain transport, has changed dramatically with the application of molecular biology methods. A superfamily of facilitated diffusion glucose-transport proteins exists (9). The mammalian forms vary from 39% to 65% sequence identity and from 50% to 75% homology between different isoforms. The family of glucose-transport proteins extends phylogenetically down to related proteins in bacteria (3), yeast (18,19,38,231), and protozoa (33,227). The high degree of conservation of their molecular structure suggests their essential role in the regulation of cellular metabolism throughout phylogeny. In mammals, glucose-transport proteins are encoded by the genes most commonly named GLUT 1 through GLUT 5 after the order of their discovery. For the purpose of this review the names GLUT 1 through 5 will refer both to the gene and to its carrier protein isoform. Their names, the sizes of the proteins tissue distribution, and the chromosomal location of the genes in humans are given in Table 5.3 (adapted from G. Bell et al.) (9).

These proteins differ from the sodium-dependent (active transport) glucose carriers, which exist in gut epithelial cells and (probably) in kidney tubule cells (106). Of the five (active transport) facilitated diffusion glucose carriers, GLUT 1 (177) (sometimes referred to as the brain-erythrocyte form) and GLUT 3 (cloned from a fetal skeletal muscle cDNA library but present most abundantly in brain [134]), are thought to be responsible for constitutive or basal cellular glucose uptake. Interestingly, although the first gene cloned for a glucose-transport protein was from a human hepatoma (177), normal liver tissue (and pancreatic B cells) express an isoform, GLUT 2 (125,238), which has a lower affinity (higher K_m) (237) for glucose. Transformed cells or those in long-term culture seem to express GLUT 1 primarily (74).

Insulin-Sensitive Glucose Transport
The GLUT 4 form predominates in insulin-responsive tissue, such as fat and muscle (17,39,80,120,121). The GLUT 4 protein translocates from intracellular membranes to the plasma membrane in response to insulin. This insulin-induced translocation appears to be the major reason for insulin-sensitive glucose uptake in fat and muscle. The basis for identification of the insulin-responsive isoform emanates from the seminal work (done independently) of Cushman (50) and Kono (230).

It is believed that the brain uses both GLUT 1 and GLUT 3 glucose carriers (22,73,134), and that GLUT 1 alone exists in the brain capillaries (22). The exact cellular and subcellular localization of different glucose carrier isoforms in the brain has not yet been examined. Recent work suggests that GLUT 3 may be expressed in glial cells and that its expression may be regulated during development (214). Until the biology of these glucose-transport proteins becomes more fully understood, it will probably not be possible to characterize adaptations in brain transport of glucose completely.

Structure of the Glucose Carrier
All glucose-transport proteins possess a similar structure. Knowledge of their structure may yield evidence about their function and help identify them. As membrane-associated proteins, glucose carriers are hydrophobic. Indeed, the

TABLE 5.3. Facilitative glucose transport proteins

Name	Size (amino acids)	Tissue distribution	Chromosome location of gene
GLUT 1	492	Erythrocyte, brain, placenta	1p35→31.3
GLUT 2	524	Liver, pancreatic β cell, kidney, small intestine	3q26
GLUT 3	496	Brain, placenta, kidney	12p13
GLUT 4	509	Skeletal muscle, heart, brown and white fat	17p13
GLUT 5	501	Small intestine	1p31

Adapted from Bell, G.I., et al. *Diabetes Care* 13(3): 198–208, 1990 (9).

predicted 12 membrane-spanning regions (177) of mammalian glucose-transport proteins are the regions in which the greatest homology exists (9). The carboxy- and aminotermini of these molecules are in the cytoplasm. Of considerable importance, these regions and the intracytoplasmic loop (between membranes spanning regions 6 and 7) and the extracellular loop (between membranes spanning regions 1 and 2, which also contains an asparagine-linked glycosylation site) are highly variable in amino acid structure between different isoforms. As a result, antibodies directed against these regions may be used to identify a particular isoform and to serve as a tool for studying its specific regulation (180,195,214,237). Similarly, it may be possible to uniquely characterize the messenger RNA for different isoforms with specific complementary oligonucleotide (cDNA or antisense RNA) sequences. Another possibility is that the variable regions may ultimately offer some clues about the unique aspects and mechanisms of regulation for different glucose carriers (e.g. insulin responsiveness).

BLOOD–BRAIN BARRIER TRANSPORT ADAPTATIONS IN DIABETES AND HYPOGLYCEMIA

Early Evidence for Regulation of Transport in Diabetes

Studies of adaptation of hexose transportation in response to altered glycemia were foreshadowed by studies of brain fuel metabolism in diabetes (211). During ketotic diabetes in animals, as in starvation, the brain slowly decreases its utilization of glucose and increases its utilization of alternate fuels, notably the ketones acetoacetate and β-hydroxybutyrate. This switch of fuels for oxidative energy metabolism occurs in both anesthetized and unanesthetized rats (20,26). Arteriovenous differences (211), which reflect effects of both transport and metabolism, and sampling of intermediary metabolites, indicated reciprocal inhibition of glucose and ketone metabolism (analogous to a glucose–fatty acid in brain during uncontrolled diabetes) (202).

Several studies have suggested that adaptation specifically to chronic hyperglycemia occurs in experimental diabetes. Using the intravenous infusion method to study flux of glucose into the brain, Gjedde and Crone (85) found that chronic hyperglycemia (streptozotocin 50 mg/kg ip 3 weeks previously) decreased the unidirectional extraction of D-glucose across the blood–brain barrier from $44 \pm 2\%$ to $25 \pm 2\%$. This appeared to result from a change in the maximum transport capacity (T_{max}) for glucose from 4.0 μmoles/g/min in control rats to 2.86 μmoles/g/min in diabetic rats. The half-saturation constant (K_m) declined from 8.6 to 6.4 mM, though this change was not statistically significant. When plasma glucose in diabetic rats was acutely lowered to normal values, the glucose-transport rate into brain was 20% below the rate seen in normal rats. These authors found no differences between diabetic and control groups in cerebral blood flow or arterial blood gases in their pentobarbital-anesthetized rats.

In similar, more extensive physiologic studies in diabetic rats (Fig. 5.1), my co-workers and I (164,165) used the BUI method to study transport of several hexoses and other metabolic substrates in streptozotocin diabetic rats (65

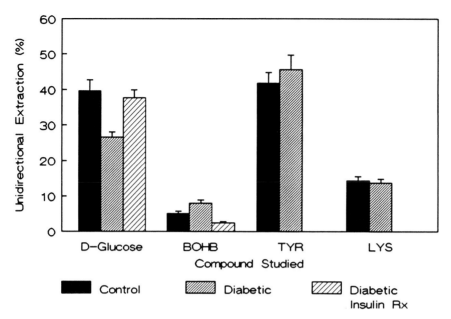

FIGURE 5.1. Blood–brain barrier (BBB) transport in streptozotocin (STZ) diabetes. STZ (65 mg/kg) was given 1–25 days earlier to produce diabetes (159). Brain transport was measured using the Brain Uptake Index (BUI) of Oldendorf (175). Single passage extraction from the circulation (mean ± SE) of D-glucose, beta-hydroxybutyrate (BOHB), L-tyrosine (TYR) and L-lysine (LYS) was compared in control (*solid bars*), untreated diabetic (*stippled bars*), and insulin-treated (7.5–10 U/kg daily for 5–7 days) diabetic rats (*striped bars*). Extraction of glucose was significantly decreased in untreated diabetic rats (p<0.01) and was restored to normal by insulin treatment. Transport of BOHB was increased in untreated diabetic rats and decreased to below control values in the insulin-treated diabetic group (p<0.05). Transport in diabetic rats of TYR and LYS, compounds using independent transport carriers, was not different from that of controls.

mg/kg; 1–25 days previously). Unidirectional extraction of D-glucose decreased from 39.6 ± 3.1% to 26.6 ± 1.4% in a single cerebral circulation passage. The maximal transport rate decreased from 1.8 to 1.0 μmoles/g/min, whereas no significant changes were observed in the half-saturation concentration constant for transport (11.5 vs. 9.0 mM). Cerebral blood flow (CBF) in ml/g/min was estimated in diabetic and control rats from the efflux constants (B) for ^3H_2O in these groups. Knowing B (min^{-1}) the volume of distribution (Vd in ml/g) for H_2O, and its blood brain extraction (E in %), Equation 1 may be used to estimate cerebral blood flow. The estimates of cerebral blood flow obtained reflect the pentobarbital-induced depression customarily observed. Later studies in unanesthetized diabetic rats showed that brain blood flow is depressed by hyperglycemia (195). Since cerebral blood flow is depressed to a similar degree by pentobarbital anesthesia in control and diabetic groups in our studies, anesthesia may have allowed more ready demonstration of transport differences by eliminating (albeit inadvertently) the potentially interfering or confounding effects of altered CBF on transport measurement. The depression of hexose transport is symmetric in that both efflux and influx of the nonmetabolized hexose analog, 3-O-methyl-D-glucose, are decreased to a similar degree (165).

$$CBF = \frac{Vd}{E} \times B \qquad (1)$$

Transport into the brain of other sugars that have a significant affinity for the glucose carrier (e.g. 2-deoxy-D-glucose, 3-O-methylglucose, galactose, xylose, and mannose) is also depressed by diabetes (165). It should be noted on the one hand that these sugars are metabolized to different extents, and via different pathways, or not at all in the case of 3-O-methylglucose. On the other hand, transport of several amino acids, which are known to use distinct carrier molecules to enter brain, is unaffected. Transport of the ketone body β-hydroxybutyrate is increased in untreated diabetic rats but depressed after insulin treatment. In addition, extraction of ^3H_2O, the reference standard for these studies, is unchanged by diabetes. Thus, transport of hexoses is uniformly and specifically affected.

We found evidence for a relationship between transport changes and prior glycemia in these studies. Insulin treatment in vivo (7.5 U/kg of PZI insulin daily for 1 week) improved D-glucose transport toward normal. In contrast, insulin added to the solution injected into the common carotid artery (10 U/ml) acutely had no effect on D-glucose extraction. Increasing glycemia by feeding sucrose to insulin-treated diabetic rats decreased D-glucose extraction. Lastly, we compared the influence of glycemia vs insulinemia on brain glucose transport by starving diabetic rats for 48 h. Starvation decreased average glucose concentrations in diabetic rats from 525 to 115 mg/dl and also normalized hexose transport.

The time course for depression of glucose transport by hyperglycemia is slow; 24 h of persistent hyperglycemia is required. Acute changes in blood glucose concentrations, whether hyperglycemia (induced by 1 g/kg intravascular dextrose 10 min before) or hypoglycemia (54 U/kg intravascular crystalline zinc insulin 1 h before) do not affect brain transport (162).

Brain Transport in Chronic Hypoglycemia

Since chronic hyperglycemia decreased glucose transport into the brain, we also investigated whether chronic hypoglycemia would have the opposite effect (162). Animals were rendered chronically hypoglycemic by three means: (1) implantation subcutaneously of an insulin-producing tumor (insulinoma); (2) implantation of an osmotic mini-pump to infuse insulin; and (3) daily injections of a long-acting insulin (protamine zinc) preparation. A fourth experimental group of animals was injected with high doses of insulin one-half to one hour before transport was studied. This last group had blood glucose values similar to those of the other, chronically hypoglycemic rats.

In chronic but not acute hypoglycemia, blood–brain barrier glucose influx was increased. Several days of consistent hypoglycemia were required to achieve this effect. Also, transport very gradually returned to normal over many days in insulinoma-implanted rats that had their tumors removed. The change in glucose transport in chronic hypoglycemia was specific, as had been shown before in studies of experimental diabetes. Thus transport of glucose and other hexoses that bind the glucose carrier (2-deoxy-D-glucose, D-xylose, D-galactose, 3-O-methyl-D-glucose, but not sucrose) was seen in several chronically hypoglycemic rat models. Other transport systems were either unaffected (e.g. large neutral amino acids or choline transport) or affected in an opposite fashion (e.g. lactate and pyruvate transport in insulinoma rats). It seems unlikely that altered cerebral blood flow, altered metabolism, or label backflux or dilution could explain these results. In particular, freeze blowing of brain to prevent post mortem metabolism of labeled hexoses still showed increased glucose extraction. Furthermore, glucose-6-phosphate, creatine-phosphate, and ATP levels in brain were not significantly lower in insulinoma-implanted rats, suggesting that the increased glucose extraction at the blood–brain barrier protected brain energy metabolism.

Specificity of Glucose Transport Alterations Questioned

Controversy has arisen over whether specific changes in transport actually occur, at least in diabetes. In large measure, this controversy relates to the observation that decreases in CBF and diffusion of L-glucose may also be present in acutely and chronically hyperglycemic rats. It has been suggested that decreases in CBF or simple diffusion might cause artifactually low estimates of D-glucose transport into brain (97,98). For example, depressed CBF would increase the flow-dependent extraction of ^3H_2O reference standard in the BUI studies mentioned above.

Duckrow et al. (65,66) used the iodoantipyrine method in unanesthetized rats to measure cerebral blood flow after chronic hyperglycemia (streptozotocin 60 mg/kg 3 weeks previously). Compared to saline-treated controls, chronically hyperglycemic rats showed decreased CBF in 5 of 17 areas measured. When streptozotocin rats were additionally administered dextrose (6 ml/kg body weight), 20 min before study, by intraperitoneal catheter, they had more marked hyperglycemia and depression of cerebral blood flow in 11 of 17 areas. These studies suggest that in unanesthetized rats hyperglycemia depresses cerebral blood flow in a regionally specific and dose-dependent manner. Significant depression of CBF was not found in anesthetized rats, presumably because anesthesia minimized these differences.

Harik and LaManna found markedly depressed CBF in awake restrained rats made acutely or chronically hyperglycemic (98) (the latter with streptozotocin). They used a double label, single pass, atrial bolus injection method to measure CBF (n-butanol) and unidirectional extraction of D-glucose and L-glucose. On average, cerebral blood flow decreased 30% after acute hyperglycemia; a further reduction of about 15% occurred with chronic hyperglycemia. Unlike Duckrow et al., Harik and colleagues found a greater depression of cerebral blood flow and less evidence for regional specificity.

Harik and LaManna also reported that L-glucose space decreases in chronic hyperglycemia (98). However the decrease is present only when one compares acute vs chronic hyperglycemia. The sole brain region affected by chronic hyperglycemia, i.e. L-glucose space, in comparison to normals was the cerebellum (28.5 ± 3.1 vs 19.5 ± 1.7 µL/g); all other regions did not significantly differ from those of normoglycemic rats. These investigators argued that no significant decrease in D-glucose transport across the blood–brain barrier occurs in diabetic rats. One potential limitation of this aspect of the work of Harik and LaManna is the absence of simultaneously studied normoglycemic control rats. The values for D-glucose transport in the four brain regions (frontal and parietal cortex, hippocampus, and cerebellum) studied in chronically (4 weeks) hyperglycemic rats were 81%, 76%, 54%, and 64% of that seen in their previously published normoglycemic controls. According to their reported data summary (147), the regions all differ significantly in glucose transport. It therefore seems likely that their own data confirm the depression of glucose transport previously observed, although the decrease is of a lesser magnitude (85,165). Also of note, unlike other investigators, Harik and colleagues found depressed D-glucose transport in acute hyperglycemia.

In a subsequent report, Duckrow (64) found no significant change in the permeability-surface area product (PS), an index of transport, for D-glucose at either 1 or 3 weeks after streptozotocin-induced diabetes. These results conflict somewhat with those in his earlier report (67), in which he observed a 15% decrease in blood–brain barrier glucose influx in experimental diabetes mellitus. Pardridge (195) has recently argued that Duckrow's study and the studies of Harik and LaManna less convincingly demonstrated a change in carrier-mediated glucose transport because they were performed at glucose concentrations that saturate the carrier-mediated mechanism (about 30 mM). Perhaps the studies of Harik (98,136) and those of Duckrow may best be understood as partially confirming a specific change in D-glucose transport, while adding new observations about the effects of diabetes on cerebral blood flow and simple diffusion.

Recent Confirmation of Glucose-Transport Changes in Diabetes

Recent findings on glucose transport in brain capillaries confirm prior work by Gjedde and our laboratory. They also begin to address the potential sites for abnormal regulation on a molecular level. Like other proteins (e.g. enzymes), if glucose carriers are affected by diabetes, several possible sites of action may be involved. The glucose carrier proteins may be changed in their number, cellular distribution, or intrinsic capacity to transport. If their number is decreased in diabetes, their synthesis might be decreased due to altered transcription or translation. Increased degradation of glucose carriers or displacement from their normal active site (the plasma membrane) could also occur. Alternatively, altered transcription or mRNA stability might occur. If the membrane milieu in which these carrier proteins are embedded is affected (e.g. decreased fluidity), their intrinsic mobility and thus transport capacity might be altered.

Choi et al. (41,42) have studied GLUT 1 mRNA levels in rats with streptozotocin diabetes. Using the rat brain cDNA to probe isolated brain microvessels from diabetic rats, they found increased steady-state levels of mRNA for GLUT 1 without any corresponding change in the transcript level of α-actin, a housekeeping gene mRNA, i.e. a gene for which mRNA transcript levels are presumed to be not regulated in this situation (41). In this paper, they also refer to results confirming depression of D-glucose extraction in streptozotocin diabetic rats using the Takasato (233) method (as described earlier, p. 62). Recently, they have reported more fully (195) on this marked decrease in blood–brain barrier D-glucose transport. Transport was assessed by the in situ brain perfusion method, and transporter protein was quantified by Western blot analysis of isolated cerebral microvessel proteins using an antibody directed against the C-terminus of GLUT 1. Choi et al. found a 44% decrease in glucose transport (unidirectional extraction) in parallel with a 44% decrease in cerebral blood flow in unanesthetized rats. In addition, they observed a $77 \pm 9\%$ decrease in GLUT 1 immunoreactivity (based on a C-terminus and presumably specific antiserum) in isolated cerebral microvessels from rats with experimental diabetes. They argue that the failure of some previous studies to find altered blood–brain barrier permeability occurred because the PS product was examined at a blood glucose concentration (30 mM) at which the glucose transporter was likely nearly saturated. Earlier work is in conflict about whether the number of glucose-transport proteins is decreased or increased in isolated cerebral microvessels of diabetic rats. The data of Matthaei et al. (157) suggested decreased glucose carriers, whereas Harik and colleagues found evidence for an increase (97). Choi et al. (41,42) conclude that the combined findings of increased mRNA for GLUT 1 and decreased GLUT 1 immunoreactivity indicate a block in translation or increased transporter degradation or some combination of the two. Whatever the explanation, these results appear to confirm definitively that blood–brain barrier transport of glucose is depressed in experimental diabetes mellitus.

Pardridge and colleagues also confirm that hyperglycemia decreases CBF in awake, unanesthetized rats. The effects of depressed transport of glucose and cerebral blood flow might doubly decrease the provision of brain fuels in some circumstances, such as cardiac arrest or stroke. How do these findings relate to the previously described BUI and intravenous transport studies in anesthetized rats? They support the correctness of the observed specific decrease in glucose transport. The earlier studies missed the depressed CBF in diabetes, probably because pentobarbital anesthesia minimized differences between diabetic and control rats. Fortuitously, the anesthesia effects permitted a clear demonstration of the specific transport changes for glucose and ketone bodies.

The Western blot data from this very exciting study need confirmation and a little caution in interpretation. The studies of the mechanisms by which transport is changed take advantage of newer molecular understanding of the glucose carrier proteins. Nonetheless, some potential limitations exist. It is clear from recent work that studies using antibodies against glucose-transport proteins may on occasion yield misleading information (222,243). It is hoped that some confirmation of the Western blot results in brain microvessels of rats with experimental diabetes (195) with several well-characterized, highly specific antisera will be done. In addition, some caution about interpretation of results of immunoreactivity even with an "ideal" (i.e. highly specific) antibody is in order. Plasma membrane glucose carriers are the only ones that are relevant to cellular glucose transport activity. Intracellular carriers are not believed to be physiologically active. Furthermore, it is increasingly apparent that both the number and the intrinsic activity (or turnover number) of transporters may be regulated (127). Despite these caveats, this study may give important new insight into the regulation of brain transport.

Cytochalasin B Binding in Isolated Brain Microvessels

Dick et al. first demonstrated the presence of glucose-transport proteins in isolated cerebral microvessels using the techniques of cytochalasin B binding and immunoblotting (Western blot analysis) with an antibody directed against the erythrocyte glucose carrier (56,50). As shown by Cushman and Wardzala (50) in studies of adipocytes and muscle tissue, the fungal metabolite cytochalasin B binds to glucose-transport proteins, and binding, which can be displaced by 500 mM D-glucose, is highly specific for these proteins.

Using this approach, Matthaei et al. (157) found that the concentration of glucose-transport proteins was reduced in isolated cerebral microvessels from streptozotocin diabetic rats. In these studies, cytochalasin B binding was measured in subcellular fractions of brain microvessels. A 43% decrease in glucose-transport proteins was found in the total microvessels from rats with untreated diabetes compared to control rats. This decrease occurred in all subfractions of vessels (50% in plasma membranes, 38% in high-density membranes, and 45% in low-density microsomes). Incubation of microvessels from control rats with supraphysiological concentrations of insulin increased cytochalasin B binding in a cycloheximide-dependent fashion. Microvessels from diabetic rats were also found to be less insulin-responsive in these studies. In other studies from this group (158) insulin increased microvessel glucose transporters present in high-density microsomes acutely, but in other subcellular fractions insulin effects only appeared after prolonged incubation (2 h).

In direct contrast to the above-mentioned findings, Harik and colleagues (97) found that cytochalasin B binding was increased by about 30% in brain microvessels from rats with streptozotocin diabetes. They argued that the alteration in cytochalasin B binding substantiated their in vivo studies, in which they found no differences in glucose-transport activity at the blood–brain barrier in experimental diabetes. They suggested that the studies by Matthaei et al. (157) may have resulted from an artifact due to sonication of the microvessels when they dispersed membranes prior to cytochalasin B studies.

A sonication artifact seems unlikely to explain the differences between these studies. It is not clear what other experimental variables might be responsible. In any case, cytochalasin B binding studies may not be considered entirely definitive, since cytochalasin binds to all glucose-transport proteins, both microsomal and plasma membrane associated, although GLUT 2 does so with a lesser affinity (2). Furthermore, since glucose-transport proteins are unevenly distributed in cells, studies in which cytochalasin binding in whole microvessels is measured may be of limited value. Plasma membrane associated glucose carriers are of most physiologic interest and correlate with cell glucose-transport activity. Photoaffinity labeling of extracellular oriented plasma membrane associated glucose carriers is a method that is being developed and may prove helpful in resolving differences between such apparently discrepant studies (34). It must also be remembered that the intrinsic activity of glucose-transport proteins may change, as well as their numbers (97,127,128). Thus although changes in transporter protein distribution or mRNA levels could explain altered glucose transport, such changes are not unequivocal evidence that the transport is in fact altered.

Changes in Transport of Other Substrates and Ions in Diabetes

Mooradian (171) used the BUI technique to study the kinetics of choline transport across the blood–brain barrier in chronically diabetic rats (> 9 weeks). The maximal transport rate for choline declined markedly (from 2.2 $\pm$ 0.8 to 0.14 $\pm$ 0.07 nmol/min/g in rats with diabetes for more than 9 weeks. Neither the K_m for transport nor the nonsaturable transport component was affected. There were no effects of diabetes of shorter duration (3 weeks) nor of acute hyperglycemia on blood–brain choline transport. In contrast to its previously described effect on glucose and β-hydroxybutyrate transport (165), insulin therapy for 5 days did not rectify the abnormal choline transport. Since choline may be an important precursor to brain acetylcholine, a neurotransmitter thought to be involved in age-related and Alzheimer's disease–related memory loss (251), this is an intriguing finding.

Mooradian has also found that dehydroascorbate, but not ascorbate, in vitro, is able to compete with glucose for entry in several tissues, including the brain (171). It is not clear, however, whether hyperglycemia could cause a deficiency of this vitamin in the brain and lead to dysfunction as a result.

Specific abnormalities in sodium transport at the blood–brain barrier in experimental diabetes have been observed by a group of Danish investigators (117,140–142). The permeability surface area product (PS), an index of blood-to-brain transport, for sodium was determined by infusing $^{24}Na^+$ intravenously for up to 15 min in diabetic and control rats. Arterial blood and brain tissue were sampled for radioactivity concentrations and a correction was made for cerebrovascular space with the protein-bound marker ^{113m}Indium. The PS decreased from 7.1 $\pm$ 1.7 (mean $\pm$ deviation standard) in the frontal cortex of control rats to 5.4 $\pm$ 0.6 $\times$ 10^{-5}/ cm^3/g/sec after 2 weeks of streptozotocin-induced diabetes (142). A similar 24% decrease occurred in occipital cortex after 2 weeks of diabetes mellitus. Chloride ($^{36}Cl^-$) and [^{3}H]sucrose transport did not differ significantly between diabetic and control rats (142), however. In a subsequent study, this group of investigators found (117) that potassium permeability was also decreased by 39%, but no difference in permeation of calcium ions into the brain was observed. Insulin treatment restores Na$^+$ transport to near-normal values within as little as a few hours (140). Changes in transport are not apparently explained by the hyperosmolarity associated with hyperglycemia, since 50% mannitol increases rather than decreases Na$^+$ transport. *Myo*-inositol treatment normalizes the deficient Na$^+$ transport, which is postulated to be caused by abnormal Na$^+$K$^+$-ATPase activity in cerebral endothelial cells (141).

It is likely that abnormal permeation of protein into the brain also occurs in animals with experimental diabetes mellitus. Stauber et al. (225) found a selective leakage of albumin, but not IgG or complement (C3), in immunohistochemical studies of the brain in streptozotocin-induced diabetes of 2 weeks duration. This leakage may be a modest effect, as studies by Williamson et al. (248) do not find enhanced [^{125}I]albumin permeation (presumably a less sensitive indicator than immunohistochemistry) into brain in animal models of diabetes, although they do find evidence for such permeation in granulation tissue and in organs (e.g. eye, kidney, and nerve) known to be susceptible to diabetic complications (Chapter 6). One study (246) has found that microvessels from fat tissue are abnormally permeable to albumin when the albumin is glycated, and that glycated albumin may even increase the permeation of nonglycated proteins through microvessels. All of these studies are consistent with the notion that in experimental animals, with very poor diabetic control the permeability of the blood–brain barrier to albumin may be affected. It is possible that these changes are relevant to the syndrome of cerebral edema that has been observed, particularly in children being treated for diabetic ketoacidosis (144,160,208,234,241).

ISOLATED CEREBRAL MICROVESSELS AND MICROVASCULAR ENDOTHELIAL CELLS AS MODEL SYSTEMS

Isolated cerebral microvessels have been used for studies of both transport and metabolism. Despite some skepticism regarding their adequacy as a model, they have proved to be very useful, although not without problems. The problems relate to several issues: the best methods for their isolation, their adequacy for metabolic studies, and the extent of isolation-induced damage. The best methods to preserve and demonstrate abnormal transport when microvessels are studied ex vivo are not fully established. Microvessels have been used to study the normal characteristics of blood–brain transport as an in vitro model system. In addition, they have also been used to study transport after in vitro perturbations (e.g. acute insulin exposure (158) or after in vivo adaptations [e.g. after induction of diabetes (157) or portocaval anastomosis (36)] have occurred. Such studies are most meaningful when particular care is taken that microvessel uptake of a radiolabeled compound is solely dependent on its transport and not on its metabolism.

Brendel et al. (29) first described isolation of metabolically active cerebral microvessels from bovine brain, using the methods of hand homogenization and nylon sieving. The oxidative metabolism of labeled glucose, pyruvate, glutamate, and oleate by the microvessels was linear for 3 h. High basal rates of oxygen consumption increased by threefold with addition of succinate to the incubated vessels.

Goldstein et al. (91) used nylon meshes followed by a 25% albumin centrifugation step and a glass bead column to separate rat brain microvessels from parenchymal tissue. Purity was quantified by 15- and 20-fold enrichment of alkaline phosphatase and γ-glutamyltranspeptidase, respectively. They demonstrated linear uptake of 2-deoxy-D-glucose, which was markedly inhibited by incubation in ice or addition of 100 mM (unlabeled) 2-deoxy-D-glucose. Rates of uptake approximated 0.25 pmol/mg protein/min. Glucose oxidation was linear for 90 min. The rate of glucose carbon oxidized to CO_2 was about 150 nmol/mg protein/h.

Hjelle et al. (111) studied bovine cerebral and retinal microvessel uptake of amino acids and showed cross competition and stereospecificity of uptake. The K_m for uptake was between 100 and 500 μM for tyrosine, leucine, and valine. One potential problem with this study is adequately separating out the kinetics of transport from metabolism, since uptake was studied over periods up to 20 min. Similarly, when Hwang et al. (115) studied labeled cystine uptake in isolated rat brain capillaries, the time course of uptake over 1 h may have reflected metabolism more than transport.

Goldstein, (90) and Betz (10) explored whether uptake of labeled hexoses reflects predominantly transport or metabolism in isolated brain microvessels. Their initial studies using varying incubation concentrations of 2-deoxy-D-glucose yielded a kinetic analysis of hexose transport, which probably reflected hexokinase flux (rate of hexose phosphorylation). In later studies, in which labeled 2-deoxy-D-glucose was incubated with microvessels at a concentration in the millimolar range, a large pool of intracellular free hexose was found. In that situation, as transport in and out of cells approach equilibrium, cellular uptake of hexose inaccurately reflects influx. These results imply that at concentrations of 2-deoxyglucose well above the K_m for hexokinase in microvessels (about 150 μM) (57), the hexose uptake reflects predominantly the activity of hexokinase rather than transport.

Another important study by Goldstein and Betz (15) illustrated the polarity of certain transport systems of the blood–brain barrier. Isolated brain microvessels were shown to possess the A-system for small, polar amino acids which transports the natural substrate alanine and the synthetic substrate aminoisobutyric acid (15). Uptake of these amino acids was found to be sodium- and energy-dependent as it is elsewhere. In contrast, the L-system transports amino acids (natural substrate example leucine, artificial substrate cycloleucine) in an equilibrium, sodium- and energy-independent fashion. Interestingly, the A-system was not found on the luminal or blood side of the blood–brain barrier. Thus, brain microvessels (and presumably endothelial cells) are asymmetric in their distribution of carrier proteins. Because of this, the study of uptake in isolated microvessels may reflect in vivo blood-to-brain transport only to the extent that the transport systems studied are equal on the blood side and the brain side. These conditions are met for glucose (135,165) and for many other, but not all, systems for transport of metabolic substrates at the blood–brain barrier.

Pardridge and his colleagues have used human brain microvessels to study the uptake of neutral amino acids (42,94,190). They have found evidence for high-affinity uptake of phenylalanine, similar to values observed for rat brain transport in vivo. Their use of nonmetabolizable amino acids analogues eliminates possible effects of metabolism. In contrast, the duration of uptake for some of the metabolizable compounds they studied may have been long enough to partly reflect metabolism. Longer duration studies additionally raise the issue of backflux of these compounds.

In very recent work (40,161), we have used 2-deoxy-D-glucose uptake at very low concentrations to study hexose uptake for up to 10 min in isolated rat and bovine brain microvessels. The use of 2-deoxy-D-glucose at concentrations far below saturation for hexokinase gives results that reflect transport not metabolism. We found that hexose transport was depressed in diabetes and increased in microvessels from insulinoma rats, findings that mirror the earlier in vivo work on blood–brain barrier transport (see above). In addition, we found that glucoregulatory hormone (e.g. dexamethasone, a synthetic glucocorticoid) depresses 2-deoxy-D-glucose transport.

Use of Endothelial Cells Cultured from Brain as a Model

A number of groups have used endothelial cells cultured from isolated brain microvessels as an in vitro model of the blood–brain barrier (23,59–61, 70,92,159,196,209). These cells are thought to form tight junctions in culture, although it is not clear whether they routinely do so uniformly and to a degree where extremely high electrical resistance can be demonstrated (168,212). Nonetheless, they will continue to serve as a developing model of the blood–brain barrier, especially as techniques for their culture improve. Drewes and colleagues (62) have shown that these cells tend to lose their responses to stimuli (e.g. phorbol esters) rather rapidly in culture. Indeed, maintenance of a highly differentiated endothelial cell phenotype with expression of endothelial and blood–brain barrier markers is often short-lived in vitro. In our own hands, endothelial cells cultured from calf brain do express these differentiated characteristics in early passage, but they lose them or express them erratically in later passage. Recent reports (55,150) suggest that co-culture of microvascular endothelial cells from brain with glial cells may be especially suitable as an in vitro model of the blood–brain barrier.

Cultured calf brain endothelial cells at early passage can show hexose transport that is responsive to glucose exposure in vitro. Thus, we have found in preliminary studies that the cellular uptake of 2-deoxy-D-glucose (at 100 nM concentrations, which reflect transport rather than hexokinase flux) is decreased or increased within a day by exposure of the cells to high or low glucose concentrations respectively. Cellular uptake of 3-O-methyl-D-glucose and glucose are similarly affected. Endothelial cells in long-term culture, however, express this regulation of hexose transport by glucose concentrations less reliably. Determination of the factors that induce or maintain the differentiated state in cultured brain endothelial cells, such as basic fibroblast growth factor or an endothelial cell–conditioned culture matrix, will be very helpful in extending the usefulness of the cultured cells for studies of metabolism and transport at the blood–brain barrier.

USE OF ISOLATED CEREBRAL MICROVESSELS TO STUDY METABOLISM

Methods for Isolation of Microvessels

A variety of methods have been used to isolate cerebral microvessels. Detailed analysis of all techniques and their nuances is beyond this article's scope. Some methodologic points, however, are pertinent to the discussion of using microvessels for metabolic studies. As mentioned above, early articles by Brendel (29) and Goldstein (91) found that isolated cerebral microvessels were able to oxidize fuels in a linear fashion for hours after their isolation. Presumably, such linearity is evidence of some metabolic integrity of the preparation. Nonetheless, Pardridge criticized the use of the isolated microvessel preparation for having unmeasurable or very low levels of ATP (187). As described in more detail below, recent work from our lab (167,228) has shown that microvessels isolated by mechanical homogenization of brain tissue followed by nylon mesh sieving do have reasonable levels of ATP. Although such a preparation often has undergone a "metabolic shock," that is initially having a low content of ATP and low ATP/ADP ratio, these energy state parameters can be markedly improved by incubation in an enriched medium such as DMEM or a balanced salt solution containing glucose (167).

Furthermore, when one compares methods of isolating cerebral microvessels, some methods are clearly superior in their combination of yield and metabolic viability, at least as judged by ATP/ADP ratio (228). The combined gentle hand homogenization, nylon mesh method seems superior in this regard. For studies of protein isolation or transport in vitro, no rigorous comparative studies have been published, so it is less clear whether one method is superior or whether different methods will yield comparable results. Given the differences in results, for example, of cytochalasin B binding in diabetic and control cerebral microvessels in studies by Matthaei et al. (157) and Harik et al. (197), this may be an important technical concern.

Energy State

One of the first papers to study the energy state of cerebral microvessels systematically was that of Lasbennes and Gayet (149). These authors compared microvessels isolated from rat brain by two methods: the first group was isolated at 4°C by hand homogenization, nylon mesh sieving and sucrose (1.2 M) sedimentation; the second group was isolated using 30 min of collagenase digestion followed by a buffered saline, 25% (w/v) bovine serum albumin medium centrifugation. ATP content was low in both groups, but clear differences were found; homogenized vessels averaged 0.43 nmol/mg protein, but enzymatically digested vessels averaged 1.51 nmol/mg protein. Similarly, the ATP/ADP ratio was 0.29 in homogenized vessels and 1.03 in enzymatically isolated microvessels. These investigators repeated Brendel's earlier experiments (29) showing that succinate markedly increased O_2 consumption by the microvessels. They interpreted these studies as indicating functional damage to microvessels, possibly including mitochondrial uncoupling. One of their major conclusions was that mechanically isolated cerebral microvessels were particularly defective in energy metabolism, and that results with such preparations must therefore be interpreted with great caution.

This conclusion about the comparative inferiority of isolated cerebral microvessels that have been produced in part by brain homogenization is suspect. Other important variables were not controlled in the Lasbennes and Gayet study (149). First, their homogenization step was at a different temperature than the collagenase digestion. Second, centrifugation in sucrose at extremely hyperosmolar concentrations, which followed their homogenization, is known to damage or disrupt the blood–brain barrier in vivo (44,69,203). Third, although the ATP/ADP ratio and ATP content were higher in enzymatically digested vessels, the values were still rather low. Furthermore, the Atkinson energy change was little different between the two tested preparations of vessels. Fourth, they did not isolate or incubate their isolated cerebral microvessels with fuels such as glucose, which may be particularly important for maintaining the energy state (see below). Last, they did not separately examine the effects of the 25% albumin centrifugation step.

Initially, studies from our laboratory (167) on microvessel energy state found that the content of ATP (in nmol/mg protein) immediately after isolation varied from 1.13 ± 0.17 to 1.81 ± 0.46 from three different animal species. These studies used mechanical (i.e. hand homogenization) disruption of brain followed by nylon mesh sieving and Percoll density centrifugation to isolate brain microvessels. Of interest, more rigorous homogenization diminished microvessel ATP only slightly, whereas incubation in tissue culture medium produced dramatic and at least equal recovery of energy state in microvessels whether they were homogenized once or twice the usual amount (167). In these studies, the ATP/ADP ratio averaged about 1.0. By comparison, cultured endothelial cells from aorta had an ATP/ADP ratio of 1.7 and endothelial cells derived from brain microvessels, 3.0. Adenosine triphosphate content was also higher in cultured endothelial cells—4.0 and 8.3 nmol/mg protein, respectively, in aorta- and brain-derived cells. Isolated cerebral microvessels have approximately a 25% greater water space so that a 20% underestimation of microvessel ATP content (expressed per milligram of protein) occurs in comparison to cultured cells. Perhaps even more important, microvessels are a mixed cell preparation, composed of endothelial cells predominantly, but also containing pericytes and some smooth muscle cells. Therefore, comparisons between microvessels and pure cell cultures are limited by these differences in composition.

Comparison of Isolation Methods

We showed in the above-mentioned work that mechanically isolated microvessels have a similar, if not superior, energy state compared to microvessels isolated by enzymatic digestion. We next wished to determine which aspects of the preparation led to the best combination of purity, yield, and energy state (ATP/ADP ratio). In these studies (228), we compared four methods commonly used for microvessel preparation: (1) homogenization and nylon mesh sieving without further purification, and this procedure followed further purification either with, (2) centrifugation in 25% albumin (albumin flotation), (3) sucrose density gradient (149), or (4) a Percoll density gradient (163). Use of a hypertonic sucrose gradient to purify microvessels consistently depressed ATP content and ATP/ADP ratio, comparable to that seen in the study of Lasbennes and Gayet (149), probably explaining their dim view of mechanical homogenization to isolate microvessels. Use of hand homogenization and nylon mesh sieving alone gave preparations with the best yield (about 1.6% of total protein), but more importantly, the best ATP/ADP ratio (mean ± SE; 2.3 ± 0.2) and ATP content (1.6 ± 0.24 nmol/mg protein. The values were at least as good as other tested methods and far superior to prior published reports. In these studies, purity of isolated brain microvessels, as gauged by marker enzyme enrichment, was highest in vessels isolated with the albumin flotation method, but the microvessel energy state (ATP/ADP ratio) was poorer using this method. These results led us to conclude that hand homogenization and nylon mesh sieving was the best method for studies in which microvessel metabolism is to be studied. In our hands, collagenase digestion isolation of microvessels has yielded a similar energy state, but at the expense of less purity and a disrupted vascular architecture. Furthermore, enzymatic digestion may have the added disadvantage that it damages or removes marker enzymes and transport systems during isolation of the microvessels (37).

Microvessel Respiration

Some specific comments are also in order regarding mitochondrial respiration and coupling in microvessel preparations. Similar to the results of prior studies, we have found (228) that succinate (5 mM) produces a threefold increase in O_2 consumption in bovine microvessels. The addition of a mitochondrial uncoupler carbonylcyanide-m-chlorophenyl hydrazone (CCCP) stimulated respiration 2.5- and 4.5-fold, respectively, in the absence and the presence of succinate. At higher doses, CCCP inhibited respiration. These results indicate that although isolated cerebral microvessels may be somewhat damaged metabolically, they can be isolated with their mitochondria in a coupled state, contrary to the interpretation of some earlier studies (149).

Importance of Glycolysis to Microvessel Energy State (ATP/ADP Ratio)

Recently, we attempted to define further the fuels and metabolic pathways that best support the energy state of isolated bovine brain microvessels (81). We found evidence that glycolysis plays a primary role and that utilization of endogenous fatty acids plays a secondary role in isolated microvessel energy metabolism. Glucose increased calf microvessel ATP/ADP (often as much as 2-fold), primarily as a result of improved ATP content (Fig. 5.2). Other fuels, including pyruvate, glutamate, hydroxybutyrate, and succinate, were ineffective. Although oxidation rates of ^{14}C-D-glucose and ^{14}C-1-L-pyruvate were similar, only glucose reliably improved or maintained microvessel energy state (ATP/ADP ratio). These studies suggest that glycolysis is crucial to energy production in microvessels. It is not certain whether these mitochondria-rich capillaries (183) normally employ glycolysis in this role in vivo. An alternative explanation is that this dependence upon glycolysis for energy production may characterize a metabolically damaged microvessel, possibly as a result of ischemia or other aspects of the isolation procedure. Whatever the explanation, these studies indicate that rates of oxidative metabolism of an exogenous fuel may not accurately predict its impact on microvessel energy state.

Insulin and Brain Microvessels

In vivo autoradiographic studies (242) first suggested that circulating insulin binds to cerebral capillaries. Frank and Pardridge (76) subsequently confirmed

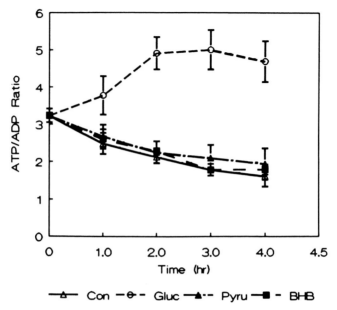

FIGURE 5.2. Effects of various fuels on brain microvessel ATP/ADP ratio. The effect of incubation with no added fuel (Con), 5 mM D-glucose (Gluc) 2 mM L-pyruvate (Pyru), or 2 mM β-hydroxybutyrate (BHB) on the ATP/ADP ratio of calf brain microvessels (78). Only glucose was capable of consistently increasing the ATP/ADP ratio, suggesting that glycolysis is an important metabolic pathway for energy generation and maintenance in isolated cerebral microvessel preparations.

that [^{125}I]iodoinsulin bound to rat microvessels with an affinity (K_d or dissociation constant) of about 9 ng/ml. Insulin binds to cerebral microvessels via specific high-affinity receptors, which have been most extensively characterized by Haskell et al. (99). The K_d for binding in their studies of neonatal porcine and adult bovine microvessels from brain was about 0.3 nM. Cross-linking studies of insulin receptors under reducing conditions showed the receptors of brain microvessels to be similar to those found in the liver, whereas receptors from nonvascular cerebral cortex contained a receptor with an α-subunit of lower molecular weight. In one study, incubation with insulin at high physiological concentrations stimulated activity of several pathways of bovine cerebral microvessel metabolism, including glucose oxidation, glucose incorporation into lipids, and cAMP phosphodiesterase within 2 h (197).

Both insulin and the insulin-like growth factors, IGF$_1$ and IGF$_2$, bind and, to varying degrees, are internalized by isolated cerebral microvessels (78). Binding of insulin appears to be modulated by development. Insulin entry into the brain appears to be higher in newborn rabbits than in adults (75), apparently as a result of increased receptor numbers on brain capillaries. Streptozotocin diabetes decreases insulin binding to isolated brain microvessels (77), and insulin treatment of these rats in vivo partly restores binding toward normal. Exposure to very high levels (100 ng/ml) of insulin appears to decrease insulin receptors on cultured brain endothelial cells in a reversible fashion (77).

A receptor-mediated transcytosis of insulin (and other hormones) across endothelial cells is believed to occur (4,93,138,139). Duffy and Pardridge (68) have suggested that brain endothelial cells may deliver insulin to the brain parenchyma in this manner, which may help to explain the unexpectedly high concentrations of insulin in brain parenchyma (102–104,151). Recent studies by Schwartz and colleagues confirm that insulin gradually enters the cerebrospinal fluid (presumably a reflection of the brain interstitium) from the peripheral circulation (217) in a receptor-mediated fashion. The role of insulin and IGFs in brain development, repair, and normal function (e.g. appetite control) is being actively explored by several groups (1,5–7,71,72,152,201, 218,249,250).

King and colleagues have found that microvascular cells (both endothelium and pericytes) from the retina are more sensitive to the action of insulin than are arterial smooth muscle and endothelial cells (137). Sensitivity to insulin or glucose may be more characteristic of nonendothelial vascular cells, including both pericytes and smooth muscle cells (124,137,229). Thus, for example, pericytes show greater effects of insulin on glucose incorporation into glycogen than other cultured vascular cells (137). Similarly, pericytes cultured from cerebral microvessels appear to be selectively affected by the aldose reductase pathway–mediated depletion of *myo*-inositol (229), a key membrane component that is thought to relate to chronic diabetic complications.

Effects of Diabetes and Hypoglycemia on Brain Microvessel Metabolism

Evidence suggests that, to some degree, the cerebral microvasculature is a target for chronic diabetic complications. Pericyte loss in brain capillaries has been observed in animal models of diabetes (178). In addition, in autopsies of humans with insulin-dependent diabetes, microvascular pathology is visible, including basement membrane thickening (126). The effects of diabetes on pericytes in brain capillaries, however, is less well established than its effects on pericytes in retinal capillaries.

Metabolic changes in brain microvessels also occur in animals with diabetes. Of particular interest is the frequent correlation between altered metabolism of a fuel in vitro by rat brain microvessels and the transport of that fuel in vivo across the blood–brain barrier (162,163,165,166). Thus compared to controls, diabetes depresses the rate of microvessel oxidation of glucose by 65%–83% and its conversion to lactate by 21%–61%. As with the transport of glucose by rat brain capillaries (Fig. 5.3) in vivo, prior glycemia was identified as an important regulatory factor for microvessel metabolism (Fig. 5.4). Thus, either insulin treatment for several days or starvation for 48 h both lowered blood glucose levels and restored microvessel glucose metabolism to normal. Similarly, 1-^{14}C-lactate oxidation was depressed in brain microvessels from diabetic rats, suggesting impaired flux through the pyruvate dehydrogenase pathway. Lactate transport in vivo, however, was not affected in diabetic rats. Restoration of glycemic control also improved flux through the pyruvate dehydrogenase pathway. This enzymatic step is an important regulatory control point for glucose metabolism since it regulates flux of glucose carbon from the glycolytic pathway into the citric acid cycle.

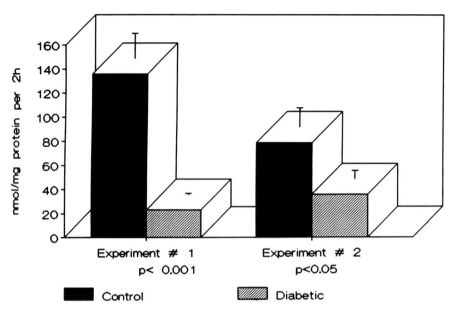

FIGURE 5.3. Effect of diabetes on rat ICMV [^{14}C]glucose converted to [^{14}C]O$_2$. Oxidation of [^{14}C]glucose to [^{14}C]O$_2$ in isolated cerebral microvessels (ICMV) from streptozotocin diabetic (*gray bars*) and control (*black bars*) rats. Results of two experiments (means ± SEM) are shown to illustrate the day-to-day variation in absolute rates of glucose oxidized to CO$_2$ and the consistent depression in microvessel glucose oxidation observed in diabetes (158).

Hingorani and Brecher (110) confirmed and extended work on the abnormal fuel metabolism of cerebral microvessels from diabetic animals in their studies of New Zealand rabbits with alloxan-diabetes (150 mg/kg). They studied isotopic oxidation of 6-^{14}C-glucose or 1-^{14}C-oleate and the incorporation of radioactivity into CO$_2$, lactate, triglycerides, cholesterol ester, and phospholipids. They found competition between the oxidation of glucose and oleate. Thus, for example, 5.5 mM glucose in a microvessel incubation mixture reduced oleate oxidation by 50%. Conversely, glucose oxidation was reduced by the addition of oleate to microvessel incubations, although lactate production remained unaffected. They concluded that the interactions between fatty acid and glucose metabolism in brain microvessels are similar, although not identical to those previously described in cardiac muscle as part of the glucose–fatty acid cycle (202). Additionally, these investigators found that neither oleate oxidation nor lactate production was significantly altered in brain microvessels from untreated diabetic rabbits.

In further metabolic studies on brain microvessels, our lab found that the oxidation of glucose and β-hydroxybutyrate were altered in a coordinated, but opposite direction in rats with diabetes and chronic hypoglycemia (subcutaneously implanted insulinoma) (166). Glucose oxidation by isolated cerebral microvessels was depressed by diabetes, as previously found, whereas chronic hypoglycemia caused increased glucose oxidation (Fig. 5.5). These findings paralleled effects on the transport of glucose in vivo across brain capillaries (162,165); i.e. in diabetes glucose transport is depressed, while in chronic hypoglycemia it is increased. No consistent changes occurred either within 1 h of insulin administration or after insulin pump treatment for 4 days. In contrast to glucose, oxidation of β-hydroxybutyrate to CO_2 by isolated cerebral microvessels was increased in diabetes, as was its transport into brain, while microvessels from insulinoma rats showed depressed oxidation of this fuel.

The mechanistic basis for these parallel effects of diabetes and chronic hypoglycemia (due to insulinoma) on the transport and metabolism of fuels by brain capillaries is unknown. It does not seem likely that local transport of glucose by microvessels could possibly determine its metabolism. To supply the whole brain with glucose, the transport carriers in microvessels must be very abundant; thus it is implausible that they would be rate-limiting for capillary metabolism, under any except extreme circumstances. Nevertheless, local capillary metabolism may well influence transport. There is considerable precedent for the idea that glucose deprivation and refeeding affect glucose transport in fibroblasts by virtue of specific metabolic pathways that regulate the transport activity (100,101,129–133,239,240). Again, the exact mechanism and pathways of metabolism that link metabolism to transport are uncertain. Different tissues may exhibit tissue-specific associations between certain metabolic pathways (or metabolites) and cellular functions like transport. Precise

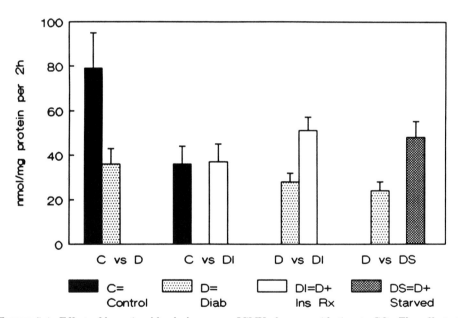

FIGURE 5.4. Effect of lowering blood glucose on ICMV glucose oxidation to CO_2. The effect of lowering blood glucose concentrations in vivo was studied on glucose oxidation to CO_2 by rat isolated cerebral microvessels. Results for each group are means ± SEM of 4–6 observations taken on separate experimental days (158). Untreated diabetic rats (D; *light gray stippled bars*) had reduced rates of glucose oxidation compared to controls (C; *black solid bars*). Microvessels from insulin-treated diabetic rats (DI; *solid white bars*) had rates of glucose oxidation similar to those of controls and greater than those of untreated diabetic rats. Similarly, microvessels from diabetic rats starved for 48 h (DS; *dark gray cross-hatched bar*) had higher rates of glucose oxidation than vessels from untreated diabetic rats. As with blood-to-brain transport of glucose, chronic changes in antecedent glycemia predicted microvessel glucose oxidation.

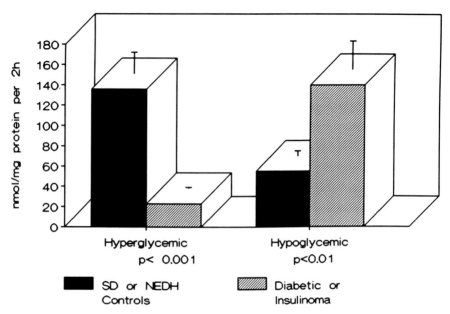

FIGURE 5.5. Hyperglycemia and hypoglycemia alter ICMV [^{14}C]glucose oxidized to [^{14}C]O$_2$. Chronic hyperglycemia and hypoglycemia in vivo alter rat brain microvessel oxidation of U-[^{14}C]glucose to [^{14}C]O$_2$ (160). Microvessels from streptozotocin diabetic rats (*gray hatched bar on left* represents mean ± SE) were isolated and compared to microvessels from their strain-matched (Sprague-Dawley, SD) controls (*black solid bar on left*). Diabetes consistently depressed oxidation of glucose. In contrast, microvessels from New England Deaconess Hospital (NEDH) rats made chronically hypoglycemic by implanting an insulinoma subcutaneously (*gray hatched bar on the right*) exhibited increased rates of glucose oxidation (p<0.01) compared to their strain-matched controls (*black solid bar on the right*).

knowledge of such control mechanisms that regulate transport might allow their deliberate, discrete induction or repression as a means of therapy.

Does the altered fuel metabolism found in experimental diabetes affect the energy state of diabetic brain microvessels? ATP content and ATP/ADP ratios of isolated cerebral microvessels were unaffected by either 1 week or 8 weeks of experimental diabetes in rats (166). Nevertheless, oxygen consumption by microvessels from diabetic rats was increased by more than one-third compared to control rat brain microvessels (Fig. 5.6). The increased oxygen consumption is probably not explained by known alterations in fuel metabolism in diabetes. While the P:O ratio (i.e. the ATP produced for each mole of oxygen consumed) would be slightly increased as a result of utilization of ketone bodies rather than glucose, this would not explain the magnitude of the observed change. The normal ATP content and ATP/ADP ratio of diabetic brain microvessels may be considered in some regards to be at the expense of the increased rate of oxygen consumption. What specific metabolic pathways contribute to the increased oxidative metabolism is unknown. One possibility is that ion homeostasis in the brain microvasculature of diabetic animals requires a higher rate of respiration. It is tempting to speculate that in poorly controlled diabetes mellitus combined with situations of fuel deprivation, such as hypoxia

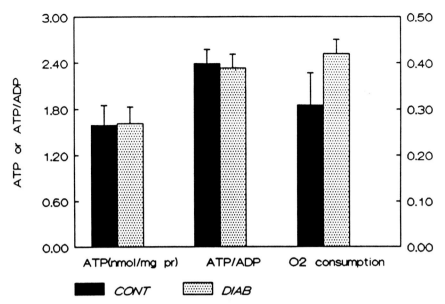

FIGURE 5.6. ATP, ATP/ADP, and O_2 consumption by diabetic and control brain microvessels. The content of ATP, ATP/ADP ratio, and rates of polarographically determined oxygen consumption were compared in several preparations of isolated brain microvessels from control (*solid black bars*; mean $\pm$ SE) and diabetic rats (160). Although ATP content and ATP/ADP ratio were unchanged by diabetes, rates of oxygen consumption were 35% greater in diabetic brain microvessels (p<0.05).

or ischemia, excessive oxygen consumption or other abnormalities of fuel utilization may produce microvascular dysfunction in brain. Future studies should address the functional consequences of this abnormal fuel metabolism on brain microvascular function.

Do Certain Metabolic Pathways Support Particular Endothelial Cell Functions?

The studies of Goldstein et al. (88) have linked oxidation of fatty acids to the rate of cellular uptake of rubidium (a potassium analog) in cerebral microvessels. They found that the rate of uptake of rubidium was dependent upon oxidative metabolism, it was inhibited by ouabain (an inhibitor of the plasma membrane Na^+K^+-ATPase), and it was increased by 40% when 0.25 mM palmitic acid was added to a microvessel suspension that already contained 5 mM glucose. This stimulation of rubidium uptake could be inhibited by 4-pentenoic acid, a somewhat nonspecific inhibitor of fatty acid oxidation. Although it may not be certain that oxidation of fatty acids is crucial to potassium uptake, the concept that flux through certain metabolic pathways is important to the maintenance or stimulation of certain cell functions is an important one. As noted earlier, based on studies in isolated brain microvessels, we have concluded that glycolysis and, secondarily, fatty acid oxidation are important for the maintenance of cellular energy state (ATP/ADP ratio).

IMPLICATIONS FOR CLINICAL MEDICINE

Diabetes Mellitus as a Cause of CNS Disease and Dysfunction

Diabetes mellitus has not traditionally been thought to cause CNS disease and dysfunction. Nevertheless, Reske-Nielsen and colleagues long ago described pathological changes in the nervous system of juvenile (type I) diabetics of long duration (206,207). Careful, quantitative analyses of cortical structure in rats with diabetes for more than one year also showed decreased brain volume and weight, as well as loss of cortical neurons (119A). Moreover, indications that chronic CNS dysfunction may be associated with diabetes, albeit often in subtle forms, is increasing. As reviewed by Mooradian (172), there are many potential causes for brain dysfunction in diabetes mellitus. These include vascular abnormalities (stroke, altered blood–brain barrier function) and metabolic disturbances (altered glycemia, ketosis, hypoxia, electrolyte and neurotransmitter changes) and the presence of other disorders such as neuropathy, hypertension, and renal failure. Since most studies have been done in experimental animals, however, their applicability to humans is uncertain.

In humans, the possible existence of a chronic encephalopathy in patients with diabetes has received increasing attention. Ryan (213) recently reviewed the neurobehavioral abnormalities associated with human diabetes and found that learning, memory, mental performance, and motor coordination may all be subtly impaired in at least a subset of patients. For children and adolescents with insulin-dependent diabetes mellitus (IDDM), age at onset and duration of diabetes are potent risk factors for neurobehavioral abnormalities. It is tempting to speculate that chronic cumulative metabolic effects, such as nonenzymatic glycation and/or repeated episodes of hypoglycemia, may play a role in this kind of impairment. In adults with diabetes, Ryan found that poor metabolic control (of diabetes) is predictive of subtle neurobehavioral performance problems. At the same time, hypoglycemia is more than twice as common with intensive insulin therapy. When manifest by coma or seizures, as seen in the feasibility phase of the Diabetes Control and Complications Trial (DCCT), hypoglycemia may cause cumulative brain damage. As Ryan points out, more systematic studies are needed to sort out the potential causes of chronic brain damage or dysfunction in diabetes.

Altered Tolerance to Hypoglycemia

Consequences of the brain transport and metabolism abnormalities seen in experimental animals may well have important implications for people with diabetes mellitus or hypoglycemia, though some caution must be taken in the extrapolation. Based on some early clinical observations (54) and later on a series of rigorous studies prospectively conducted, it has become clear that the threshold for symptoms of hypoglycemia varies depending on average recent glycemic control (24,220). However, the time course and extent of the adaptations so far observed vary considerably, partly based on technique used to study them, partly because of small but important differences in experimental conditions. For example, the recent work of Jakobsen et al. (118), shows that brain parenchymal glucose metabolism in diabetic animals first increases and then decreases. Changes in cerebral blood flow may depend upon the degree of hyperglycemia and are insignificant in most studies with less extreme hyperglycemia. In addition, human and animal models of diabetes are frequently inappropriately compared. Thus, most studies on diabetic rats have been with administration of moderate to high doses of streptozotocin, a pancreatic B-cell toxin that induces hypoinsulinemia and marked hyperglycemia. High doses of the drug produce a model like that of untreated type I diabetes. One last caveat is that human brains are extraordinarily complex and heterogeneous—indeed, the brain is legitimately considered the most heterogeneous organ in the body.

Given these cautions, it is appropriate to speculate how animal data *may* apply to patients with diabetes. In light of the finding that chronic hyperglycemia represses glucose transport across the blood–brain barrier in the rat, it is reasonable to propose that a similar phenomenon in humans accounts for the fact that patients with poorly controlled diabetes have a poor tolerance for acute lowering of blood glucose levels to normal, often experiencing CNS symptoms and responses associated with frank hypoglycemia (24,54). Conversely, it seems similarly reasonable to conclude that the increased efficiency of blood-to-brain glucose transfer that occurs in animals after hyperinsulinemic hypoglycemia may help explain the extraordinary tolerance to moderate hypoglycemia of intensively treated diabetic people, such as those self-administering insulin via an insulin pump (220). Figure 5.7 schematically depicts the effects of altered blood-to-brain glucose transport on the availability of glucose to the brain and brain cellular glucose metabolism. It should be emphasized that only when transport is rate-limiting for brain metabolism, as occurs in hypoglycemia and stroke, or when high metabolic demand for glucose exists (e.g. seizures), will modulations in brain glucose transport affect cellular supply and metabolism.

Potential Benefits to Adaptation of Brain Glucose Transport

There may be a potential teleologic benefit from adaptation of the brain transport mechanisms for glucose. Decreased transport may limit "glucose toxicity" to the brain (210). At least in extreme hyperglycemia, decreased use of glucose as a fuel by brain cells occurs. The mass action effect of hyperglycemia may be mitigated by downregulation of transport, which may thus curtail potentially toxic processes such as nonenzymatic glycation or flux through the aldose reductase pathway in the brain. Over time, the latter biochemical reactions and their consequences to cell function may be deleterious to brain function.

It also seems teleologically appropriate for the brain to enhance its efficiency to extract glucose, its major fuel, in response to chronic glucose lowering. It remains to be seen whether such adaptation occurs in chronically hypoglycemic humans such as those with type I (Von Gierke's) glycogen storage disease. It is remarkable, nonetheless, that patients with this and other disorders associated with chronic hypoglycemia tolerate glucose values that are quite low without obvious clinical symptoms. In our studies of rats with insulin-producing tumors or implanted insulin pumps, greater tolerance of hypoglycemia was certainly observed (162). Similarly, patients given intensive in-

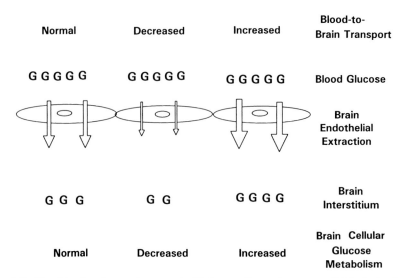

FIGURE 5.7. Blood-brain glucose transport efficiency alters glucose available to brain when transport is rate-limiting for brain energy metabolism. This figure schematically depicts how modulation of glucose transport at the blood–brain barrier may affect brain interstitial glucose levels and brain cellular glucose metabolism, e.g. ATP or lactate generation. *Left:* reduced efficiency of glucose extraction at the blood–brain barrier, as might occur in uncontrolled diabetes. When glucose levels in the blood are lowered, decreased transport at the blood–brain barrier lowers concentrations of glucose in brain interstitial fluid and therefore reduces glucose available for cellular glucose metabolism in brain cells. *Middle:* normal transport (shown for contrast). *Right:* effect of increased blood-to-brain glucose transport such as may occur with chronic hyperinsulinemia. In this situation, increased transport at the blood–brain barrier makes more glucose available for brain cellular glucose metabolism. Normally, cellular glucose metabolism in the brain is *not* limited by the rate of entry across the blood–brain barrier. On the other hand, when glucose levels are reduced (as in hypoglycemia or stroke), cellular metabolism in the brain could be influenced by blood–brain barrier transport efficiency.

sulin treatment also adapt to tolerate low glucose levels asymptomatically. These adaptations may be incomplete, however, and remain only partially protective.

Diabetes and Stroke Damage—Does Altered Transport Contribute?

Diabetes increases the frequency and severity of stroke (145,175), for reasons that are incompletely understood. There is considerable evidence in both animals and humans to suggest that elevated blood glucose is toxic to the brain during a stroke (116,143,146,169,198–200,244). Inducing marked hyperglycemia just prior to a stroke has been shown to increase the extent of brain damage in several experimental models of global brain ischemia (116,198). Even relatively mild hyperglycemia predicts greater stroke damage in animals and humans, and this worsened damage is not obviously explained by more severe atherosclerosis.

A possible brain toxin during ischemia is the lactic acid that is produced by anaerobic metabolism of glucose. During a stroke, lactic acid accumulates inside brain cells, lowers their intracellular pH, and causes cell death (143,219,223). Inducing hypoglycemia protects against glucose-mediated stroke damage (219,223). Administration of substances that either block glucose entry into the brain or inhibit glycolysis also protects against glucose toxicity (169). Immature animals that have not yet undergone the developmental increased efficiency of blood-to-brain glucose transport also appear to be less susceptible to toxicity during experimental ischemia. Taken together, these observations suggest that adaptations in glucose transport at either the blood–brain barrier or the brain parenchymal cell membrane may also have the potential to modify glucose toxicity to the brain during stroke.

In recent unpublished preliminary studies, we have found that hyperglycemia combined with hyperinsulinemia (rats either given a 50% glucose infusion or combined treatment with dexamethasone and sucrose) increases blood–brain glucose transport in vivo. These findings contrast with results seen in streptozotocin diabetes (hypoinsulinemic rats). The combination of hyperglycemia and hyperinsulinemia is common in those with marked insulin resistance or as a result of insulin therapy in some with type II diabetes. If hyperglycemic hyperinsulinemia-induced increased brain glucose transport seen in rats also occurs in humans, one can envision the following maladaptive consequences: First, the course of global brain ischemia might be worsened in such hyperinsulinemic and hyperglycemic people, based on studies in animals. Indeed, it seems likely, that the combination of increased transport of glucose plus increased plasma levels could be doubly toxic in the generation of intracellular lactic acid during severe ischemia. The second consequence of increased brain glucose transport in hyperglycemic (and hyperinsulinemic patients) could be increased flux through pathways leading to nonenzymatic glycation or polyol formation. If these pathways are significant in brain in people and contribute to subtle cognitive deficits, upregulation of glucose transport at the blood–brain barrier when combined with hyperglycemia could increase their potential for long-term brain damage.

Increased blood-to-brain (blood–brain barrier) transport of glucose increases the glucose available to the brain interstitium. At any given plasma glucose level, more glucose would then be made available to brain neurons and glia for metabolism. Normally, however, this would *not* be expected to affect brain energy metabolism or generation of lactic acid. This is so because blood–brain barrier transport of glucose does not usually limit brain metabolism. Excess glucose could efflux from the brain or be metabolized via low-affinity pathways (e.g. aldose reductase). However, as Pardridge (187) has clearly indicated, in some situations blood–brain barrier transport of glucose limits brain metabolism.

One additional caveat may be needed in applying the reasoning that increased glucose transport may worsen stroke damage. Glucose does not always worsen the damage of ischemia; it may even protect, particularly in focal brain ischemia or in the ischemic penumbra surrounding an area of dense stroke damage. Presumably areas of brain protected by glucose are less severely hypoxic and use glucose to generate ATP oxidatively rather than cause excessive lactate generation. Thus, in several animal models of focal cerebral ischemia, even rather extreme acute hyperglycemia not only does not exacerbate necrosis of brain cells it also protects against severe ischemic damage (82,253). Moreover, in cellular models of NMDA (a glutamate receptor subclass thought to be involved in stroke and hypoglycemia-induced brain damage) toxicity to cultured cerebellar granule cells, Henneberry and colleagues have elegantly shown that glucose protects against cell damage (45,107–109,179). They have also found that corticosterone in high doses, presumably by downregulating granule cell glucose influx, diminishes the protective effect of glucose on NMDA-induced damage.

Despite these cautions, increasing evidence suggests that even mild diabetes is associated with more severe stroke damage and poorer recovery. Certainly, more extensive vascular disease could explain why even mild hyperglycemia is associated with worse stroke damage. Nonetheless, there is some evidence that diabetes causes more severe stroke damage in people who have similar degrees of atherosclerosis. More importantly, severity of atherosclerosis is clearly not a factor in experimental brain ischemia.

Pulsinelli et al. stratified patients in a small study and found that blood glucose concentrations in excess of 120 mg/dl predicted poorer recovery from stroke (199). Recently, another group has found that blood glucose at the time of stroke in excess of 155 mg/dl predicts poorer stroke outcome (146). One interpretation of these studies is that a more severe stroke produces greater stress-related hyperglycemia. Because animal data suggest that even modest hyperglycemia may increase brain cellular lactate levels and damage, it is also possible that glucose causes, rather than reflects, more severe brain damage.

It is a little difficult to imagine why a very slight increase above normal blood glucose values would be toxic based simply on mass action. It is in part for this reason that involvement of other adaptations that may be synergistically deleterious, such as increased blood–brain glucose influx from hyperinsulinemia, remains an attractive hypothesis, as it would magnify the effect of mild hyperglycemia. Clearly, many other adaptations—in blood flow, in brain metabolism, in generation of factors augmenting recovery or repair—are also possibilities. Further examination of these factors and the many others that may modify stroke damage in diabetes is in order. Diabetes is very prevalent, and the prevalence is increasing as our population ages. Despite the marked improvement in hypertension therapy, stroke remains an extremely common cause of morbidity and mortality. Older women with diabetes and hypertension are particularly predisposed to stroke, as shown by the Framingham study, among others (145).

Diabetes and Stroke Damage—Does Altered Vascular Metabolism Contribute?

Cerebral microvessels in untreated diabetes have greater than a one-third increase in oxygen consumption (166), which certainly seems likely to affect vascular tolerance of hypoxia. Increased vascular oxygen consumption in the face of decreased oxygen availability might thus create a cellular energy failure. The consequences could include altered vascular tone, ionic disequilibrium, or release of endothelial cell products that exacerbate stroke damage by some other mechanism. Just as the brain may suffer from dysfunction related to acute fuel deprivation, so may its vasculature. Brain blood vessels are generally accorded a resistance to ischemia. Indeed, the fact that one can isolate cerebral microvessels at all, after imposing what is surely a marked ischemic/hypoxic insult, indicates this hardiness in the face of fuel deprivation. In diabetes, the brain microvessels show a gradual adaptation toward use of ketone bodies or other fuels and away from the oxidation of glucose. This could also affect the response to ischemia in vivo, which might be particularly important in situations in which rapid institution of tight glycemic control after very poor control was accomplished.

The peculiar dependence of cerebral microvessels (in vitro at least) upon glycolysis as a major source for ATP is also potentially relevant to the issue of stroke damage. Since microvessels upon isolation are clearly rendered hypoxic, they may even serve as a reasonable model of the effects of ischemia upon function and metabolism. If the observations in calf microvessels also apply to humans, glucose may be an important fuel to minimize the microvessel cellular loss of ATP. Such loss has been tied to endothelial dysfunction and cellular death in other models (110a).

Other metabolic abnormalities may also occur in the vasculature of diabetic people and animals. It is tempting, though perhaps premature, to speculate that altered glycemia and/or insulinemia in vivo may affect a variety of important vascular cell functions. Certainly the recent observation that endothelin [a potent vasoconstrictor that may alter microcirculatory flow in brain (245)] production by endothelial cells in culture is affected by glucose exposure in vitro (252) is intriguing in this light. Endothelin concentrations in plasma are also elevated in people with diabetes (232). Elegant studies by Cohen and colleagues (43,235,236) have indicated that vascular prostanoid metabolism and contractile responses to vascular agonists are altered by diabetes. Similarly, Deykin and co-workers have found that the production of HETE derivatives of arachidonic acid are abnormal in cultured porcine aortic endothelial cells exposed to high glucose concentrations (32). It remains to be shown whether these latter observations also apply to microvascular endothelial cells from the brain.

SUMMARY

The blood–brain barrier is comprised structurally of a continuous layer of endothelial cells whose tight junctions form a seamless barrier between the bloodstream and the brain. The barrier function of cerebral endothelium is augmented by the high content of degradative enzymes in brain capillaries. The endothelium of the brain is also a gatekeeper, regulating entry of nutrients and ions in a dynamic fashion. Recent cloning of several glucose-transport proteins will permit a molecular understanding of the mechanisms involved in this regulation.

In uncontrolled diabetes, depression of blood-to-brain transport of glucose occurs at any given glucose concentration, whereas in chronic hypoglycemia glucose transport is increased. These changes are specific in that other transport systems are unaffected or are affected differently, e.g. ketone body transport is increased in untreated diabetes. Transport of choline into brain is reduced after long-standing diabetes, and transport of ions (sodium and potassium) appears to be specifically altered, probably related to changes in the activity of the Na^+K^+-ATPase in brain endothelium. Abnormal increases in permeability to proteins may also occur. Recent studies suggest that insulin, and possibly other glucoregulatory hormones, may also be capable of slowly modulating brain glucose entry.

Many physiologic effects of diabetes on the brain have been observed in animal studies, including alterations in cerebral blood flow and cerebral glucose metabolism. The precise effects may be complex, and they may depend upon the severity of diabetes and its duration. Some confusion may have arisen methodologically in studies on brain transport because of multiple effects and their complexity. Recent evidence suggests that abnormal synthesis of glucose-transport proteins may be responsible, at least in part, for the specific depression of blood–brain barrier transport of glucose in experimental diabetes. The mechanisms for altered cerebral blood flow and brain metabolism changes are less well understood. The change in simple diffusion of substrates into the brain as a result of hyperglycemia is a finding that also needs further definition.

Brain microvessels have substantial ATP concentrations but are in some regards legitimately considered "metabolically shocked." Low initial ATP values are probably due to the procedures required for their isolation. Incubation of such isolated microvessels in an enriched medium containing glucose restores their content of ATP when it is low. The major metabolic pathway responsible for this restoration of ATP appears to be glycolysis. Oxidation of fatty acids may serve as a secondary source of ATP in isolated brain microvessels, especially when they are fuel deprived. Fat oxidation may specifically contribute to regulation of potassium transport in microvessels.

The oxidation of metabolic substrates by the cerebral microvasculature tends to parallel transport of the same substrates. In diabetes, glucose oxidation is depressed; in chronic hypoglycemia, glucose oxidation by isolated cerebral microvessels is increased. Isolated brain microvessels from diabetic rats consume oxygen at a rate that is one-third greater than that of nondiabetic controls, although the content of ATP and the ATP/ADP ratio of cerebral microvessels is unchanged by diabetes.

Clinical correlates of the altered brain transport and metabolism observed in animals with experimental diabetes are speculative. Three pathophysiological states in humans are of particular relevance: excessive brain damage after stroke, altered tolerance to glucose lowering in insulin-treated diabetes, and the mild, chronic encephalopathy observed in some patients with long-standing diabetes.

Finally, it should be emphasized that investigation of the metabolism of the brain microvasculature is a relatively new field. Basic scientific advances in research on vascular transport and metabolism of the brain have been quickly applied to clinical neurology and diabetes care, particularly to altered tolerance of acute glucose lowering in diabetes. As with any clinical application of all basic scientific information, some caution is warranted. The advances described here are probably important to human diabetes; nonetheless, a full understanding of how diabetes affects the brain will require more research—both of a basic and a clinical nature.

ACKNOWLEDGMENTS

The work described in this chapter was supported by Public Health Service grants RO1 NS22213, PO1 NS17493, The Juvenile Diabetes Foundation International, the Oregon affiliate of the American Diabetes Association, and the Medical Research Foundation of Oregon. The author gratefully acknowledges the efforts of many colleagues in accomplishing this research, and in particular the editorial assistance of Dr. Keith Tornheim and Dr. Neil Ruderman.

REFERENCES

1. ADAMO, M., RAIZADA, M. K., and LEROITH, D. Insulin and insulin-like growth factor receptors in the nervous system. *Mol. Neurobiol.* 3: 71–100, 1989.
2. AXELROD, J. D., and PILCH, P. F. Unique cytochalasin B binding characteristics of the hepatic glucose carrier. *Biochemistry* 22: 2222–2227, 1983.
3. BALDWIN, S. A., and HENDERSON, P. J. F. Homologies between sugar transporters from eukaryotes and prokaryotes. *Annu. Rev. Physiol.* 51: 459–571, 1989.
4. BANSKOTA, N. K., CARPENTER, J. L., and KING, G. L. Processing and release of insulin and insulin-like growth factor I by macro- and microvascular endothelial cells. *Endocrinology* 119: 1904–1913, 1986.
5. BASKIN, D. G., FIGLEWICZ, D. P., WOODS, S. C., PORTE, D., JR., and DORSA, D. M. Insulin in the brain. *Annu. Rev. Physiol.* 49: 335–347, 1987.
6. BASKIN, D. G., PORTE, D., JR., GUEST, K., and DORSA, D. M. Regional concentrations of insulin in the rat brain. *Endocrinology* 112: 898–903, 1983.
7. BASKIN, D. G., STEIN, L. J., IKEDA, H., WOODS, S. C., FIGLEWICZ, D. P., PORTE, D., JR., GREENWOOD, M. R., and DORSA, D. M. Genetically obese Zucker rats have abnormally low brain insulin content. *Life Sci.* 36: 627–633, 1985.
8. BECK, D. W., VINTERS, H. V., HART, M. N., and CANCILLA, P. A. Glial cells influence polarity of the blood-brain barrier. *J. Neuropathol. Exp. Neurol.* 43: 219–224, 1984.
9. BELL, G. I., KAYANO, T., BUSE, J. B., BURANT, C. F., TAKEDA, J., LIN, D., FUKUMOTO, H., and SEINO, S. Molecular biology of mammalian glucose transporters. *Diabetes Care* 13: 198–208, 1990.
10. BETZ, A. L., CSEJTEY, J., and GOLDSTEIN, G. W. Hexose transport and phosphorylation by capillaries isolated from rat brain. *Am. J. Physiol.* 236: 96–102, 1979.
11. BETZ, A. L., GILBOE, D. D., and DREWES, L. R. Effects of anoxia on net uptake and unidirectional transport of glucose into the isolated dog brain. *Brain Res.* 67: 307–316, 1974.
12. BETZ, A. L., GILBOE, D. D., and DREWES, L. R. Accelerative exchange diffusion kinetics of glucose between blood and brain and its relation to transport during anoxia. *Biochim, Biophys. Acta* 401: 416–428, 1975.
13. BETZ, A. L., GILBOE, D. D., and DREWES, L. R. Kinetics of unidirectional leucine transport into brain: effects of isoleucine, valine, and anoxia. *Am. J. Physiol.* 228: 895–900, 1975.
14. BETZ, A. L., GILBOE, D. D., YUDILEVICH, D. L., and DREWES, L. R. Kinetics of unidirectional glucose transport into the isolated dog brain. *Am. J. Physiol.* 225: 586–592, 1973.
15. BETZ, A. L., and GOLDSTEIN, G. W. Polarity of the blood-brain barrier: neutral amino acid transport into isolated brain capillaries. *Science* 202: 225–227, 1978.
16. BETZ, A. L., IANNOTTI, F., and HOFF, J. T. Ischemia reduces blood-to-brain glucose transport in the gerbil. *J. Cereb. Blood Flow Metab.* 3: 200–206, 1983.
17. BIRNBAUM, M. J. Identification of a novel gene encoding an insulin-responsive glucose transporter protein. *Cell* 57: 305–315, 1989.
18. BISSON, L. F., and FRAENKEL, D. G. Involvement of kinases in glucose and fructose uptake by *Saccharomyces cerevisiae*. *Proc. Natl. Acad. Sci USA* 80: 1730–1734, 1983.
19. BISSON, L. F., NEIGEBORN, L., CARLSON, M., and FRAENKEL, D. G. The SNF3 gene is required for high-affinity glucose transport in *Saccharomyces cerevisiae*. *J. Bacteriol.* 169: 1656–1662, 1987.
20. BLACKSHEAR, P. J., and ALBERTI, K. G. Experimental diabetic ketoacidosis. Sequential changes of metabolic intermediates in blood, liver, cerebrospinal fluid and brain after acute insulin deprivation in the streptozotocin-diabetic rat. *Biochem. J.* 138: 107–117, 1974.
21. BLASBERG, R. G., PATLAK, C. S., and FENSTERMACHER, J. D. Selection of experimental conditions for the accurate determination of blood–brain transfer constants from single-time experiments: a theoretical analysis. *J. Cereb. Blood Flow Metab.* 3: 215–225, 1983.

22. BOADO, R. J., and PARDRIDGE, W. M. The brain-type glucose transporter mRNA is specifically expressed at the blood-brain barrier. *Biochem. Biophys. Res. Commun.* 166: 174–179, 1990.

23. BOWMAN, P. D., ENNIS, S. R., RAREY, K. E., BETZ, A. L., and GOLDSTEIN, G. W. Brain microvessel endothelial cells in tissue culture: a model for study of blood-brain barrier permeability. *Ann. Neurol.* 14: 396–402, 1983.

24. BOYLE, P. J., SCHWARTZ, N. S., SHAH, S. D., CLUTTER, W. E., and CRYER, P. E. Plasma glucose concentrations at the onset of hypoglycemic symptoms in patients with poorly controlled diabetes and in nondiabetics. *N. Engl. J. Med.* 318: 1487–1492, 1988.

25. BRADBURY, M. W. *The Concept of a Blood-Brain Barrier.* New York: John Wiley & Sons, 1979.

26. BRADBURY, M. W. The structure and function of the blood-brain barrier. *Federation Proc.* 43: 186–190, 1984.

27. BRAUN, L. D., CORNFORD, E. M., and OLDENDORF, W. H. Newborn rabbit blood-brain barrier is selectively permeable and differs substantially from the adult. *J. Neurochem.* 34: 147–152, 1980.

28. BRAY, G. A., TEAGUE, R. J., and LEE, C. K. Brain uptake of ketones in rats with differing susceptibility to dietary obesity. *Metabolism* 36: 27–30, 1987.

29. BRENDEL, K. E., MEEZAN, E., and CARLSON, E. C. Isolated brain microvessels: a purified, metabolically active preparation from bovine cerebral cortex. *Science* 185: 953–955, 1974.

30. BRIGHTMAN, M. W., and REESE, T. S. Junctions between intimately apposed cell membranes in the vertebrate brain. *J. Cell Biol.* 40: 648–677, 1969.

31. BRIGHTMAN, M. W., REESE, T. S., and FEDER, N. Assessment with the electron microscope of the permeability to peroxidase of cerebral endothelium and epithelium in mice and sharks. In: *Capillary Permeability,* edited by C. Crone and N. A. Lassen. New York: Academic, 1970, pp. 468–476.

32. BROWN, M. L., JAKUBOWSKI, J. A., LEVENTIS, L. L., and DEYKIN, D. Elevated glucose alters eicosanoid release from porcine aortic endothelial cells. *J. Clin. Invest.* 82: 2136–2141, 1988.

33. CAIRNS, B. R., COLLARD, M. W., and LANDFEAR, S. M. Developmentally regulated gene from Leishmania encodes a putative membrane transport protein. *Proc. Natl. Acad. Sci. USA* 86: 7682–7686, 1989.

34. CALDERHEAD, D. M., and LIENHARD, G. E. Labeling of glucose transporters at the cell surface in 3T3-L1 adipocytes. Evidence for both translocation and a second mechanism in the insulin stimulation of transport. *J. Biol. Chem.* 263: 12171–12174, 1988.

35. CANCILLA, P. A., and DEBAULT, L. E. Neutral amino acid transport properties of cerebral endothelial cells in vitro. *J. Neuropathol. Exp. Neurol.* 42: 191–199, 1983.

36. CARDELLI CANGIANO, P., CANGIANO, C., JAMES, J. H., JEPPSSON, B., BRENNER, W., and FISCHER, J. E. Uptake of amino acids by brain microvessels isolated from rats after portacaval anastomosis. *J. Neurochem.* 36: 627–632, 1981.

37. CARDELLI CANGIANO, P., FIORI, A., CANGIANO, C., BARBERINI, F., ALLEGRA, P., PERESEMPIO, V., and STROM, R. Isolated brain microvessels as in vitro equivalents of the blood-brain barrier: selective removal by collagenase of the A-system of neutral amino acid transport. *J. Neurochem.* 49: 1667–1675, 1987.

38. CELENZA, J. L., MARSHALL-CARLSON, L., and CARLSON, M. The yeast SNF3 gene encodes a glucose transporter homologous to the mammalian protein. *Proc. Natl. Acad. Sci. USA* 85: 2130–2134, 1988.

39. CHARRON, M. J., BROSIUS, F. C., III. ALPER, S. L., and LODISH, H. F. A glucose transport protein expressed predominately in insulin-responsive tissues. *Proc. Natl. Acad. Sci. USA* 86: 2535–2539, 1989.

40. CHIPKIN, S. R., and MCCALL, A. L. Dexamethasone decreases hexose uptake by isolated cerebral microvessels. *Proc. Soc. Neurosci.* 15: 820, 1989.

41. CHOI, T. B., BOADO, R. J., and PARDRIDGE, W. M. Blood-brain barrier glucose transporter mRNA is increased in experimental diabetes mellitus. *Biochem. Biophys. Res. Commun.* 164: 375–380, 1989.

42. CHOI, T. B., and PARDRIDGE, W. M. Phenylalanine transport at the human blood-brain barrier. Studies with isolated human brain capillaries. *J. Biol. Chem.* 261: 6536–6541, 1986.

43. COHEN, R. A., TESFAMARIAM, B., WEISBROD, R. M., and ZITNAY, K. M. Adrenergic denervation in rabbits with diabetes mellitus. *Am. J. Physiol.* 259 (*Heart Circ. Physiol.* 28): H55–H61, 1990.

44. CORKEY, B. E. Analysis of acyl-coenzyme A esters in biological samples. *Methods Enzymol.* 166: 55–70, 1988.

45. Cox, J. A., Lysko, P. G., and Henneberry, R. C. Excitatory amino acid neurotoxicity at the N-methyl-D-aspartate receptor in cultured neurons: role of the voltage-dependent magnesium block. *Brain Res.* 499: 267–272, 1989.

46. Cremer, J. E., Braun, L. D., and Oldendorf, W. H. Changes during development in transport processes of the blood-brain barrier. *Biochim. Biophys. Acta* 448: 633–637, 1976.

47. Cremer, J. E., Cunningham, V. J., Pardridge, W. M., Braun, L. D., and Oldendorf, W. H. Kinetics of blood-brain barrier transport of pyruvate, lactate and glucose in suckling, weanling and adult rats. *J. Neurochem.* 33: 439–445, 1979.

48. Crone, C. Facilitated transfer of glucose from blood into brain tissue. *J. Physiol. (Lond.)* 181: 103–113, 1965.

49. Crone, C. The permeability of brain capillaries to non-electrolytes. *Acta Physiol. Scand.* 64: 407–417, 1965.

50. Cushman, S. W., and Wardzala, L. J. Potential mechanism of insulin action on glucose transport in the isolated rat adipose cell. Apparent translocation of intracellular transport systems to the plasma membrane. *J. Biol. Chem.* 255: 4758–4762, 1980.

51. Dallman, P. R., and Spirito, R. A. Brain response to protein undernutrition. Mechanism of preferential protein retention. *J. Clin. Invest.* 51: 2175–2180, 1972.

52. Debault, L. E., and Cancilla, P. A. Induction of gamma-glutamyl transpeptidase in isolated cerebral endothelial cells. *Adv. Exp. Med. Biol.* 131: 79–88, 1980.

53. Debault, L. E., and Cancilla, P. A. Gamma-glutamyl transpeptidase in isolated brain endothelial cells: induction by glial cells in vitro. *Science* 207: 653–655, 1980.

54. Defronzo, R. A., Hendler, R., and Christensen, N. Stimulation of counterregulatory hormonal responses in diabetic man by a fall in glucose concentration. *Diabetes* 29: 125–131, 1980.

55. Dehouck, M. P., Meresse, S., Delorme, P., Fruchart, J. C., and Cecchelli, R. An easier, reproducible, and mass-production method to study the blood-brain barrier in vitro. *J. Neurochem.* 54: 1798–1801, 1990.

56. Dick, A. P., Harik, S. I., Klip, A., and Walker, D. M. Identification and characterization of the glucose transporter of the blood-brain barrier by cytochalasin B binding and immunological reactivity. *Proc. Natl. Acad. Sci. USA* 81: 7233–7237, 1984.

57. Djuricic, B. M., and Mrsulja, B. B. Brain microvessel hexokinase: kinetic properties. *Experientia* 35: 169–171, 1979.

58. Djuricic, B. M., Rogac, L., Spatz, M., Rakic, L. M., and Mrsulja, B. B. Brain microvessels. I. Enzymic activities. *Adv. Neurol.* 20: 197–205, 1978.

59. Dorovini Zis, K., Bowman, P. D., Betz, A. L., and Goldstein, G. W. Hyperosmotic arabinose solutions open the tight junctions between brain capillary endothelial cells in tissue culture. *Brain Res.* 302: 383–386, 1984.

60. Dorovini Zis, K., Bowman, P. D., Betz, A. L., and Goldstein, G. W. Formation of a barrier by brain microvessel endothelial cells in culture. *Federation Proc.* 46: 2521–2522, 1987.

61. Dorovini Zis, K., Bowman, P. D., Betz, A. L., and Goldstein, G. W. Hyperosmotic urea reversibly opens the tight junctions between brain capillary endothelial cells in cell culture. *J. Neuropathol. Exp. Neurol.* 46: 130–140, 1987.

62. Drewes, L. R., Broderius, M. A., and Gerhart, D. Z. Phorbol ester stimulates hexose uptake by brain microvessel endothelial cells. *Brain Res. Bull.* 21: 771–776, 1988.

63. Drewes, L. R., Gilboe, D. D., and Betz, A. L. Metabolic alterations in brain during anoxic-anoxia and subsequent recovery. *Arch. Neurol.* 29: 385–390, 1973.

64. Duckrow, R. B. Glucose transfer into rat brain during acute and chronic hyperglycemia. *Metab. Brain Dis.* 3: 201–209, 1988.

65. Duckrow, R. B., Beard, D. C., and Brennan, R. W. Regional cerebral blood flow decreases during hyperglycemia. *Ann. Neurol.* 17: 267–272, 1985.

66. Duckrow, R. B., Beard, D. C., and Brennan, R. W. Regional cerebral blood flow decreases during chronic and acute hyperglycemia. *Stroke* 18: 52–58, 1987.

67. Duckrow, R. B., and Bryan, R. M., Jr. Regional cerebral glucose utilization during hyperglycemia. *J. Neurochem.* 48: 989–993, 1987.

68. Duffy, K. R., and Pardridge, W. M. Blood-brain barrier transcytosis of insulin in developing rabbits. *Brain Res.* 420: 32–38, 1987.

69. Ennis, S. R., and Betz, A. L. Sucrose permeability of the blood-retinal and blood-brain barriers. Effects of diabetes, hypertonicity, and iodate. *Invest. Ophthalmol. Vis. Sci.* 27: 1095–1102, 1986.

70. Estrada, C., Bready, J., Berliner, J., and Cancilla, P. A. Choline uptake by cerebral capillary endothelial cells in culture. *J. Neurochem.* 54: 1467–1473, 1990.

71. Figlewicz, D. P., Ikeda, H., Hunt, T. R., Stein, L. J., Dorsa, D. M., Woods, S. C., and

PORTE, D., JR. Brain insulin binding is decreased in Wistar Kyoto rats carrying the 'fa' gene. *Peptides* 7: 61–65, 1986.

72. FIGLEWICZ D. P., STEIN, L. J., WEST, D., PORTE, D., JR., and WOODS, S. C. Intracisternal insulin alters sensitivity to CCK-induced meal suppression in baboons. *Am. J. Physiol.* 250 (*Regulatory Integrative Comp. Physiol.* 19): R856–R866, 1986.

73. FLIER, J. S., MUECKLER, M., MCCALL, A. L., and LODISH, H. F. Distribution of glucose transporter messenger RNA transcripts in tissues of rat and man. *J. Clin. Invest.* 79: 657–661, 1987.

74. FLIER, J. S., MUECKLER, M. M., USHER, P., and LODISH, H. F. Elevated levels of glucose transport and transporter messenger RNA are induced by ras or src oncogenes. *Science* 235: 1492–1495, 1987.

75. FRANK, H. J., JANKOVIC VOKES, T., PARDRIDGE, W. M., and MORRIS, W. L. Enhanced insulin binding to blood-brain barrier in vivo and to brain microvessels in vitro in newborn rabbits. *Diabetes* 34: 728–733, 1985.

76. FRANK, H. J., and PARDRIDGE, W. M. Insulin binding to brain microvessels. *Adv. Metab. Disorders* 10: 291–302, 1983.

77. FRANK, H. J., PARDRIDGE, W. M., JANKOVIC VOKES, T., VINTERS, H. V., and MORRIS, W. L. Insulin binding to the blood-brain barrier in the streptozotocin diabetic rat. *J. Neurochem.* 47: 405–411, 1986.

78. FRANK, H. J., PARDRIDGE, W. M., MORRIS, W. L., ROSENFELD, R. G., and CHOI, T. B. Binding and internalization of insulin and insulin-like growth factors by isolated brain microvessels. *Diabetes* 35: 654–661, 1986.

79. FREEDMAN, L. S., and SAMUELS, S. Sparing of the brain in neonatal undernutrition: amino acid transport and incorporation into brain and muscle. *Science* 207: 902–904, 1980.

80. FUKUMOTO, H., KAYANO, T., BUSE, J. B., EDWARDS, Y., PILCH, P. F., BELL, G. I., and SEINO, S. Cloning and characterization of the major insulin-responsive glucose transporter expressed in human skeletal muscle and other insulin-responsive tissues. *J. Biol. Chem.* 264: 7776–7779, 1989.

81. GAPOSCHKIN, C. G., TORNHEIM, K., SUSSMAN, I., RUDERMAN, N. B., and MCCALL, A. L. Glucose is required to maintain ATP/ADP ratio of isolated bovine cerebral microvessels. *Am. J. Physiol.* 258 (*Endocrinol. Metab.* 21): E543–E547, 1990.

82. GINSBERG, M. D., and BUSTO, R. Rodent models of cerebral ischemia. *Stroke* 20: 1627–1642, 1989.

83. GJEDDE, A. Rapid steady-state analysis of blood-brain glucose transfer in rat. *Acta Physiol. Scand.* 108: 331–339, 1980.

84. GJEDDE, A., and CRONE, C. Induction processes in blood-brain transfer of ketone bodies during starvation. *Am. J. Physiol.* 229: 1165–1169, 1975.

85. GJEDDE, A., and CRONE, C. Blood-brain glucose transfer: repression in chronic hyperglycemia. *Science* 214: 456–457, 1981.

86. GOLDMANN, E. E. Die Aussere under innere Sekretion des Gesunden und kranken Organismus im lichte der "vitalen färbung." *Beitr. Z. Klin. Chir.* 64: 192–265, 1909.

87. GOLDMANN, E. E. *Vitalfärbung am zentral Nervensystem. Beitrag zur Physiologie des Plexus choriordeus und der Hirnhaute.* Berlin: Abh. Preuss. Akad. Wiss., Phys. Math. Kl., No. 1, pp. 1–60, 1913.

88. GOLDSTEIN, G. W. Relaxation of potassium transport to oxidative metabolism in isolated brain capillaries. *J. Physiol. (Lond.)* 286: 185–195, 1979.

89. GOLDENSTEIN, G. W., BETZ, A. L., BOWMAN, P. D., and DOROVINI ZIS, K. In vitro studies of the blood-brain barrier using isolated brain capillaries and cultured endothelial cells. *Ann. NY. Acad. Sci.* 481: 202–213, 1986.

90. GOLDSTEIN, G. W., CSEJTEY, J., and DIAMOND, I. Carrier mediated glucose transport in capillaries isolated from rat brain. *J. Neurochem.* 28: 725–728, 1977.

91. GOLDSTEIN, G. W., WOLINSKY, J. S., CSEJTEY, J., and DIAMOND, I. Isolation of metabolically active capillaries from rat brain. *J. Neurochem.* 25: 715–717, 1975.

92. GUILLOT, F. L., AUDUS, K. L., and RAUB, T. J. Fluid-phase endocytosis by primary cultures of bovine brain microvessel endothelial cell monolayers. *Microvasc. Res.* 39: 1–14, 1990.

93. HACHIYA, H. L., HALBAN, P. A., and KING, G. L. Intracellular pathways of insulin transport across vascular endothelial cells. *Am. J. Physiol.* 255 (*Cell Physiol.* 24): C459–C464, 1988.

94. HARGREAVES, K. M., and PARDRIDGE, W. M. Neutral amino acid transport at the human blood-brain barrier. *J. Biol. Chem.* 263: 19392–19397, 1988.

95. HARIK, S. I. Blood-brain barrier sodium/potassium pump: modulation by central noradrenergic innervation. *Proc. Natl. Acad. Sci. USA* 83: 4067–4070, 1986.

96. HARIK, S. I., DOULL, G. H., and DICK, A. P. Specific ouabain binding to brain microvessels and choroid plexus. *J. Cereb. Blood Flow Metab.* 5: 156–160, 1985.

97. HARIK, S. I., GRAVINA, S. A., and KALARIA, R. N. Glucose transporter of the blood-brain barrier and brain in chronic hyperglycemia. *J. Neurochem.* 51: 1930–1934, 1988.

98. HARIK, S. I., and LAMANNA, J. C. Vascular perfusion and blood-brain glucose transport in acute and chronic hyperglycemia. *J. Neurochem.* 51: 1924–1929, 1988.

99. HASKELL, J. F., MEEZAN, E., and PILLION, D. J. Identification of the insulin receptor of cerebral microvessels. *Am. J. Physiol.* 248 (*Endocrinol. Metab.* 11): E115–E125, 1985.

100. HASPEL, H. C., BIRNBAUM, M. J., WILK, E. W., and ROSEN, O. M. Biosynthetic precursors and in vitro translation products of the glucose transporter of human hepatocarcinoma cells, human fibroblasts, and murine preadipocytes. *J. Biol. Chem.* 260: 7219–7225, 1985.

101. HASPEL, H. C., WILK, E. W., BIRNBAUM, M. J., CUSHMAN, S. W., and ROSEN, O. M. Glucose deprivation and hexose transporter polypeptides of murine fibroblasts. *J. Biol. Chem.* 261: 6778–6789, 1986.

102. HAVRANKOVA, J., BROWNSTEIN, M., and ROTH, J. Insulin and insulin receptors in rodent brain. *Diabetologia* 20: 268–273, 1981.

103. HAVRANKOVA, J., ROTH, J., and BROWNSTEIN, M. J. Concentrations of insulin and insulin receptors in the brain are independent of peripheral insulin levels. Studies of obese and streptozotocin-treated rodents. *J. Clin. Invest.* 64: 636–642, 1979.

104. HAVRANKOVA, J., SCHMECHEL, D., ROTH, J., and BROWNSTEIN, M. Identification of insulin in rat brain. *Proc. Natl. Acad. Sci. USA* 75: 5737–5741, 1978.

105. HAWKINS, R. A., MANS, A. M., and BIEBUYCK, J. F. The passage of neutral amino acids across the blood-brain barrier of individual brain structures in normal and encephalopathic rats. *Biochem. Soc. Trans.* 8: 609–610, 1980.

106. HEDIGER, M. A., IKEDA, T., COADY, M., GUNDERSEN, C. B., and WRIGHT, E. M. Expression of size-selected mRNA encoding the intestinal Na/glucose cotransporter in *Xenopus laevis* oocytes. *Proc. Natl. Acad. Sci. USA* 84: 2634–2637, 1987.

107. HENNEBERRY, R. C. The role of neuronal energy in the neurotoxicity of excitatory amino acids. *Neurobiol. Aging* 10: 611–613 (discussion), 1989.

108. HENNEBERRY, R. C., NOVELLI, A., COX, J. A., and LYSKO, P. G. Neurotoxicity at the N-methyl-D-aspartate receptor in energy-compromised neurons. An hypothesis for cell death in aging and disease. *Ann. N. Y. Acad. Sci.* 568: 225–233, 1989.

109. HENNEBERRY, R. C., NOVELLI, A., VIGANO, M. A., REILLY, J. A., COX, J. A., and LYSKO, P. G. Energy-related neurotoxicity at the NMDA receptor: a possible role in Alzheimer's disease and related disorders. *Prog. Clin. Biol. Res.* 317: 143–156, 1989.

110. HINGORANI, V., and BRECHER, P. Glucose and fatty acid metabolism in normal and diabetic rabbit cerebral microvessels. *Am. J. Physiol.* 252 (*Endocrinol. Metab.* 15): E648–E653, 1987.

110a. HINSHAW, D. B., ARMSTRONG, B. C., BEALS, T. G., and HYSLOP, P. A. A cellular model of endothelial cell ischemia. *J. Surg. Res.* 44: 527–537, 1988.

111. HJELLE, J. T., BAIRD LAMBERT, J., CARDINALE, G., SPECTOR, S., and UDENFRIEND, S. Isolated microvessels: the blood-brain barrier in vitro. *Proc. Natl. Acad. Sci. USA* 75: 4544–4548, 1978.

112. HOLMES, C. S., HAYFORD, J. T., GONZALEZ, J. L., and WEYDERT, J. A. A survey of cognitive functioning at difference glucose levels in diabetic persons. *Diabetes Care* 6: 180–185, 1983.

113. HOLMES, C. S., and RICHMAN, L. C. Cognitive profiles of children with insulin-dependent diabetes. *J. Dev. Behav. Pediatr.* 6: 323–326, 1985.

114. HOLMES, C. S., TSALIKIAN, E., and YAMADA, T. Blood glucose control and visual and auditory attention in men with insulin-dependent diabetes. *Diabetic Med.* 5: 634–639, 1988.

115. HWANG, S. M., WEISS, S., and SEGAL, S. Uptake of L-[35S]cystine by isolated rat brain capillaries. *J. Neurochem.* 35: 417–424, 1980.

116. INAMURA, K., OLSSON, Y., and SIESJO, B. K. Substantia nigra damage induced by ischemia in hyperglycemic rats. A light and electron microscopic study. *Acta Neuropathol. (Berlin)* 75: 131–139, 1987.

117. JAKOBSEN, J., KNUDSEN, G. M., and JUHLER, M. Cation permeability of the blood-brain barrier in streptozotocin-diabetic rats. *Diabetologia* 30: 409–413, 1987.

118. JAKOBSEN, J., NEDERGAARD, M., AARSLEW JENSEN, M., and DIEMER, N. H. Regional brain glucose metabolism and blood flow in streptozotocin-induced diabetic rats. *Diabetes* 39: 437–440, 1990.

119. JAKOBSEN, J., NEDERGAARD, M., AARSLEW-JENSEN, M., and DIEMER, N. H. Regional brain glucose metabolism and blood flow in streptozotocin-induced diabetic rats. *Diabetes* 39: 437–440, 1990.

120. JAMES, D. E., BROWN, R., NAVARRO, J., and PILCH, P. F. Insulin-regulating tissues express a unique insulin-sensitive glucose transport protein. *Nature* 333: 183–185, 1988.

121. JAMES, D. E., STRUBE, M., and MUECKLER, M. Molecular cloning and characterization of an insulin-regulatable glucose transporter. *Nature* 338: 83–87, 1989.

122. JAMES, J. H., ESCOURROU, J., and FISCHER, J. E. Blood-brain neutral amino acid transport activity is increased after portacaval anastomosis. *Science* 200: 1395–1397, 1978.

123. JAMES, J. H., and FISCHER, J. E. Transport of neutral amino acids at the blood-brain barrier. *Pharmacology* 22: 1–7, 1981.

124. JIALAL, I., CRETTAZ, M., HACHIYA, H. L., KAHN, C. R., MOSES, A. C., BUZNEY, S. M., and KING, G. L. Characterization of the receptors for insulin and the insulin-like growth factors on micro- and macrovascular tissues. *Endocrinology* 117: 1222–1229, 1985.

125. JOHNSON, J. H., NEWGARD, C. B., MILBURN, J. L., LODISH, H. F., and THORENS, B. The high K_m glucose transporter of islets of Langerhans is functionally similar to the low affinity transporter of liver and has an identical primary sequence. *J. Biol. Chem.* 265: 6548–6551, 1990.

126. JOHNSON, P. C., BRENDEL, K., and MEEZAN, E. Thickened cerebral cortical capillary basement membranes in diabetics. *Arch. Pathol. Lab. Med.* 106: 214–217, 1982.

127. KAHN, B. B., and CUSHMAN, S. W. Subcellular translocation of glucose transporters: role in insulin action and its perturbation in altered metabolic states. *Diabetes/Metab. Rev.* 1: 203–227, 1985.

128. KAHN, B. B., and CUSHMAN, S. W. Mechanism for markedly hyperresponsive insulin-stimulated glucose transport activity in adipose cells from insulin-treated streptozotocin diabetic rats. Evidence for increased glucose transporter intrinsic activity. *J. Biol. Chem.* 262: 5118–5124, 1987.

129. KALCKAR, H. M. Regulation of hexose transport-carrier activity in cultured animal fibroblasts: another confrontation with cellular recycling requiring oxidative energy generation. *Trans. N. Y. Acad. Sci.* 41: 83–86, 1983.

130. KALCKAR, H. M., CHRISTOPHER, C. W., and ULLREY, D. Uncouplers of oxidative phosphorylation promote derepression of the hexose transport system in cultures of hamster cells. *Proc. Natl. Acad. Sci. USA* 76: 6453–6455, 1979.

131. KALCKAR, H. M., and ULLREY, D. B. Hexose uptake regulation mediated through aerobic pathways: schism in a fibroblast mutant. *Federation Proc.* 43: 2242–2245, 1984.

132. KALCKAR, H. M., and ULLREY, D. B. Further clues concerning the vectors essential to regulation of hexose transport, as studied in fibroblast cultures from a metabolic mutant. *Proc. Natl. Acad. Sci. USA* 81: 1126–1129, 1984.

133. KALCKAR, H. M., ULLREY, D. B., and LAURSEN, R. A. Effects of combined glutamine and serum deprivation on glucose control of hexose transport in mammalian fibroblast cultures. *Proc. Natl. Acad. Sci. USA* 77: 5958–5961, 1980.

134. KAYANO, T., FUKUMOTO, H., EDDY, R. L., FAN, Y. S., BYERS, M. G., SHOWS, T. B., and BELL, G. I. Evidence for a family of human glucose transporter-like proteins. Sequence and gene localization of a protein expressed in fetal skeletal muscle and other tissues. *J. Biol. Chem.* 263: 15245–15248, 1988.

135. KENNEDY, A., FRANK, R. N., MANCINI, M. A., and LANDE, M. Collagens of the retinal microvascular basement membrane and of retinal microvascular cells in vitro. *Exp. Eye Res.* 42: 177–199, 1986.

136. KIKANO, G. E., LAMANNA, J. C., and HARIK, S. I. Brain perfusion in acute and chronic hyperglycemia in rats. *Stroke* 20: 1027–1031, 1989.

137. KING, G. L., BUZNEY, S. M., KAHN, C. R., HETU, N., BUCHWALD, S., MACDONALD, S. G., and RAND, L. I. Differential responsiveness to insulin of endothelial and support cells from micro- and macrovessels. *J. Clin. Invest.* 71: 974–979, 1983.

138. KING, G. L., and JOHNSON, S. M. Receptor-mediated transport of insulin across endothelial cells. *Science* 227: 1583–1586, 1985.

139. KING, G. L., JOHNSON, S. M., and JIALAL, I. Processing and transport of insulin by vascular endothelial cells. Effects of sulfonylureas on insulin receptors. *Am. J. Med.* 79: 43–47, 1985.

140. KNUDSEN, G. M., and JAKOBSEN, J. Blood-brain barrier permeability to sodium. Modification by glucose or insulin. *J. Neurochem.* 52: 174–178, 1989.

141. KNUDSEN, G. M., JAKOBSEN, J., BARRY, D. I., COMPTON, A. M., and TOMLINSON, D. R. Myo-inositol normalizes decreased sodium permeability of the blood-brain barrier in streptozotocin diabetes. *Neuroscience* 29: 773–777, 1989.

142. KNUDSEN, G. M., JAKOBSEN, J., JUHLER, M., and PAULSON, O. B. Decreased blood-brain barrier permeability to sodium in early experimental diabetes. *Diabetes* 35: 1371–1373, 1986.

143. KRAIG, R. P., PULSINELLI, W. A., and PLUM, F. Hydrogen ion buffering during complete brain ischemia. *Brain Res.* 342: 281–290, 1985.

144. KRANE, E. J., ROCKOFF, M. A., WALLMAN, J. K., and WOLFSDORF, J. I. Subclinical brain

swelling in children during treatment of diabetic ketoacidosis. *N. Engl. J. Med.* 312: 1147–1151, 1985.

145. KULLER, L. H., DORMAN, J. S., and WOLF, P. A. Cerebrovascular disease and diabetes. In: *Diabetes in America—Diabetes data compiled 1984,* edited by M. I. Harris and R. F. Hamman. Bethesda: U.S. Department of Health and Human Services, 1985, pp. 18-1–18-18.

146. KUSHNER, M., NENCINI, P., REIVICH, M., RANGO, M., JAMIESON, D., FAZEKAS, F., ZIMMERMAN, R., CHAWLUK, J., ALAVI, A., and ALVES, W. Relation of hyperglycemia early in ischemic brain infarction to cerebral anatomy, metabolism, and clinical outcome. *Ann. Neurol.* 28: 129–135, 1990.

147. LAMANNA, J. C., and HARIK, S. I. Regional comparisons of brain glucose influx. *Brain Res.* 326: 299–305, 1985.

148. LAMANNA, J. C., and HARIK, S. I. Regional studies of blood-brain barrier transport of glucose and leucine in awake and anesthetized rats. *J. Cereb. Blood Flow Metab.* 6: 717–723, 1986.

149. LASBENNES, F., and GAYET, J. Capacity for energy metabolism in microvessels isolated from rat brain. *Neurochem. Res.* 9: 1–10, 1984.

150. LATERRA, J., GUERIN, C., and GOLDSTEIN, G. W. Astrocytes induce neural microvascular endothelial cells to form capillary-like structures in vitro. *J. Cell. Physiol.* 144: 204–215, 1990.

151. LE ROITH, D., HENDRICKS, S. A., LESNIAK, M. A., RISHI, S., BECKER, K. L., HAVRANKOVA, J., ROSENZWEIG, J. L., BROWNSTEIN, M. J., and ROTH, J. Insulin in brain and other extrapancreatic tissues of vertebrates and nonvertebrates. *Adv. Metab. Disorders* 10: 303–340, 1983.

152. LOWE, W. L., JR., BOYD, F. T., CLARKE, D. W., RAIZADA, M. K., HART, C., and LEROITH, D. Development of brain insulin receptors: structural and functional studies of insulin receptors from whole brain and primary cell cultures. *Endocrinology* 119: 25–35, 1986.

153. MANS, A. M., BIEBUYCK, J. F., and HAWKINS, R. A. Ammonia selectively stimulates neutral amino acid transport across blood-brain barrier. *Am. J. Physiol.* 245 (*Cell Physiol.*): C74–77, 1983.

154. MANS, A. M., BIEBUYCK, J. F., SAUNDERS, S. J., KIRSCH, R. E., and HAWKINS, R. A. Tryptophan transport across the blood-brain barrier during acute hepatic failure. *J. Neurochem.* 33: 409–418, 1979.

155. MANS, A. M., BIEBUYCK, J. F., SHELLY, K., and HAWKINS, R. A. Regional blood-brain barrier permeability to amino acids after portacaval anastomosis. *J. Neurochem.* 38: 705–717, 1982.

156. MANS, A. M., DEJOSEPH, M. R., DAVIS, D. W., and HAWKINS, R. A. Brain energy metabolism in streptozotocin-diabetes. *Biochem. J.* 249: 57–62, 1988.

157. MATTHAEI, S., HORUK, R., and OLEFSKY, J. M. Blood-brain glucose transfer in diabetes mellitus. Decreased number of glucose transporters at blood-brain barrier. *Diabetes* 35: 1181–1184, 1986.

158. MATTHAEI, S., OLEFSKY, J. M., and HORUK, R. Biochemical characterization and subcellular distribution of the glucose transporter from rat brain microvessels. *Biochim. Biophys. Acta* 905: 417–425, 1987.

159. MAXWELL, K., BERLINER, J. A., and CANCILLA, P. A. Stimulation of glucose analogue uptake by cerebral microvessel endothelial cells by a product released by astrocytes. *J. Neuropathol. Exp. Neurol.* 48: 69–80, 1989.

160. McALOON, J., CARSON, D., and CREAN, P. Cerebral oedema complicating diabetic ketoacidosis. *Acta Paediatr. Scand.* 79: 115–117, 1990.

161. McCALL, A. L. Effects of diabetes and hypoglycemia on brain microvessel hexose transport. *Diabetes* 40: 1991 (abstract).

162. McCALL, A. L., FIXMAN, L. B., FLEMING, N., TORNHEIM, K., CHICK, W., and RUDERMAN, N. B. Chronic hypoglycemia increases brain glucose transport. *Am. J. Physiol.* 251 (*Endocrinol. Metab.* 14): E442–E447, 1986.

163. McCALL, A. L., GOULD, J. B., and RUDERMAN, N. B. Diabetes-induced alterations of glucose metabolism in rat cerebral microvessels. *Am. J. Physiol.* 247 (*Endocrinol. Metab.* 10): E462–E467, 1984.

164. McCALL, A. L., MILLINGTON, W., TEMPLE, S., and WURTMAN, R. J. Altered transport of hexoses across the blood-brain barrier in diabetes. *Diabetes* 28: 1979 (abstract).

165. McCALL, A. L., MILLINGTON, W. R., and WURTMAN, R. J. Metabolic fuel and amino acid transport into the brain in experimental diabetes mellitus. *Proc. Natl. Acad. Sci. USA* 79: 5406–5410, 1982.

166. McCALL, A. L., SUSSMAN, I., TORNHEIM, K., CORDERO, R., and RUDERMAN, N. B. Effects of

hypoglycemia and diabetes on fuel metabolism by rat brain microvessels. *Am. J. Physiol.* 254 (*Endocrinol. Metab.* 17): E272–E278, 1988.

167. MCCALL, A. L. VALENTE, J., CORDERO, R., RUDERMAN, N. B., and TORNHEIM, K. Metabolic characterization of isolated cerebral microvessels: ATP and ADP concentrations. *Microvasc. Res.* 35: 325–333, 1988.

168. MERESSE, S., DEHOUCK, M.-P., DELORME, P., BENSAID, M., TAUBER, J.-P., DELBART, C., FRUCHART, J.-C., and CECCHELLI, R. Bovine brain endothelial cells express tight junctions and monoamine oxidase activity in long-term culture. *J. Neurochem.* 53: 1363–1371, 1989.

169. MILLER, L. P., VILLENEUVE, J. B., and OLDENDORF, W. H. Pretreatment with 3-O-methyl-D-glucose or 2-deoxy-D-glucose attenuates the post-mortem rise in rat brain lactate. *Neurochem. Res.* 11: 489–495, 1986.

170. MOORADIAN, A. D. Blood-brain barrier choline transport is reduced in diabetic rats. *Diabetes* 36: 1094–1097, 1987.

171. MOORADIAN, A. D. Effect of ascorbate and dehydroascorbate on tissue uptake of glucose. *Diabetes* 36: 1001–1004, 1987.

172. MOORADIAN, A. D. Diabetes and the central nervous system. *Endo. Rev.* 9: 346–356, 1988.

173. MOORADIAN, A. D. Metabolic fuel and amino acid transport into the brain in experimental hypothyroidism. *Acta Endocrinol. (Copenh.)* 122: 156–162, 1990.

174. MOORE, T. J., LIONE, A. P., SUGDEN, M. C., and REGEN, D. M. Beta-hydroxybutyrate transport in rat brain: developmental and dietary modulations. *Am. J. Physiol.* 230: 619–630, 1976.

175. MORTEL, K. F., MEYER, J. S., SIMS, P. A., and MCCLINTIC, K. Diabetes mellitus as a risk factor for stroke. *South. Med. J.* 83: 904–911, 1990.

176. MRSULJA, B. B., DJURICIC, B. M., MRSULJA, B. J., ROGAC, L., SPATZ, M., and KLATZO, L. Brain microvessels. II. Effect of ischemia and dihydroergotoxin on enzymic activities. *Adv. Neurol.* 20: 207–213, 1978.

177. MUECKLER, M., CARUSO, C., BALDWIN, S. A., PANICO, M., BLENCH, I., MORRIS, H. R., ALLARD, W. J., LIENHARD, G. E., and LODISH, H. F. Sequence and structure of a human glucose transporter. *Science* 229: 941–945, 1985.

178. MUKAI, N., HORI, S., and POMEROY, M. Cerebral lesions in rats with streptozotocin-induced diabetes. *Acta Neuropathol. (Berlin)* 51: 79–84, 1980.

179. NOVELLI, A., REILLY, J. A., LYSKO, P. G., and HENNEBERRY, R. C. Glutamate becomes neurotoxic via the N-methyl-D-aspartate receptor when intracellular energy levels are reduced. *Brain Res.* 451: 205–212, 1988.

180. OKA, Y., ASANO, T., SHIBASAKI, Y., KASUGA, M., KANAZAWA, Y., and TAKAKU, F. Studies with antipeptide antibody suggest the presence of at least two types of glucose transporter in rat brain and adipocyte. *J. Biol. Chem.* 263: 13432–13439, 1988.

181. OLDENDORF, W. H. Measurement of brain uptake of radiolabeled substances using a tritiated water internal standard. *Brain Res.* 24: 372–376, 1970.

182. OLDENDORF, W. H. Brain uptake of radiolabeled amino acids, amines, and hexoses after arterial injection. *Am. J. Physiol.* 221: 1629–1639, 1971.

183. OLDENDORF, W. H., CORNFORD, M. E., and BROWN, W. J. The large apparent work capability of the blood-brain barrier: a study of the mitochondrial content of capillary endothelial cells in brain and other tissues of the rat. *Ann. Neurol.* 1: 409–417, 1977.

184. OWEN, O. E., MORGAN, A. P., KEMP, H. G., SULLIVAN, J. M., HERRERA, M. G., and CAHILL, G. F., JR. Brain metabolism during fasting. *J. Clin. Invest.* 46: 1589–1595, 1967.

185. PARDRIDGE, W. M Inorganic mercury: selective effects on blood-brain barrier transport systems. *J. Neurochem.* 27: 333–335, 1976.

186. PARDRIDGE, W. M. Regulation of amino acid availability to brain: selective control mechanisms for glutamate. In: *Glutamic Acid: Advances in Biochemistry and Physiology*, edited by L. J. Filer, Jr., S. Garattini, M. R. Kare, W. A. Reynolds, and R. J. Wurtman. New York: Raven, 1979, pp. 125–137.

187. PARDRIDGE, W. M. Brain metabolism: a perspective from the blood-brain barrier. *Physiol. Rev.* 63: 1481–1535, 1983.

188. PARDRIDGE, W. M. Receptor-mediated peptide transport through the blood-brain barrier. *Endocrinol. Rev.* 7: 314–330, 1986.

189. PARDRIDGE, W. M. Recent advances in blood-brain barrier transport. *Annu. Rev. Pharmacol. Toxicol.* 28: 25–39, 1988.

190. PARDRIDGE, W. M., and CHOI, T. B. Neutral amino acid transport at the human blood-brain barrier. *Federation Proc.* 45: 2073–2078, 1986.

191. PARDRIDGE, W. M., CONNOR, J. D., and CRAWFORD, I. L. Permeability changes in the blood-brain barrier: causes and consequences. *CRC. Crit. Rev. Toxicol.* 3: 159–199, 1975.

192. PARDRIDGE, W. M., CRAWFORD, I. L., and CONNOR, J. D. Permeability changes in the blood-

brain barrier induced by nortriptyline and chlorpromazine. *Toxicol. Appl. Pharmacol.* 26: 49–57, 1973.

193. PARDRIDGE, W. M., LANDAW, E. M., MILLER, L. P., BRAUN, L. D., and OLDENDORF, W. H. Carotid artery injection technique: bounds for bolus mixing by plasma and by brain. *J. Cereb. Blood Flow Metab.* 5: 576–583, 1985.

194. PARDRIDGE, W. M., and OLDENDORF, W. H. Transport of metabolic substrates through the blood-brain barrier. *J. Neurochem.* 28: 5–12, 1977.

195. PARDRIDGE, W. M., TRIGUERO, D., and FARREL, C. R. Downregulation of blood-brain barrier glucose transporter in experimental diabetes. *Diabetes* 39: 1040–1044, 1990.

196. PARDRIDGE, W. M., TRIGUERO, D., YANG, J., and CANCILLA, P. A. Comparison of in vitro and in vivo models of drug transcytosis through the blood-brain barrier. *J. Pharmacol. Exp. Ther.* 253: 884–891, 1990.

197. PILLION, D. J., HASKELL, J. F., and MEEZAN, E. Cerebral cortical microvessels: an insulin-sensitive tissue. *Biochem. Biophys. Res. Commun.* 104: 686–692, 1982.

198. PULSINELLI, W., WALDMAN, S., SIGSBEE, B., RAWLINSON, D., SCHERER, P., and PLUM, F. Experimental hyperglycemia and diabetes mellitus worsen stroke outcome. *Trans. Am. Neurol. Assoc.* 105: 21–24, 1980.

199. PULSINELLI, W. A., LEVY, D. E., SIGSBEE, B., SCHERER, P., and PLUM, F. Increased damage after ischemic stroke in patients with hyperglycemia with or without established diabetes mellitus. *Am. J. Med.* 74: 540–544, 1983.

200. PULSINELLI, W. A., WALDMAN, S., RAWLINSON, D., and PLUM, F. Moderate hyperglycemia augments ischemic brain damage: a neuropathologic study in the rat. *Neurology* 32: 1239–1246, 1982.

201. RAIZADA, M. K., SHEMER, J., JUDKINS, J. H., CLARKE, D. W., MASTERS, B. A., and LEROITH, D. Insulin receptors in the brain: structural and physiological characterization. *Neurochem. Res.* 13: 297–303, 1988.

202. RANDLE, P. J., GARLAND, P. B., HALES, C. N., and NEWSHOLME, E. A. The glucose-fatty acid cycle. Its role in insulin sensitivity and the metabolic disturbances of diabetes mellitus. *Lancet 1:* 785–789, 1963.

203. Rapoport, S. I. *Blood-Brain Barrier in Physiology and Medicine.* New York: Raven, 1976.

204. REESE, T. S., and KARNOVSKY, M. J. Fine structural localization of blood-brain barrier to exogenous peroxidase. *J. Cell Biol.* 34: 207–217, 1967.

205. REGEN, D. M., CALLIS, J. T., and SUGDEN, M. C. Studies of cerebral beta-hydroxybutyrate transport by carotid injection; effects of age, diet and injectant composition. *Brain Res.* 271: 289–299, 1983.

206. RESKE NIELSEN, E., and LUNDBAEK, K. Pathological changes in the central and peripheral nervous system of young long-term diabetics. II. The spinal cord and peripheral nerves. *Diabetologia* 4: 34–43, 1968.

207. RESKE NIELSEN, E., LUNDBAEK, K., GREGERSEN, G., and HARMSEN, A. Pathological changes in the central and peripheral nervous system of young long-term diabetics. The terminal neuro-muscular apparatus. *Diabetologia* 6: 98–103, 1970.

208. ROSENBLOOM, A. L. Intracerebral crises during treatment of diabetic ketoacidosis. *Diabetes Care* 13: 22–33, 1990.

209. ROSENFELD, R. G., PHAM, H., KELLER, B. T., BORCHARDT, R. T., and PARDRIDGE, W. M. Demonstration and structural comparison of receptors for insulin-like growth factor-I and -II (IGF-I and -II) in brain and blood-brain barrier. *Biochem. Biophys. Res. Commun.* 149: 159–166, 1987.

210. ROSSETTI, L. GIACCARI, A., and DEFRONZO, R. A. Glucose toxicity. *Diabetes Care* 13: 610–630, 1990.

211. RUDERMAN, N. B., ROSS, P. S., BERGER, M., and GOODMAN, M. N. Regulation of glucose and ketone-body metabolism in brain of anaesthetized rats. *Biochem. J.* 138: 1–10, 1974.

212. RUTTEN, M. J., HOOVER, R. L., and KARNOVSKY, M. J. Electrical resistance and macromolecular permeability of brain endothelial monolayer cultures. *Brain Res.* 425: 301–310, 1987.

213. RYAN, C. M. Neurobehavioral complications of type I diabetes. Examination of possible risk factors. *Diabetes Care* 11: 86–93, 1988.

214. SADIQ, F., HOLTZCLAW, L., CHUNDU, K., MUZZAFAR, A., and DEVASKAR, S. The ontogeny of the rabbit brain glucose transporter. *Endocrinology* 126: 2417–2424, 1990.

215. SARNA, G. S., BRADBURY, M. W., and CAVANAGH, J. Permeability of the blood-brain barrier after portocaval anastomosis in the rat. *Brain Res.* 138: 550–554, 1977.

216. SARNA, G. S., BRADBURY, M. W., CREMIER, J. E., LAI, J. C., and TEAL, H. M. Brain metabolism and specific transport at the blood-brain barrier after portocaval anastomosis in the rat. *Brain Res.* 160: 69–83, 1979.

217. SCHWARTZ, M. W., SIPOLS, A., KAHN, S. E., LATTEMANN, D. F. TABORSKY, G. J., JR,. BERMAN,

R. N., Woods, S. C., and Porte, D., Jr. Kinetics and specificity of insulin uptake from plasma into cerebrospinal fluid. *Am. J. Physiol.* 259 (*Endocrinol. Metab.* 22): E378–E383, 1990.

218. Shemer, J., Raizada, M. K., Masters, B. A., Ota, A., and Leroith, D. Insulin-like growth factor I receptors in neuronal and glial cells. Characterization and biological effects in primary culture. *J. Biol. Chem.* 262: 7693–7699, 1987.

219. Siesjo, B. K. Mechanisms of ischemic brain damage. *Crit. Care Med.* 16: 954–963, 1988.

220. Simonson, D. C., Tamborlane, W. V., Defronzo, R. A., and Sherwin, R. S. Intensive insulin therapy reduces counterregulatory hormone responses to hypoglycemia in patients with type I diabetes. *Ann. Intern. Med.* 103: 184–190, 1985.

221. Sistonen, L., Holtta, E., Lehvaslaiho, H., Lehtola, L., and Alitalo, K. Activation of the *neu* tyrosine kinase induces the *fos/jun* transcription factor complex, the glucose transporter and ornithine decarboxylase. *J. Cell Biol.* 109: 1911–1919, 1989.

222. Slot, J. W., Moxley, R., Geuze, H. J., and James, D. E. No evidence for expression of the insulin-regulatable glucose transporter in endothelial cells. *Nature* 346: 369–371, 1990.

223. Smith, M. L., von Hanwehr, R., and Siesjo, B. K. Changes in extra- and intracellular pH in the brain during and following ischemia in hyperglycemic and in moderately hypoglycemic rats. *J. Cereb. Blood Flow Metab.* 6: 574–583, 1986.

224. Smith, Q. R. Quantitation of blood-brain barrier permeability. In: *Implications of the Blood-Brain Barrier and Its Manipulation—Volume I, Basic Science Aspects,* edited by E. A. Neuwelt. New York: Plenum, 1988, pp. 85–118.

225. Stauber, W. T., Ong, S.-H., and McCuskey, R. S. Selective extravascular escape of albumin into the cerebral cortex of the diabetic rat. *Diabetes* 30: 500–503, 1981.

226. Steele, R. D. Blood-brain barrier transport of the alpha-keto acid analogs of amino acids. *Federation Proc.* 45: 2060–2064, 1986.

227. Stein, D. A., Cairns, B. R., and Landfear, S. M. Developmentally regulated transporter in Leishmania is encoded by a family of clustered genes. *Nucleic Acids Res.* 18: 1549–1557, 1990.

228. Sussman, I., Carson, M. P., McCall, A. L., Schultz, V., Ruderman, N. B., and Tornheim, K. Energy state of bovine cerebral microvessels: comparison of isolation methods. *Microvasc. Res.* 35: 167–178, 1988.

229. Sussman, I., Carson, M. P., Schultz, V., Wu, X. P., McCall, A. L. Ruderman, N. B., and Tornheim, K. Chronic exposure to high glucose decreases myo-inositol in cultured cerebral microvascular pericytes but not in endothelium. *Diabetologia* 31: 771–775, 1988.

230. Suzuki, K., and Kono, T. Evidence that insulin causes translocation of glucose transport activity to the plasma membrane from an intracellular storage site. *Proc. Natl. Acad. Sci. USA* 77: 2542–2545, 1980.

231. Szkutnicka, K., Tschopp, J. F., Andrews, L., and Cirillo, V. P. Sequence and structure of the yeast galactose transporter. *J. Bacteriol.* 171: 4486–4493, 1989.

232. Takahashi, K., Ghatei, M. A., Lam, H. C., O'Halloran, D. J., and Bloom, S. R. Elevated plasma endothelin in patients with diabetes mellitus. *Diabetologia* 33: 306–310, 1990.

233. Takasato, Y., Rapoport, S. I., and Smith, Q. R. An in situ brain perfusion technique to study cerebrovascular transport in the rat. *Am. J. Physiol.* 247 (*Heart Circ. Physiol.* 16): H484–H493, 1984.

234. Taubin, H., and Matz, R. Cerebral edema, diabetes insipidus, and sudden death during the treatment of diabetic ketoacidosis. *Diabetes* 17: 108–109, 1968.

235. Tesfamariam, B., Brown, M. L., Deykin, D., and Cohen, R. A. Elevated glucose promotes generation of endothelium-derived vasoconstrictor prostanoids in rabbit aorta. *J. Clin. Invest.* 85: 929–932, 1990.

236. Tesfamariam, B., Jakubowski, J. A., and Cohen, R. A. Contraction of diabetic rabbit aorta caused by endothelium-derived PGH_2-TxA_2. *Am. J. Physiol.* 257 (*Heart Circ. Physiol.* 26): H1327–H1333, 1989.

237. Thorens, B., Lodish, H. F., and Brown, D. Differential localization of two glucose transporter isoforms in rat kidney. *Am. J. Physiol.* 259 (*Cell Physiol.* 28): C286–C294, 1990.

238. Thorens, B., Sarkar, H. K., Kaback, H. R., and Lodish, H. F. Cloning and functional expression in bacteria of a novel glucose transporter present in liver, intestine, kidney, and beta-pancreatic islet cells. *Cell* 55: 281–290, 1988.

239. Ullrey, D. B., and Kalckar, H. M. The nature of regulation of hexose transport in cultured mammalian fibroblasts: aerobic "repressive" control by D-glucosamine. *Arch. Biochem. Biophys.* 209: 168–174, 1981.

240. ULLREY, D. B., and KALCKAR, H. M. Schism and complementation of hexose-mediated transport regulation as illustrated in a fibroblast mutant lacking phosphoglucose-isomerase. *Biochem. Biophys. Res. Commun.* 107: 1532–1538, 1982.
241. VAN DER MEULEN, J. A., KLIP, A., and GRINSTEIN, S. Possible mechanism for cerebral oedema in diabetic ketoacidosis. *Lancet* 2: 306–308, 1987.
242. VAN HOUTEN, M., and POSNER, B. I. Insulin binds to brain blood vessels in vivo. *Nature* 282: 623–625, 1979.
243. VILARO, S., PALACIN, M., PILCH, P. F., TESTAR, X., and ZORZANO, A. Expression of an insulin-regulatable glucose carrier in muscle and fat endothelial cells. *Nature* 342: 798–800, 1989.
244. WARNER, D. S., SMITH, M. L., and SIESJO, B. K. Ischemia in normo- and hyperglycemic rats: effects on brain water and electrolytes. *Stroke* 18: 464–471, 1987.
245. WILLETTE, R. N., SAUERMELCH, C., EZEKIEL, M., FEUERSTEIN, G., and OHLSTEIN, E. H. Effect of endothelin on cortical microvascular perfusion in rats. *Stroke* 21: 451–458, 1990.
246. WILLIAMS, S. K., DEVENNY, J. J., and BITENSKY, M. W. Micropinocytic ingestion of glyco-sylated albumin by isolated microvessels: possible role in pathogenesis of diabetic microangiopathy. *Proc. Natl. Acad. Sci. USA* 78: 2393–2397, 1981.
247. WILLIAMS, S. K., GILLIS, J. F., MATTHEWS, M. A., WAGNER, R. C., and BITENSKY, M. W. Isolation and characterization of brain endothelial cells: morphology and enzyme activity. *J. Neurochem.* 35: 374–381, 1980.
248. WILLIAMSON, J. R., CHANG, K., TILTON, R. G., PRATER, C., JEFFREY, J. R., WEIGEL, C., SHERMAN, W. R., EADES, D. M., and KILO, C. Increased vascular permeability in spontaneously diabetic BB/W rats and in rats with mild versus severe streptozotocin-induced diabetes. Prevention by aldose reductase inhibitors and castration. *Diabetes* 36: 813–821, 1987.
249. WOODS, S. C., and PORTE, D., JR. The role of insulin as a satiety factor in the central nervous system. *Adv. Metab. Disorders* 10: 457–468, 1983.
250. WOODS, S. C., PORTE, D., JR., BOBBIONI, E., IONESCU, E., SAUTER, J. F., ROHNER JEANRE-NAUD, I., and JEANRENAUD, B. Insulin: its relationship to the central nervous system and to the control of food intake and body weight. *Am. J. Clin Nutr.* 42: 1063–1071, 1985.
251. WURTMAN, R. J., BLUSZTAJN, J. K., ULUS, I. H., COVIELLA, I. L., BUYUKUYSAL, R. L., GROWDON, J. H., and SLACK, B. E. Choline metabolism in cholinergic neurons: implications for the pathogenesis of neurodegenerative diseases. *Adv. Neurol.* 51: 117–125, 1990.
252. YAMAUCHI, T., OHNAKA, K., TAKAYANAGI, R., UMEDA, F., and NAWATA, H. Enhanced secretion of endothelin-1 by elevated glucose levels from cultured bovine aortic endothelial cells. *FEBS Lett.* 267: 16–18, 1990.
253. ZASSLOW, M. A., PEARL, R. G., SHUER, L. M., STEINBERG, G. K., LIEBERSON, R. E., and LARSON, C. P. Hyperglycemia decreases acute neuronal ischemic changes after middle cerebral artery occlusion in cats. *Stroke* 20: 519–523, 1989.

II

POLYOLS, *myo*-INOSITOL, AND SIGNAL TRANSDUCTION

6

Mechanisms of Glucose- and Diabetes-Induced Vascular Dysfunction

JOSEPH R. WILLIAMSON, CHARLES KILO, AND RONALD G. TILTON

Vascular dysfunction manifested by increased vascular permeability, impaired autoregulation of blood flow, and increased glomerular filtration rate develops early after the onset of poorly controlled diabetes in humans and animals. Several lines of evidence are consistent with the hypothesis that these functional changes predispose the vasculature to injury by risk factors independent of diabetes (such as hypertension and hyperlipemia), and it is the interaction between vascular injury by these risk factors and diabetes-induced vascular dysfunction that culminates in the vascular complications of diabetes. A corrolary of this hypothesis is that elucidation of the metabolic imbalances that mediate glucose/diabetes–induced vascular dysfunction is pivotal to understanding the pathogenesis of diabetic vascular disease. Recent observations in animal models (which will be discussed in this chapter) suggest the following sequence of events (Fig. 6.1). Elevated glucose levels increase flux of glucose via the sorbitol pathway, which increases the ratio of $NADH/NAD^+$ (as a consequence of increased oxidation of sorbitol to fructose). This change in cytoplasmic redox state causes an elevation of triose phosphates (which are among the most reactive naturally occurring nonenzymatic glycation agents) and has an impact on two pathways of lipid metabolism, resulting in accumulation of amphipathic lipids—i.e. 1,2-diacyl-sn-glycerol (DAG) and long-chain fatty acyl esters, which modulate the activity of several important enzymes (i.e. Na^+K^+-ATPase, Ca^{2+}-ATPase, and protein kinase C) linked to glucose- and diabetes-induced vascular dysfunction.

In the first part of this chapter we will briefly review manifestations of vascular dysfunction in diabetic humans and animals. We will then consider several hypotheses that have been proposed to explain the pathogenesis of these vascular functional abnormalities. Lastly, we will examine evidence from a variety of in vivo and in vitro studies that address each of these hypotheses.

VASCULAR DYSFUNCTION IN DIABETES

Vascular dysfunction in diabetic humans and animals is manifested by both hemodynamic alterations and by increased permeation of the vasculature by plasma constituents. Such functional changes are closely linked to structural

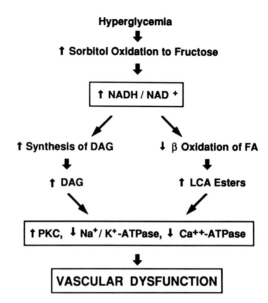

FIGURE 6.1. Pathogenesis of glucose- and diabetes-induced vascular dysfunction.

vascular alterations that culminate in organ failure in some tissues, i.e. renal failure, loss of vision, and cardiovascular complications of atherosclerotic disease of arteries. While the nature of the relationship between these functional and structural changes in the vasculature remains unclear, the fact that they are such closely coupled phenomena suggests that they share some pathogenetic mechanisms in common.

Hemodynamic Changes

Perhaps the best-documented functional vascular change in both diabetic humans and animals is the increase in glomerular filtration rate (GFR), which develops shortly after the onset of poorly controlled diabetes (Fig. 6.2) (3,4,16,17,29,42,50,52,80,91,95,98–100,119,142,143). This increase in GFR has been attributed to an imbalance in the resistance of the afferent and efferent glomerular arterioles, which results in an increase in transcapillary glomerular filtration pressure (95,143). In animal models of diabetes this increase in GFR is accompanied by an increase in renal blood flow (3,4,50,52,80, 98,100,119,142) attributable to a net decrease in overall resistance of afferent and efferent arterioles (95,143). The decreased GFR associated with end-stage human diabetic kidney disease is, in contrast, the consequence of a decrease in filtration surface area due to mesangial expansion (114).

Although there is relatively good agreement among investigators regarding diabetes-induced hemodynamic and filtration changes in the kidney, discordant results have been reported on retinal blood flow changes in diabetic humans and in animal models of diabetes. Increased blood flow, no change in blood flow, decreased blood flow, and increased blood flow in some regions of the retinal vasculature with decreased blood flow in other areas have been reported by various investigators (32,46,47,64,65,110,112,113). These discordant observations may be attributed in part to methodological differences for assessing blood flow and to differences in severity and duration of diabetes and, in humans, to differences in the severity of vascular disease. Despite the discordance in these observations, they are (overall) indicative of diabetes-induced hemodynamic alterations in the retina as well as in the kidney. Much less information is available regarding the relationship of diabetes-induced blood flow changes in the retina to those in the kidney and in other tissues. Acquisition of such information would be facilitated by methodology that provides assessments of blood flow concurrently in multiple tissues. We have recently employed radiolabeled microspheres, injected into the left ventricle, to assess blood flow in multiple tissues of rats with diabetes induced by injection of streptozotocin. As shown in Figure 6.3 in rats with diabetes of 4–8 weeks duration, blood flow (assessed by injection of 15 μm [85]Sc-microspheres) is markedly increased in anterior and posterior uveal vessels as well as in the retina, in peripheral nerve, and kidney (98,100,119). In general, blood flow in diabetic animals is preferentially increased in tissues that correspond to sites of marked vascular structural changes and/or clinically significant complications in diabetic humans.

Increased Vascular Permeation by Plasma Constituents

In diabetic humans and rats the transcapillary escape rate (whole body) for radiolabeled albumin is significantly increased, attesting to an increase in overall vascular albumin permeation (93,94,126). By the use of fluorescein angiography it has been shown that leakage of fluorescein-labeled albumin from retinal vessels is increased in diabetics and is especially pronounced in new vessels arising (most commonly) from the optic disc and the adjoining retina (63,65). Increased albumin permeation in other tissues of human diabetics is

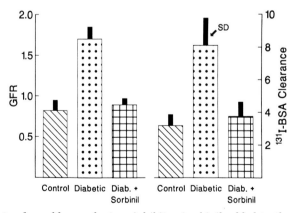

FIGURE 6.2. Effects of an aldose reductase inhibitor (sorbinil added to the diet to provide a daily dose of 0.2 mmol/kg body weight/day) on glomerular filtration rate and on renal clearance of [^{131}I] BSA (mg plasma/kidney/min) in male Sprague-Dawley rats with streptozotocin-induced diabetes of 2 months duration.

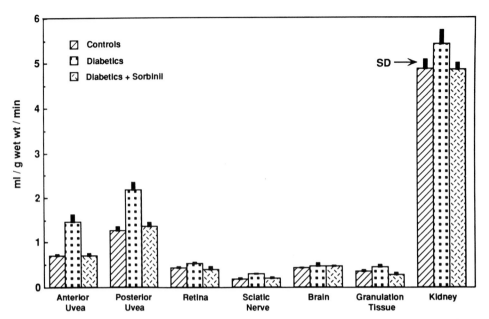

FIGURE 6.3. Effects of an aldose reductase inhibitor (sorbinil added to the diet to provide a daily dose of 0.2 mmol/kg body weight/day) on regional blood flow in male Sprague-Dawley rats with streptozotocin-induced diabetes of 2 months duration.

manifested in the kidney by albuminuria (81,83,95,122), and in peripheral nerve by an increase in albumin concentration in endoneurial fluid (89).

Vascular albumin permeation in rats with spontaneous diabetes, as well as in those with streptozotocin-induced diabetes, is, like blood flow, preferentially increased in tissues that are sites of clinically significant complications in human subjects, i.e. eyes, peripheral nerve, kidney (i.e. albuminuria), and aorta [(99,100,119,130,131); Fig. 6.4].

In view of evidence that new vessels arising from the optic disc and adjoining retina of poorly controlled human diabetics appear to be more susceptible (than vessels present before the onset of diabetes) to the impact of the diabetic milieu on vascular function, we have investigated the effects of diabetes on blood flow and vascular albumin permeation in newly formed subcutaneous granulation tissue vessels in which angiogenesis is induced by: (1) implanting fabric under the skin (57,100,119,131), or (2) removal of a circle of skin followed by insertion of a plastic chamber (135,139) as described in the skin chamber granulation tissue model presented below. In the subcutaneous granulation tissue model, vascular albumin permeation is markedly increased in the newly formed vessels in diabetic rats (57,100,119,131), despite a minimal change, or no change at all, in albumin permeation in neighboring vessels within overlying skin or underlying muscle (Fig. 6.5), which give rise to the new vessels. Blood flow and vascular albumin permeation are markedly increased in granulation tissue in the skin chamber model (in nondiabetic rats) following topical application of glucose to the vessels during angiogenesis (135,139). In this model there is no increase in systemic blood glucose levels.

These observations indicate that newly formed vessels are indeed much more susceptible to injury in the diabetic milieu than older vessels present before the onset of diabetes. They also indicate that elevated tissue glucose levels, in the absence of systemic hormonal and metabolic imbalances associated with the diabetic milieu, are sufficient to induce vascular dysfunction (135).

The greater susceptibility of new granulation tissue vessels to the impact of the diabetic milieu on vascular function, relative to that of vessels present before the onset of diabetes, is consistent with the more pronounced leakage of fluorescein from new vessels arising from the optic disc and retina (vs neighboring retinal and optic disc vessels present before the onset of diabetes) in human diabetics (63,65).

Relevance of Vascular Dysfunction to End-Stage Vascular Disease in Human Diabetics

Since animal models of diabetes have not been observed to develop end-stage vascular complications characteristic of those observed in human diabetics, it is appropriate to question the relevance of structural and functional changes in the animal model to the end-stage vascular complications in human subjects. It is important to note in this regard that many diabetic humans also do not develop end-stage vascular (structural changes) disease affecting the kidney and the eyes (Fig. 6.6), despite evidence that a high percentage of them develop "background" vascular structural changes in the retina (i.e. microaneurysms and capillary basement membrane thickening), kidney (glomerular

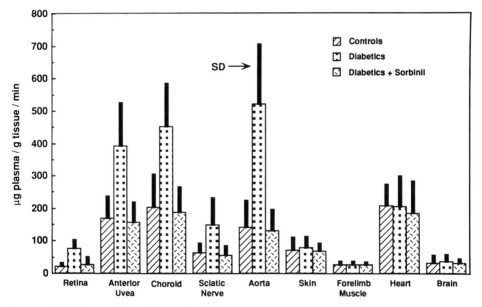

FIGURE 6.4. Effects of an aldose reductase inhibitor (sorbinil added to the diet to provide a daily dose of 0.2 mmol/kg body weight/day) on regional plasma clearance of [131I]BSA in male Sprague-Dawley rats with streptozotocin-induced diabetes of 2 months duration.

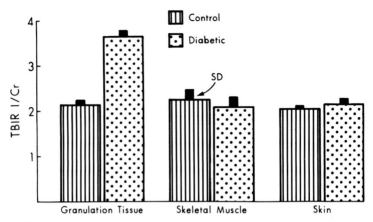

FIGURE 6.5. Effects of diabetes on vascular albumin permeation in vessels of skin, muscle, and (subcutaneous) granulation tissue. Note the absence of any effect of diabetes, under these conditions, on albumin permeation in vessels of skeletal muscle and skin, which give rise to the new granulation tissue vessels. The index of vascular albumin permeation is the tissue-to-blood isotope ratio of ^{51}Cr-labeled red cells to [^{131}I]BSA albumin (131).

capillary basement membrane thickening and mesangial expansion identical to that occurring in animal models of diabetes), and other tissues (i.e. thickening of skeletal muscle capillary basement membranes) (56,96,102,111, 115,117). Such observations suggest that (*1*) risk factors independent of the diabetic milieu play an important role in the development of end-stage (as opposed to background) diabetic vascular disease, and (*2*) the metabolic imbalances and functional derangements (i.e. hemodynamic and vascular permeability changes) induced by diabetes might act by increasing the vulnerability of the vasculature to injury by these risk factors. A list of such risk factors would include hypertension and hyperlipemia, both of which have been linked to acceleration of atherosclerotic vascular disease in nondiabetics as well as diabetics (106,107), and to acceleration of retinopathy (14,34,64) and nephropathy in diabetics (25,35,49,53,55). Dietary protein intake also has been linked to the pathogenesis of diabetic nephropathy (82).

    In view of the importance of hypertension as an independent risk factor in the pathogenesis of end-stage diabetic vascular disease (1,14,26, 27,62,76,78,81), we would emphasize that impaired autoregulation (implied by increases in GFR and in blood flow to the eyes, kidneys, and peripheral nerves, in the absence of any change in arterial blood pressure) may play a permissive, but critical, role in increasing the vulnerability of the microvasculature to the effects of systemic (arterial) hypertension. Thus the evidence of increased blood flow in several tissues of diabetic rats, in the absence of an increase in arterial blood pressure, implies microvascular hypertension in the affected vasculatures. Such tissues may be at especially high risk to injurious effects of arterial hypertension. While the importance of hypertension as a risk factor in the pathogenesis of end-stage diabetic vascular disease is clear, not all investigators are in agreement regarding the role of increased glomerular pressure in *initiating* diabetic nephropathy (3).

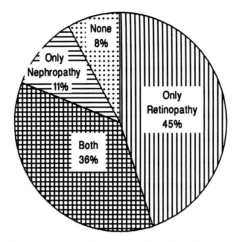

FIGURE 6.6.   Prevalence of retinopathy and nephropathy after 20 years of type I diabetes [From Sterky and Wall (115).]

HYPOTHESES FOR THE PATHOGENESIS OF DIABETIC VASCULAR DISEASE

Numerous hypotheses have been proposed to explain the pathogenesis of diabetic vascular disease. None of these hypotheses is mutually exclusive and, in view of evidence attesting to the multifactorial nature of the pathogenesis of diabetic vascular disease, it is conceivable that many of the mechanisms postulated by these hypotheses may contribute to the onset and progression of early and/or late vascular changes. Leading hypotheses to explain how metabolic imbalances mediate complications of diabetes currently favor (*1*) increased metabolism of glucose via the sorbitol pathway (36,44,45,59,138), (*2*) glucose-induced increased de novo synthesis of diacylglycerol and associated activation of protein kinase C (30,31,67,68,139), and (*3*) increased nonenzymatic glycation of cellular and extracellular constituents, which is caused by elevated glucose levels and/or increased levels of glucose-derived metabolites (10,11). Evidence that the metabolic imbalances postulated by each of these hypotheses contribute to, or may be the consequence of, an increase in the ratio of NADH/NAD$^+$ suggests a (unifying) fourth hypothesis that an increase in the ratio of NADH/NAD$^+$ may play a key role in the pathogenesis of vascular complications of diabetes (135,136,139).

Increased Metabolism of Glucose by the Sorbitol Pathway

Metabolism of glucose via the sorbitol pathway is considered to consist of two reactions, although products of the pathway (i.e. fructose) can be further metabolized by various pathways. In the first reaction (Fig. 6.7) glucose is reduced to sorbitol by the enzyme aldose reductase, with the cofactor NADPH serving as the hydrogen donor. This reaction is, for practical purposes, irreversible. In the second reaction sorbitol is oxidized to fructose by the enzyme sorbitol (polyol) dehydrogenase, with the cofactor NAD$^+$ serving as the hydrogen acceptor.

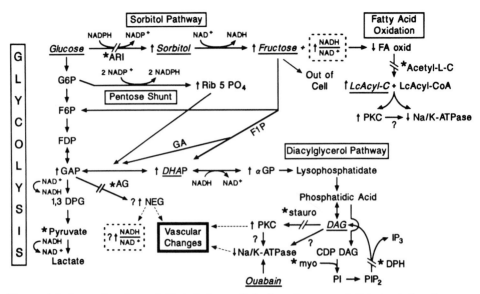

FIGURE 6.7. Interrelated metabolic imbalances linked to glucose- and diabetes-induced vascular dysfunction. Pharmacologic interventions that prevent glucose-induced vascular dysfunction are indicated by an asterisk and include aldose reductase inhibitors (ARI), aminoguanidine (AG), staurosporine (stauro), pyruvate, *myo*-inositol (myo), diphenhydramine (DPH), and acetyl-L-carnitine (Acetyl-L-C). FA, free fatty acid; LcAcyl-C, long-chain acylcarnitine; LcAcyl-CoA, long-chain acyl coenzyme A; NEG, nonenzymatic glycation. *Substances that mimic glucose effects on vascular function are italicized and underlined.*

A variety of sugars can be metabolized by this pathway. Galactose is of particular interest since several diabetes-like complications (neuropathy, capillary basement membrane thickening, retinal microaneurysms, increased regional blood flow, and increased GFR) are observed in animals fed galactose-supplemented diets (5,21,36,39,41,45,99,103,104,118). It is noteworthy, however, that galactitol, the reduction product of galactose, is a poor substrate for polyol dehydrogenase. Therefore tissue levels of galactitol are much higher in galactose-fed rats than sorbitol levels in corresponding tissues of diabetic rats, and vascular dysfunction induced by galactose would appear to be mediated by metabolic imbalances resulting from reduction of galactose to galactitol (dulcitol).

At normal plasma glucose levels intracellular concentrations of free glucose are relatively low in most tissues (since the K_m of hexokinase for glucose is quite low relative to the rate of glucose uptake), and little glucose is metabolized by the sorbitol pathway. However, in (non-insulin-requiring) tissues freely permeable to glucose, intracellular free glucose concentrations may approach those in the extracellular space, and substantial amounts of glucose may be metabolized by the sorbitol pathway, e.g. up to 33% of total glucose utilization in the lens (43) and 11% in human red cells (86).

Several metabolic consequences of increased polyol pathway metabolism have been implicated in the pathogenesis of functional and structural changes associated with diabetic cataracts and neuropathy, the two complications in which the role of polyol pathway–linked metabolic imbalances have been investigated most extensively.

Osmotic Stress Linked to Accumulation of Intracellular Sorbitol
According to the "osmotic stress" hypothesis, diabetic cataracts are the consequence of swelling of lens epithelial cells caused by accumulation of osmotically significant amounts of polyol. Swelling of the epithelial cells then initiates a cascade of metabolic imbalances culminating in rupture of epithelial cells and formation of cataracts. The osmotic hypothesis is based primarily on two lines of evidence: (*1*) the accumulation of millimolar concentrations of sorbitol in the lens of diabetic animals (and of galactitol in galactose-fed animals) and in lenses incubated in the presence of "diabetic" glucose levels in vitro, and (*2*) observations that elevation of the osmolarity of incubation media prevents a variety of metabolic abnormalities in lenses incubated at elevated glucose levels in vitro (59–61). While the osmotic hypothesis is consistent with a considerable body of experimental data on the lens, its role in the pathogenesis of diabetic cataracts is questioned (74), and it is generally considered to be untenable as an explanation for the pathogenesis of diabetic complications in most other tissues in which sorbitol concentrations never exceed the micromolar range and in which no evidence of cellular swelling is evident by electron microscopy.

Redox Imbalances Associated with Reduction of Glucose to Sorbitol and/or Oxidation of Sorbitol to Fructose
Increased Ratio of $NADP^+/NADPH$. Several investigators have reported evidence of an increase in ratio of $NADP^+$ to NADPH in lenses of diabetic rats and rats fed galactose-enriched diets. Since levels of reduced glutathione, which are dependent on the ratio of $NADP^+/NADPH$, are of critical importance in protecting the lens from oxidative damage, it is postulated that increased oxidation of NADPH to $NADP^+$ associated with an increase in the rate of reduction of glucose to sorbitol (Fig. 6.7) may increase the susceptibility of the lens to injury by oxidative mechanisms (74). It is of interest in this regard that diabetes does appear to increase the susceptibility of the lens to oxidative injury (74) and that various antioxidants have been reported to prevent the development of diabetes-induced cataracts.

There is little evidence regarding changes in reduced glutathione levels in the vasculature of tissues subject to late complications. It is of interest, however, that Carroll et al. have reported that reduced glutathione levels are not decreased in peripheral nerve of diabetic rats (18).

Increased $NADH/NAD^+$. An increase in the ratio of $NADH/NAD^+$ resulting from increased oxidation of sorbitol to fructose may cause a variety of metabolic imbalances that lead to vascular dysfunction. It is noteworthy that evidence of marked glucose- and diabetes-induced increases in cytosolic $NADH/NAD^+$ (manifested by an increase in lactate/pyruvate and/or in $NADH/NAD^+$) has been observed in a variety of tissues of diabetic animals, as well as in tissues from normal animals incubated with elevated glucose levels in vitro [(13,22,54,58,70,73,105,123–125,129); Table 6.1]. Although the increased ratio of $NADH/NAD^+$ in the lens (22,58,70,125) is linked to increased polyol

TABLE 6.1. Tissues manifesting glucose- and diabetes-induced increased NADH/NAD$^+$ and/or increased lactate/pyruvate

1. Liver	5. Red blood cells
2. Skeletal muscle	6. Lens
3. Diaphragm	7. Retina
4. Islets of Langerhans	8. Granulation tissue
	9. Glomeruli
	10. Endoneurium

For tissues in the right-hand column the changes in NADH/NAD$^+$ and lactate/pyruvate are all linked to increased flux of glucose via the sorbitol pathway (see text).

pathway activity, the relationship of these redox changes to the pathogenesis of diabetic cataracts remains unclear. Nevertheless, several lines of evidence (discussed below) in animal models of diabetes are consistent with an important role for an increase in the ratio of NADH/NAD$^+$ in mediating diabetes-induced vascular dysfunction.

Metabolic imbalances that could result from an increase in the ratio of NADH/NAD$^+$ include the following: (*1*) an increase in levels of tissue triose phosphate (highly reactive nonenzymatic glycating agents); (*2*) increased reduction of dihydroxyacetone phosphate to α-glycerophosphate, the first step in one pathway for de novo synthesis of diacylglycerol (Fig. 6.7); (*3*) impaired synthesis of *myo*-inositol (cyclization of D-glucose-6-phosphate to L-*myo*-inositol-1-phosphate requires NAD$^+$ as a cofactor) (72,77); and (*4*) impaired beta oxidation of fatty acids [(28,84); the second step of beta oxidation of fatty acids is inhibited by an increase in the intramitochondrial ratio of NADH/NAD$^+$]. The mechanisms by which these metabolic imbalances may mediate glucose-induced vascular injury is discussed below.

Increased Fructose Levels
Increased tissue fructose levels associated with increased oxidation of sorbitol to fructose in the second step of the polyol pathway have been reported in the lens, retina, and peripheral nerve of diabetic rats (9,45,48,58,97,128). Since fructose and its phosphorylated derivatives are much more reactive glycating agents than glucose (116), it has been suggested that increased tissue levels of fructose associated with increased sorbitol pathway metabolism may contribute to tissue damage by nonenzymatic fructosylation of tissue constituents. The potential importance of this mechanism remains unclear.

Decreased Tissue myo-*Inositol Levels, Altered Phosphatidyl Inositol Metabolism, and Decreased Na$^+$K$^+$-ATPase Activity Associated with Increased Polyol Pathway Metabolism of Glucose*
Numerous investigators have reported evidence that *myo*-inositol levels and Na$^+$K$^+$-ATPase activity are decreased and electrophysiological activity is impaired in peripheral nerve of diabetic animals (44,45,138). All of these alterations are prevented in diabetic rats that were (*1*) fed *myo*-inositol-supplemented diets which, however, have no effect on nerve sorbitol levels (44, 45,138) or (*2*) given aldose reductase inhibitors, which normalize endoneurial

myo-inositol as well as sorbitol levels (44,45,138). In view of discordant obser-vations regarding changes in *myo*-inositol levels in peripheral nerve and other tissues of diabetic humans and animals (37,38,44,45,71,75), it may be that although absolute *myo*-inositol levels are not decreased, they may be decreased (1) relative to plasma glucose levels and/or other metabolic imbalances asso-ciated with the diabetic milieu, or (2) in small discrete pools critical for main-tenance of normal phosphatidyl inositol metabolism and turnover and for maintenance of Na^+K^+-ATPase activity (109,138). It is noteworthy that im-paired glucose- and diabetes-induced Na^+K^+-ATPase activity has been re-ported in virtually all tissues affected by diabetic complications, including lens, peripheral nerve, cultured retinal capillary endothelial cells, and isolated glo-meruli (23,24,68,109,138,140), as well as in the aorta (obtained from normal rabbits) exposed to elevated glucose levels in vitro (109,138).

Increased De Novo Synthesis of Diacylglycerol and Associated Activation of Protein Kinase C

Evidence of glucose-induced increased de novo synthesis and/or levels of dia-cylglycerol and associated activation of protein kinase C have recently been reported in retinal vascular endothelial cells and aortic endothelial and smooth muscle cells cultured in vitro (67,68), in the heart (90), in glomeruli isolated from diabetic rats (30,31), and in granulation tissue exposed to elevated glu-cose levels (139). Since many cellular functions are mediated by activation of protein kinase C, and since several of these functions in vascular cells appear to be deranged in diabetes, these observations suggest that vascular compli-cations of diabetes may be initiated-mediated by activation of protein kinase C as a consequence of hyperglycemia-induced increases in de novo synthesis of diacylglycerol. Note that this hypothesis postulates activation of protein ki-nase C, whereas the hypothesis of Greene et al. (Chapter 7) postulates that protein kinase C activity is diminished by diabetes (44,45).

Increased Nonenzymatic Glycation

The demonstration of increased amounts of early and late products of nonen-zymatic glycation (Chapters 11–14) in virtually all tissues of diabetic humans and animals, together with evidence of alterations in functional properties of these glycation products, has generated a great deal of interest in the possi-bility that nonenzymatic glycation of vascular constituents may play an im-portant role in the pathogenesis of vascular complications of diabetes. Evi-dence for a role of nonenzymatic glycation in the pathogenesis of vascular dysfunction will be discussed below.

ANIMAL MODELS FOR ASSESSING DIABETES-INDUCED VASCULAR DYSFUNCTION

One of the major obstacles to elucidating the nature of the metabolic imbal-ances that mediate vascular dysfunction associated with diabetes has been the lack of suitable animal models in which to investigate putative metabolic changes and vascular dysfunction. Although the effects of a variety of pharmacologic interventions can be examined on vascular function in tissues (in animals) that are sites of complications in humans, pharmacologic agents often have multiple effects, and it is difficult to determine which of the multiple systemic metabolic and hormonal imbalances associated with the diabetic milieu is of importance in the pathogenesis of vascular dysfunction. While many of these problems can be circumvented by studies of vascular cells cultured in vitro, such studies cannot resolve the role of specific metabolic imbalances observed in cultured cells in mediating vascular dysfunction in vivo.

We have recently made use of a skin chamber granulation tissue model (which can be employed in both nondiabetic and diabetic rats) to circumvent some of the limitations inherent in conventional in vivo and in vitro studies of vascular metabolism and function (54,135,139). After a 2 cm circle of skin is removed from either side of the back of an anesthetized rat, plastic chambers are sewn in place, with the skin overlapping the flanged base (to prevent re-epithelialization of the granulation tissue forming inside the chamber) (Fig. 6.8). Granulation tissue forms spontaneously in the chamber from fibroblasts and vessels at the surface of the exposed fascia. The plastic chambers are equipped with stainless-steel caps that can be readily removed for repeated applications of test substances—i.e. substrates, hormones, pharmacologic agents, etc.—to the new granulation tissue vessels as they form in the chamber. Thus, it is possible to add "tissue culture media" that differ in their content

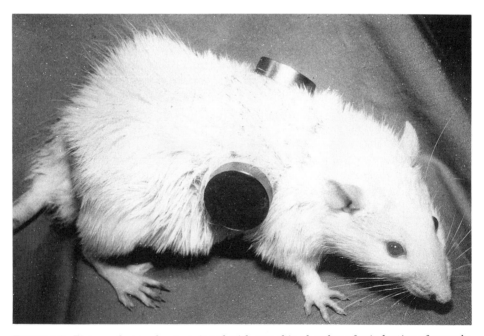

FIGURE 6.8. Picture of normal rat equipped with two skin chambers for induction of granulation tissue. The stainless-steel caps are readily removable for topical application of metabolites, hormones, and/or pharmacologic agents.

of a single component (test substance) to the control and test chambers and assess the impact of the test substance on vascular function in vivo. Vascular permeation by macromolecules and blood flow are assessed by injection of radiolabeled albumin and radiolabeled microspheres, respectively. The granulation tissue can then be removed for metabolic studies and/or chemical analyses. Correlative studies of vascular function and metabolism in these tissue chamber vessels, together with corresponding studies of vascular function and metabolism in tissues (of the same animal) that are sites of vascular complications in human diabetics, have yielded several new insights into the nature of the metabolic imbalances that mediate vascular dysfunction in diabetes. These observations form the basis for much of the remaining discussion.

EVIDENCE LINKING INCREASED SORBITOL PATHWAY METABOLISM TO GLUCOSE-INDUCED VASCULAR DYSFUNCTION

Among the criteria for implicating increased polyol pathway metabolism in the pathogenesis of any complication of diabetes, Kinoshita (60) has suggested that the complication should be (1) prevented by two or more structurally different inhibitors of aldose reductase, (2) manifested in animals fed a galactose-enriched diet, and (3) prevented in galactose-fed animals by aldose reductase inhibitors.

Several lines of evidence from a variety of experimental animal models fulfill these criteria, attesting to an important role (in animal models) for increased polyol pathway metabolism in the pathogenesis of vascular dysfunction associated with diabetes.

Effects of Aldose Reductase Inhibitors

Inhibition of diabetes-induced vascular dysfunction by several structurally different inhibitors of aldose reductase has been observed by most, but not all, investigators. Among the indices of diabetes-induced vascular dysfunction that are improved by aldose reductase inhibitors are increased GFR, albuminuria, and proteinuria [(4,7,8,42,79,99,119); Fig. 6.9]; increased blood flow in the kidney, ocular tissues, and peripheral nerve (4,119); and increased vascular permeability in ocular tissues, peripheral nerve, aorta, and granulation tissue (99,119,131,135). The apparent lack of efficacy of aldose reductase inhibitors in preventing diabetes-induced increases in GFR and albuminuria (33,114) reported by some investigators may be explained by differences in the amount and/or intrinsic efficacy of aldose reductase inhibitors administered, the frequency and method of administration of the inhibitors, the duration and severity of diabetes, and the methodological differences in assessment of vascular function.

Inhibition by aldose reductase inhibitors of vascular dysfunction in the retina of diabetic rats is of particular interest in view of evidence that these agents also prevent structural changes in retinal vessels of diabetic rats (19,20), as well as galactose-fed rats (41,103,104). In contrast, two recent reports indicate that these compounds fail to prevent glomerular capillary base-

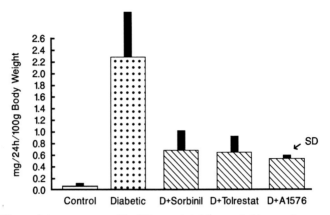

FIGURE 6.9. Effects of three structurally different inhibitors of aldose reductase (added to the diet to provide a daily dose of 0.2 mmol of sorbinil and tolrestat and 0.02 mmol of AL-1576/kg body weight/day) on 24 h urinary ablumin excretion in male Sprague-Dawley rats with strep-tozotocin diabetes of 2 months duration.

ment membrane thickening in diabetic rats (93,121). The apparently discordant effects of aldose reductase inhibitors on early vascular functional and structural changes in the eyes versus the kidneys raise important questions regarding the nature of the relationship(s) (*1*) between early functional and early structural vascular changes associated with diabetes, and (*2*) of early (functional and structural) vascular changes to late (end-stage) vascular disease (responsible for loss of vision or renal function, and for atherosclerotic vascular disease).

Galactose Models

Although several investigators have described early vascular structural changes, i.e. retinal capillary basement membrane thickening, in rats and dogs fed galactose-enriched diets (39,41,103,104,132), there are relatively few reports addressing vascular functional changes in galactose-fed animals. We have observed vascular functional changes in rats fed galactose-enriched diets identical to those in tissues of diabetic rats (21,99,118). These vascular changes include increased blood flow and/or increased albumin permeation in ocular tissues, peripheral nerve, aorta, granulation tissue, and kidney. Increases in GFR and in urinary albumin and IgG excretion are comparable to those in diabetic rats. Increases in GFR and in renal plasma/blood flow in galactose-fed rats have also been observed by other investigators (5,88). The demonstration of these vascular functional changes in galactose-fed rats, together with the finding that all of them are prevented by aldose reductase inhibitors (5,21,88,99,118), provides strong support for the conclusion that corresponding vascular changes in diabetic rats are the consequence of increased flux of glucose via the sorbitol pathway.

Sorbitol Loading Experiments

Although sorbitol penetrates cell membranes rather slowly, exposure of cells and tissues to millimolar extracellular concentrations of sorbitol for several hours to several days has been shown to mimic polyol pathway–linked alterations in cell metabolism (2,40,66,141). In addition, exposure of skin chamber granulation tissue to sorbitol induces vascular dysfunction identical to that in granulation tissue exposed to high levels of glucose and galactose (133). These observations are consistent with the hypothesis that polyol pathway–linked vascular dysfunction results from oxidation of sorbitol to fructose rather than from reduction of glucose to sorbitol, as discussed below.

Sorbitol Pathway–Associated Metabolic Imbalances Linked to Glucose-Induced Vascular Dysfunction

Imbalances in myo-Inositol/phosphatidylinositol Metabolism and Impaired Na^+K^+-ATPase Activity

Levels of myo-inositol have been reported to be decreased in peripheral nerve, lens, retina, retinal pigment epithelium, and glomeruli from rats shortly after the onset of poorly controlled diabetes (44,45,71,100). Not all investigators have observed a decrease in tissue myo-inositol levels in diabetic humans or animals (37,38,48,71,100,128,131). It is of interest that although myo-inositol levels are not decreased in the aorta of diabetic animals (71,100), Simmons and Winegrad (109) have reported that decreased Na^+K^+-ATPase activity induced by elevated glucose levels during incubation of rabbit aorta in vitro is prevented by addition of an aldose reductase inhibitor or by raising myo-inositol levels in the incubation medium. Similarly, treatment with aldose reductase inhibitors prevents the decrease in myo-inositol levels in glomeruli isolated from diabetic rats. Aldose reductase inhibitors completely prevent, and diets supplemented with 0.5%, 1%, and 2% myo-inositol decrease (in a dose-dependent manner), but do not completely normalize, diabetes-induced increases in GFR and urinary albumin excretion, as well as increased blood flow and vascular albumin permeation in ocular tissues, peripheral nerve, granulation tissue, and aorta (100). Both aldose reductase inhibitors and myo-inositol–supplemented diets normalize myo-inositol levels in endoneurium of sciatic nerve (100,119). These observations raise the possibility that hemodynamic and vascular filtration changes associated with diabetes are linked to relative or absolute decreases in tissue levels of myo-inositol and an associated decrease in Na^+K^+-ATPase activity. This interpretation is supported by evidence that glucose-induced increases in blood flow and vascular albumin permeation in skin chamber granulation tissue are prevented both by aldose reductase inhibitors and by myo-inositol (even though tissue myo-inositol levels are not decreased), and by evidence that exposure of skin chamber granulation tissue to ouabain in the presence of 5 mM glucose causes vascular dysfunction like that induced by glucose and by diabetes (unpublished observations).

Increased Ratio of NADH/NAD+

Several lines of evidence are consistent with the likelihood that metabolic imbalances associated with an increase in the ratio of NADH/NAD+ (resulting from increased oxidation of sorbitol to fructose) play an important role in mediating glucose/diabetes–induced vascular dysfunction. As noted earlier in this section, an increase in this ratio has been demonstrated in the lens of diabetic rats and in lenses of normal rats incubated in vitro in the presence of elevated glucose levels. An increase in the lactate/pyruvate ratio of human red cells incubated in the presence of elevated glucose levels, sorbitol, or xylitol attests to a corresponding change in redox state (2,40,123). The prevention of these changes in red cells by an aldose reductase inhibitor (40,123) indicates that they are linked to increased metabolism of glucose by the polyol pathway. Similarly, Kawamura et al. (54) have found that incubation of skin chamber granulation tissue (removed from chambers in normal rats) in 50 vs 5 mM glucose in vitro also is associated with an increase in the lactate/pyruvate ratio, which is attenuated by an inhibitor of aldose reductase.

If glucose-induced vascular dysfunction in granulation tissue is indeed linked to an increase in NADH/NAD$^+$ resulting from increased oxidation of sorbitol to fructose (rather than to an increase in NADP$^+$/NADPH associated with reduction of glucose to sorbitol), then exposure of skin chamber granulation tissue to increased sorbitol levels (in the absence of elevated tissue glucose levels) should induce vascular dysfunction comparable to that induced by increased tissue glucose levels. This is indeed the case, as noted earlier (133). If these sorbitol-induced increases in blood flow and vascular albumin permeation are in some way the consequence of an increase in NADH/NAD$^+$ linked to increased oxidation of sorbitol to fructose, then they should not be prevented by co-administration of an aldose reductase inhibitor with the sorbitol, but they should be prevented by an intervention that would normalize the ratio NADH/NAD$^+$. Normalization of this ratio should be favored by co-administration of pyruvate (with sorbitol), which will reoxidize NADH to NAD$^+$ via the lactate dehydrogenase reaction. Indeed, vascular dysfunction is induced in skin chamber granulation tissue vessels by topical sorbitol application and is prevented by co-administration of pyruvate, but it is unaffected by aldose reductase inhibitors [(133); unpublished observations].

The interpretation that these effects of pyruvate on sorbitol-induced vascular dysfunction are linked to normalization of the ratio NADH/NAD$^+$ is con-

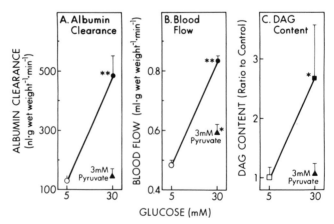

FIGURE 6.10. Effects of glucose and of pyruvate on albumin clearance, blood flow, and diacylglycerol levels in granulation tissue after 10 days of twice daily instillation of glucose and/or pyruvate in normal rats. [From Wolf et al. (139).]

sistent with observations that pyruvate (but not inhibitors of aldose reductase) also prevents sorbitol-induced changes in red cell glycolytic metabolites whose levels are related to the NADH/NAD$^+$ ratio. Thus exposure of human red cells to sorbitol or xylitol in vitro causes marked elevations in the ratio of lactate/pyruvate, triose phosphates, and α-glycerophosphate levels (2,40,123). These changes are prevented in cells incubated with sorbitol + pyruvate (2).

EVIDENCE LINKING INCREASED DE NOVO SYNTHESIS OF DIACYLGLYCEROL AND ACTIVATION OF PROTEIN KINASE C TO GLUCOSE-INDUCED VASCULAR DYSFUNCTION

Several observations in the skin chamber granulation tissue model attest to a role for increased diacylglycerol levels and associated activation of protein kinase C in mediating glucose-induced vascular dysfunction, especially increased vascular albumin permeation. First, increased vascular albumin permeation in skin chamber granulation tissue exposed to 30 mM glucose is accompanied by a ~2.7× increase in granulation tissue levels of 1,2-diacyl-sn-glycerol (139). This increase in diacylglycerol levels is prevented by coadministration of 3 mM pyruvate with glucose, which also prevents the vascular dysfunction induced by glucose (Fig. 6.10). The increased vascular albumin permeation, but not the increased blood flow, induced by 30 mM glucose also is prevented by co-administration of staurosporine (Fig. 6.11), an inhibitor of protein kinase C. In addition, exposure of skin chamber granulation tissue to a phorbol ester (i.e. exogenous diacylglycerol) induces increased vascular albumin permeation in the absence of elevated tissue glucose levels. Likewise, exposure of skin chamber granulation tissue to 1-monoolein (which inhibits catabolism of endogenous diacylglycerol, and presumably increases tissue levels of endogenous diacylglycerol) in buffer containing 5 mM glucose also in-

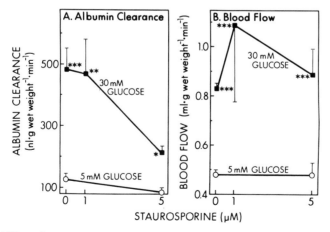

FIGURE 6.11. Effect of staurosporine, a protein kinase C inhibitor, on albumin clearance and blood flow in granulation tissue from skin chambers exposed to 5 or 30 mM D-glucose (twice daily) for 10 days [From Wolf et al. (139).]

duces increased vascular albumin permeation and blood flow comparable to corresponding changes induced by 30 mM glucose. The increased vascular albumin permeation (but not increased blood flow) induced by 1-monoolein is attenuated by co-administration of staurosporine. The apparent failure of staurosporine to prevent glucose-induced increases in blood flow may be accounted for by a variety of factors related to the experimental conditions in the skin chamber model, rather than constituting evidence that glucose-induced increases in blood flow are not linked to activation of protein kinase C. In any case, these observations support a role for increased diacylglycerol levels and activation of protein kinase C in mediating glucose- and diabetes-induced vascular permeability changes. Further studies are required to determine what role, if any, changes in diacylglycerol levels and protein kinase C activity may play in glucose- and diabetes-induced hemodynamic changes.

EVIDENCE LINKING GLUCOSE-INDUCED VASCULAR DYSFUNCTION TO
INCREASED NONENZYMATIC GLYCATION

Evidence linking glucose- and diabetes-induced vascular dysfunction to nonenzymatic glycation is limited to observations that increased vascular albumin permeation in animal models of diabetes is markedly attenuated by treatment with aminoguanidine, a nucleophilic hydrazine compound. This compound has been postulated to prevent the formation of end products of nonenzymatic glycation by combining with intermediate glycation products (10). If this is indeed the sole mechanism by which aminoguanidine prevents vascular dysfunction (induced by glucose), then the prevention of diabetes-induced increased vascular albumin permeation in ocular tissues, peripheral nerve, and aorta by aminoguanidine (51,120) constitutes strong evidence for a role of nonenzymatic glycation in mediating these vascular function changes. On the other hand, in view of evidence that aminoguanidine also inhibits diamine oxidase activity (6), there is concern that aminoguanidine may have other, as yet unrecognized, effects (independent of interaction with glycation products) which might mediate its effects in vivo, including those on glucose- and diabetes-induced vascular dysfunction.

In this regard, prevention of glucose- and sorbitol-induced vascular dysfunction in skin chamber granulation tissue vessels by aminoguanidine (unpublished observations) is somewhat surprising since in the sorbitol-treated granulation tissue, there is no elevation of tissue glucose levels, and in the case of the glucose-treated tissues, the total duration of elevated glucose levels (maximum of 30 mM glucose) was only ~40 h. Thus these observations raise questions regarding the nature of the glycation agents and products, particularly in tissues exposed to sorbitol in the absence of any elevation of glucose.

Since triose phosphate levels are increased in granulation tissue exposed to 50 mM glucose in vitro (54), and since triose phosphates are highly reactive glycating agents (116), it is conceivable that glycation of intracellular constituents by triose phosphates may play a role in the pathogenesis of vascular functional changes induced by hyperglycemia. Two other highly reactive glycating agents, fructose-3-phosphate and 3-deoxyglucosone, are polyol pathway–linked metabolites (117). The accumulation of these metabolites in the lenses of diabetic rats is prevented by sorbinil.

INTERACTIONS BETWEEN INCREASED SORBITOL PATHWAY METABOLISM,
INCREASED GLYCOLYSIS, INCREASED TISSUE DIACYLGLYCEROL LEVELS,
AND INCREASED NONENZYMATIC GLYCATION IN THE PATHOGENESIS OF
GLUCOSE/DIABETES-INDUCED VASCULAR DYSFUNCTION

Evidence reviewed in this chapter indicates that virtually all manifestations of vascular dysfunction in ocular tissues, peripheral nerve, aorta, kidney, and granulation tissue can be prevented or markedly attenuated in rats with diabetes of 6–8 weeks duration by treatment with aminoguanidine or *myo*-inositol–supplemented diets as well as by aldose reductase inhibitors. Likewise, glucose-induced vascular dysfunction (identical to that in all of the above tissues in diabetic rats) in skin chamber granulation tissue can be prevented by such diverse pharmacologic agents as aldose reductase inhibitors, *myo*-inositol, pyruvate, aminoguanidine, staurosporine, a histamine receptor antagonist (diphenhydramine), and acetyl-L-carnitine (134,135,137,139; unpublished observations). These findings clearly have important implications regarding both the pathogenesis and the treatment of diabetic vascular complications.

One implication of these observations is that the pathogenesis of diabetic complications may not be the consequence of a single metabolic imbalance, but rather of one or more cascades of metabolic imbalances, correction of any one of which can enable the affected vasculature to maintain normal function as manifested by blood flow and vascular albumin permeation. Obviously, elucidation of the nature of the relationship(s) of the individual metabolic imbalances [comprising the cascade(s)] to each other is critical to understanding the pathogenesis of diabetic complications as well as to development of rational therapeutic interventions to prevent their onset and progression. One feature that most of these metabolic imbalances appear to share in common is that they either contribute to or are the consequence of an increase in the ratio $NADH/NAD^+$, as depicted in Figures 6.2 and 6.7. According to the sequence of events depicted in these figures, two cascades of metabolic imbalances resulting from an increase in $NADH/NAD^+$ (resulting from increased oxidation of sorbitol to fructose) would lead to increased de novo synthesis of diacylglycerol on the one hand and to impaired beta oxidation of fatty acids on the other. Partially oxidized fatty acids then accumulate as long-chain acyl esters of carnitine and CoA (28,84). These long-chain acyl esters and diacylglycerol are potent modulators of protein kinase C, Na^+K^+-ATPase, and Ca^+-ATPase, among other enzymes (28). Changes in the activity of these enzymes have been linked to a variety of physiological and pathophysiological vascular changes.

At present it is unclear how/whether the prevention of glucose-induced vascular dysfunction by aminoguanidine and the glucomimetic effects of galactose on vascular dysfunction can be reconciled with the cascade of metabolic imbalances depicted in Figure 6.7. One possible explanation for the effects of aminoguanidine is that it might prevent nonenzymatic glycation of nucleoproteins (12,69), which has been reported to result in single strand breaks in DNA. Single strand DNA breaks are known to activate the repair enzyme poly(ADP ribose) synthase, which degrades NAD^+ to nicotinamide, thereby decreasing total NAD^+ and, presumably, the ratio of $NAD^+/NADH$. This is thought to be the mechanism of injury causing necrosis of beta cells by streptozotocin (which induces single strand DNA breaks by a different mechanism) (108,127). This latter explanation would be consistent with the importance of an imbalance in the redox state in the mediation of glucose-induced vascular dysfunction. By preventing damage to nucleoproteins, aminoguanidine would prevent activation of poly(ADP ribose) synthetase and degradation of NAD^+.

The difficulty in reconciling the effects of galactose with the cascade of metabolic imbalances depicted in Figure 6.7 is that galactitol is a poor substrate for polyol dehydrogenase, and therefore its oxidation to tagatose is considered to be minimal in most tissues. Thus, the very slow rate of catabolism of galactitol, coupled with the greater affinity of aldose reductase for galactose than for glucose, presumably accounts for the observation that galactitol levels in tissues of galactose-fed rats may be $\sim$10–20$\times$ the levels of sorbitol in corresponding tissues of severely diabetic animals. At present we can only speculate on the following possibilities: (*1*) that very high levels of galactitol may, at some point, have an impact on the cascade of metabolic imbalances depicted in Figure 6.7, or (*2*) that the increase in pentose shunt activity associated with reduction of galactose to galactitol might have an impact on de novo diacylglycerol synthesis and/or fatty acid oxidation, among other processes.

SUMMARY—FUTURE DIRECTIONS

In summary, evidence reviewed in this chapter is consistent with the hypothesis that a more reduced cytosolic redox state plays an important role in mediating glucose- and diabetes-induced vascular dysfunction. Further studies are needed to assess the impact of the more reduced cytosolic redox state on diacylglycerol levels/synthesis and fatty acid oxidation, as well as on the nature of the metabolic imbalances that mediate diabetes-like complications in galactose-fed animals. Additional studies also are indicated to examine the important therapeutic implication of these observations that a polypharmacological intervention with agents that have different mechanisms of action, (i.e. in which an aldose reductase inhibitor, *myo*-inositol, acetyl-L-carnitine, and aminoguanidine are given concurrently) may be far more efficacious than any one of these pharmacologic agents given alone, in delaying or preventing the onset of late complications of diabetes.

ACKNOWLEDGMENTS

This research was supported by grants from the National Institutes of Health (EY 06600, HL 30678, and DK 20579) and by the Kilo Diabetes and Vascular Research Foundation.

REFERENCES

1. ANDERSON, S., RENNKE, H. G., GARCIA, D. L., BRENNER, B. M., RILEY, S. L., and SANDSTROM, D. J. Short and long term effects of antihypertensive therapy in the diabetic rat. *Kidney Int.* 36: 526–536, 1989.
2. ASAKURA, T., ADACHI, K., MINAKAMI, S., and YOSHIKAWA, H. Non-glycolytic sugar metabolism in human erythrocytes. I. Xylitol metabolism. *J. Biochem. (Tokyo)* 62: 184–193, 1967.
3. BANK, N., KLOSE, R., AYNEDJIAN, H. S., NGUYEN, D., and SABLAY, L. B. Evidence against increased glomerular pressure initiating diabetic nephropathy. *Kidney Int.* 31: 898–905, 1987.
4. BANK, N., MOWER, P., AYNEDJIAN, H. S., WILKES, B. M., and SILVERMAN, S. Sorbinil prevents glomerular hyperperfusion in diabetic rats. *Am. J. Physiol.* 256 *(Renal Fluid Electrolyte Physiol.* 25) F1000–F1006, 1989.
5. BANK, N., COCO, M., and AYNEDJIAN, H. S. Galactose feeding causes glomerular hyperperfusion: Prevention by aldose reductase inhibition. *Am. J. Physiol.* 256 *(Renal Fluid Electrolyte Physiol.* 25) F994–F999, 1989.
6. BEAVEN, M. A. *Factors Regulating Availability of Histamine at Tissue Receptors.* In: *Pharmacology of Histamine Receptors,* edited by Ganellin, C. R., and Parsons, M. E., eds) London: John Wright & Sons, 1982, pp. 103–145.
7. BEYER-MEARS, A., CRUZ, E., EDELIST, T., and VARAGIANNIS, E. Diminished proteinuria in diabetes mellitus by sorbinil, an aldose reductase inhibitor. *Pharmacology* 32: 52–60, 1986.
8. BEYER-MEARS, A., MURRAY, F. T., DEL VAL, M., CRUZ, E., and SCIADINI, M. Reversal of proteinuria by sorbinil, an aldose reductase inhibitor in spontaneously diabetic BB rats. *Pharmacology* 36: 111–119, 1988.
9. BIANCHI, R., BERTI-MATTERA, L. N., FIORI, M. G., and EICHBERG, J. Correction of altered metabolic activities in sciatic nerves of streptozotocin-induced diabetic rats: effect of ganglioside treatment. *Diabetes* 39: 782–788, 1990.
10. BROWNLEE, M., CERAMI, A., and VLASSARA, H. Advanced glycosylation end products in tissue and the biochemical basis of diabetic complications. *N. Engl. J. Med.* 318: 1315–1321, 1988.
11. BROWNLEE, M., CERAMI, A., and VLASSARA, H. Advanced products of nonenzymatic glycosylation and the pathogenesis of diabetic vascular disease. *Diabetes/Metab. Rev.* 4, 437–451, 1988.
12. BUCALA, R., MODEL, P., and CERAMI, A. Modification of DNA by reducing sugars: a possible mechanism for nucleic acid aging and age-related dysfunction in gene expression. *Proc. Natl. Acad. Sci. USA* 81: 105–109, 1984.
13. BUSE, M. G., WEIGAND, D. A., PEELER, D., and HEDDEN, M. P. The effect of diabetes and the redox potential on amino acid content and release by isolated rat hemidiaphragms. *Metabolism* 29: 605–616, 1980.
14. CAIRD, F. I., PIRIE, A., and RAMSEL, T. G. *Diabetes and the Eye.* Oxford: Blackwell Scientific Publications, 1968, pp. 112–113.
15. CALDWELL, G., and KOHNER, E. M. Diabetic retinopathy and nephropathy—are they related? *J. Diabetic Complications* 3: 137–138, 1989.
16. CARBONELL, L. F., SALOM, M. G., GARCIA-ESTAN, J., SALAZAR, F. J., UBEDA, M., and QUESADA, T. Hemodynamic alterations in chronically conscious unrestrained diabetic rats. *Am. J. Physiol.* 252 *(Heart Circ. Physiol.* 21): H900–H905, 1987.
17. CARNEY, S. L., WONG, N. L. M., and DIRKS, J. H. Acute effects of streptozotocin diabetes on rat renal function. *J. Lab. Clin. Med.* 93, 950–961, 1979.
18. CARROLL, P. B., THORNTON, B., and GREENE, D. A. Glutathione redox state is not the link between polyol pathway activity and myo-inositol—related Na^+-K^+-ATPase defect in experimental diabetic neuropathy. *Diabetes* 35: 1282–1285, 1986.
19. CHAKRABARTI, S., and SIMA, A. A. F. Effect of aldose reductase inhibition and insulin treatment on retinal capillary basement membrane thickening in BB rats. *Diabetes* 38: 1181–1186, 1989.
20. CHANDLER, M. L., SHANNON, W. A., and DESANTIS, L. Prevention of retinal capillary basement membrane thickening in diabetic rats by aldose reductase inhibitors. *Invest. Ophthalmol. Vis. Sci.* 25: 159, 1984.
21. CHANG, K., TOMLINSON, M., JEFFREY, J. R., TILTON, R. G., SHERMAN, W. R., ACKERMANN, K. E., BERGER, R. A., CICERO, T. J., KILO, C., and WILLIAMSON, J. R. Galactose ingestion increases vascular permeability and collagen solubility in normal male rats. *J. Clin. Invest.* 79: 367–373, 1987.
22. CHENG, H.-M., GONZALEZ, R. G., VON SALTZA, I., CHYLACK, L. T., JR., and HUTSON, N. J.

Glucose flux and the redox state of pyridine dinucleotides in the rat lens. *Exp. Eye Res.* 46: 947–952, 1988.

23. COHEN, M. P., DASMAHAPATRA, A., and SHAPIRO, E. Reduced glomerular sodium/potassium adenosine triphosphatase activity in acute streptozocin diabetes and its prevention by oral sorbinil. *Diabetes* 34: 1071–1074, 1985.

24. COHEN, M. P., and KLEPSER, H. Glomerular Na$^+$-K$^+$-ATPase activity in acute and chronic diabetes and with aldose reductase inhibition. *Diabetes* 37: 558–562, 1988.

25. COLLINS, V. R., DOWSE, G. K., FINCH, C. F., ZIMMET, P. Z., and LINNANE, A. W. Prevalence and risk factors for micro- and macroalbuminuria in diabetic subjects and entire population of Nauru. *Diabetes* 38: 1602–1610, 1989.

26. COOPER, M. E., ALLEN, T. J., MACMILLAN, P., BACH, L., JERUMS, G., and DOYLE, A. E. Genetic hypertension accelerates nephropathy in the streptozotocin diabetic rat. *Am. J. Hypertens.* 1: 5–10, 1988.

27. COOPER, M. E., ALLEN, T. J., O'BRIEN, R. C., MACMILLAN, P. A., CLARKE, B., JERUMS, G., and DOYLE, A. E. Effects of genetic hypertension on diabetic nephropathy in the rat— functional and structural characteristics. *J. Hypertens.* 6: 1009–1016, 1988.

28. CORR, P. B., GROSS, R. W., and SOBEL, B. E. Amphipathic metabolites and membrane dysfunction in ischemic myocardium. *Circ. Res.* 55: 135–154, 1984.

29. CRAVEN, P. A., CAINES, M.A., and DERUBERTIS, F. R. Sequential alterations in glomerular prostaglandin and thrombaxane synthesis in diabetic rats: relationship to the hyperfiltration of early diabetes. *Metabolism* 36: 95–103, 1987.

30. CRAVEN, P. A., and DERUBERTIS, F. R. Protein kinase C is activated in glomeruli from streptozotocin diabetic rats: Possible mediation by glucose. *J. Clin. Invest.* 83: 1667–1675, 1989.

31. CRAVEN, P. A., DAVIDSON, C. M., and DERUBERTIS, F. R. Increase in diacylglycerol mass in isolated glomeruli by glucose from de novo synthesis of glycerolipids. *Diabetes* 39: 667–674, 1990.

32. CUNHA-VAZ, J. G., FONSECA, J. R., DE ABREU, J. R. F., and LIMA, J. J. P. Studies on retinal blood flow. II. Diabetic retinopathy. *Arch. Ophthalmol.* 96: 809–811, 1978.

33. DANIELS, B. S., and HOSTETTER, T. H. Aldose reductase inhibition and glomerular abnormalities in diabetic rats. *Diabetes* 38: 981–986, 1989.

34. DECKERT, T., SIMONSEN, S. E., and POULSEN, J. E. Prognosis of proliferative retinopathy in juvenile diabetes. *Diabetes* 16: 728–733, 1967.

35. DUNN, F. L. Hyperlipidemia in diabetes mellitus. *Diabetes/Metab. Rev.* 6: 47–61, 1990.

36. DVORNIK, D. *Aldose Reductase Inhibition: An Approach to the Prevention of Diabetic Complications,* edited by D. Porte. New York: McGraw-Hill, 1987.

37. DYCK, P. J., SHERMAN, W. R., HALLCHER, L. M., SERVICE, F. J., O'BRIEN, P. C., GRINA, L. A., PALUMBO, P. J., and SWANSON, C. J. Human diabetic endoneurial sorbitol, fructose, and *myo*-inositol related to sural nerve morphometry. *Ann. Neurol.* 8: 590–596, 1980.

38. DYCK, P. J., ZIMMERMAN, B. R., VILEN, T. H., MINNERATH, S. R., KARNES, J. L., YAO, J. K., and PODUSLO, J. F. Nerve glucose, fructose, sorbitol, *myo*-inositol, and fiber degeneration and regeneration in diabetic neuropathy. *N. Engl. J. Med.* 319: 542–548, 1988.

39. ENGERMAN, R. L., and KERN, T. S. Experimental galactosemia produces diabetic-like retinopathy. *Diabetes* 33: 97–100, 1984.

40. FRANGOS, M., SMITH, S., SANTIAGO, J., and KILO, C. Sorbitol-induced imbalances in glycolysis in human erythrocytes are reduced by pyruvate. *Diabetes* 39: 274A, 1990.

41. FRANK, R. N., KERN, J. R., KENNEDY, A., and FRANK, K. W. Galactose-induced retinal capillary basement membrane thickening: prevention by sorbinil. *Invest. Ophthalmol. Vis. Sci.* 24: 1519–1524, 1983.

42. GOLDFARB, S., SIMMONS, D. A., and KERN, K. Amelioration of glomerular hyperfiltration in acute experimental diabetes by dietary *myo*-inositol and by an aldose reductase inhibitor. *Trans. Assoc. Am. Physicians* 99: 67–72, 1986.

43. GONZALEZ, R. G., BARNETT, P., AGUAYO, J., CHANG, H.-M., and CHYLACK, L. T., JR. Direct measurement of polyol pathway activity in the ocular lens. *Diabetes* 33: 196–199, 1984.

44. GREENE, D. A., LATTIMER, S. A., and SIMA, A. A. F. Are disturbances of sorbitol, phosphoinositide, and Na$^+$-K$^+$-ATPase regulation involved in pathogenesis of diabetic neuropathy? *Diabetes* 37: 688–693, 1988.

45. GREENE, D. A., LATTIMER, S. A., and SIMA, A. A. F. Pathogenesis and prevention of diabetic neuropathy. *Diabetes/Metab. Rev.* 4: 201–221, 1988.

46. GRUNWALD, J. E., RIVA, C. E., BRUCKER, A. J., SINCLAIR, S. H., and PETRIG, B. L. Altered retinal vascular response to 100% oxygen breathing in diabetes mellitus. *Ophthalmology* 91: 1447–1452, 1984.

47. GRUNWALD, J. E., RIVA, C. E., SINCLAIR, S. H., BRUCKER, A. J., and PETRIG, B. L. Laser doppler velocimetry study of retinal circulation in diabetes mellitus. *Arch. Ophthalmol.* 104: 991–996, 1986.

48. HALE, P. J., NATTRASS, M., SILVERMAN, S. H., SENNIT, C., PERKINS, C. M., UDEN, A., and SUNDKVIST, G. Peripheral nerve concentrations of glucose, fructose, sorbitol and *myo*-inositol in diabetic and non-diabetic patients. *Diabetologia* 30: 464–467, 1987.

49. HEIFETS, M., DAVIS, T. A., TEGTMEYER, E., and KLAHR, S. Exercise training ameliorates progressive renal disease in rats with subtotal nephrectomy. *Kidney Int.* 32: 815–820, 1987.

50. HOSTETTER, T. H., TROY, J. L., and BRENNER, B. M. Glomerular hemodynamics in experimental diabetes mellitus. *Kidney Int.* 19: 410–415, 1981.

51. IDO, Y., CHANG, K., OSTROW, E., ALLISON, W., KILO, C., and TILTON, R. G. Aminoguanidine prevents regional blood flow increases in streptozotocin-diabetic rats. *Diabetes* 39: 93A, 1990.

52. JENSEN, P. K., CHRISTIANSEN, J. S., STEVEN, K., and PARVING, H.-H. Renal function in streptozotocin-diabetic rats. *Diabetologia* 21: 409–414, 1981.

53. KASISKE, B. L., O'DONNELL, M. P., CLEARY, M. P., and KEANE, W. F. Treatment of hyperlipidemia reduces glomerular injury in obese Zucker rats. *Kidney Int.* 33: 667–672, 1988.

54. KAWAMURA, T., SMITH, S., and WILLIAMSON, J. R. Glucose-induced metabolic changes in tissue chamber granulation tissue. *Diabetes* 39: 192A, 1990.

55. KEANE, W. F., KASISKE, B. L., and O'DONNELL, M. P. Hyperlipidemia and the progression of renal disease. *Am. J. Clin. Nutr.* 47: 157–160, 1988.

56. KILO, C., VOGLER, N., and WILLIAMSON, J. R. Muscle capillary basement membrane changes related to aging and to diabetes mellitus. *Diabetes* 21: 881–905, 1972.

57. KILZER, P., CHANG, K., MARVEL, J., ROWOLD, E., JAUDES, P., ULLENSVANG, S., KILO, C., and WILLIAMSON, J. R. Albumin permeation of new vessels is increased in diabetic rats. *Diabetes* 34: 333–336, 1985.

58. KINOSHITA, J. H., FUKUSHI, S., KADOR, P., and MEROLA, L. O. Aldose reductase in diabetic complications of the eye. *Metabolism* 28: 462–469, 1979.

59. KINOSHITA, J. H., KADOR, P. F., and DATILES, M. Aldose reductase in diabetic cataracts. *JAMA* 246: 257–261, 1981.

60. KINOSHITA, J. H. Concept of aldose reductase and diabetic cataracts. pp. 82–84, In: Cogan, D. G., moderator. Aldose Reductase and Complications of Diabetes. *Ann. Intern. Med.* 82: 82–91, 1984.

61. KINOSHITA, J. H., and NISHIMURA, C. The involvement of aldose reductase in diabetic complications. *Diabetes/Metab. Rev.* 4: 323–337, 1988.

62. KNOWLER, W. C., BENNETT, P. H., and BALLINTINE, E. J. Increased incidence of retinopathy in diabetics with elevated blood pressure: a six-year follow-up study in Pima Indians. *N. Engl. J. Med.* 302: 645–650, 1980.

63. KOHNER, E. M., DOLLERY, C. T., PATERSON, J. W., and OAKLEY, N. W. Arterial fluorescein studies in diabetic retinopathy. *Diabetes* 16: 1–10, 1967.

64. KOHNER, E. M., and OAKLEY, N. W. Diabetic retinopathy. *Metabolism* 24: 1085–1102, 1975.

65. KOHNER, E. M. The problems of retinal blood flow in diabetes. *Diabetes* 25: 839–844, 1976.

66. LATTIMER, S. A., DIAZ, T. C., DELMONTE, M., and GREENE, D. A. Extracellular polyols acutely lower *myo*-inositol content and uptake in human retinal pigment epithelial cells. *Diabetes* 38: 94A, 1989.

67. LEE, T.-S., Saltsman, K. A., Ohashi, H., and KING, G. L. Activation of protein kinase C by elevation of glucose concentration: Proposal for a mechanism in the development of diabetic vascular complications. *Proc. Natl. Acad. Sci. USA* 86: 5141–5145, 1989.

68. LEE, T. S., MacGREGOR, L. C., FLUHARTY, S. J., and KING, G. L. Differential regulation of protein kinase C and (Na,K)-adenosine triphosphatase activities by elevated glucose levels in retinal capillary endothelial cells. *J. Clin. Invest.* 83: 90–94, 1989.

69. LORENZI, M., MONTISANO, D. F., TOLEDO, S., and BARRIEUX. High glucose induces DNA damage in cultured human endothelial cells. *J. Clin. Invest.* 77: 322–325, 1986.

70. LOU, M. F., DICKERSON, J. R., JR., GARADI, R., and YORK, B. M., JR. Glutathione depletion in the lens of galactosemic and diabetic rats. *Exp. Eye Res.* 46: 517–530, 1988.

71. LOY, A., LURIE, K. G., GHOSH, A., WILSON, J. M., MacGREGOR, L. C., and MATSCHINSKY, F. M. Diabetes and the *myo*-inositol paradox. *Diabetes* 39: 1305–1312, 1990.

72. MAEDA, T., and EISENBERG, F., JR. Purification, structure, and catalytic properties of l-*myo*-inositol-1-phosphate synthase from rat testis. *J. Biol. Chem.* 255: 8458–8464, 1980.

73. MALAISSE, W. J., HUTTON, J. C., KAWAZU, S., HERCHUELZ, A., VALVERDE, I., and SENER, A. The stimulus-secretion coupling of glucose-induced insulin release. XXXV. The links between metabolic and cationic events. *Diabetologia* 16: 331–341, 1979.

74. MALONE, J. I., LOWITT, S., and COOK, W. R. Nonosmotic diabetic cataracts. *Pediatr. Res.* 27: 293–296, 1990.

75. MARANO, C. W., and MATSCHINSKY, F. M. Biochemical manifestations of diabetes mellitus in microscopic layers of the cornea and retina. *Diabetes/Metab. Rev.* 5: 1–15, 1989.

76. MATHIESEN, E. R., RONN, B., JENSEN, T., STOMR, B., and DECKERT, T. Relationship between blood pressure and urinary albumin excretion in development of microalbuminuria. *Diabetes* 39: 245–249, 1990.

77. MAUCK, L. A., WONG, Y. H., and SHERMAN, W. R. L-*myo*-inositol 1-phosphate synthase: Purification to homogeneity from bovine testis and partial characterization. *Biochemistry* 19: 3623–3629, 1980.

78. MAUER, S. M., STEFFES, M. W., AZAR, S., SANDBERG, K. S., and BROWN, D. M. The effects of Goldblatt hypertension on development of the glomerular lesions of diabetes mellitus in the rat. *Diabetes* 27: 738–744, 1978.

79. McCALEB, M. L., SREDY, J., MILLEN, J., ACKERMAN, D. M., and DVORNIK, D. Prevention of urinary albumin excretion in 6 month streptozocin-diabetic rats with the aldose reductase inhibitor tolrestat. *J. Diabetic Complications* 2: 16–18, 1988.

80. MICHELS, L. D., DAVIDMAN, M., and KEANE, W. F. Determinants of glomerular filtration and plasma flow in experimental diabetic rats. *J. Lab. Clin. Sci.* 98: 869–885, 1981.

81. MOGENSEN, C. E., SCHMITZ, A., and CHRISTENSEN, C. K. Comparative renal pathophysiology relevant to IDDM and NIDDM patients. *Diabetes/Metab. Rev.* 4: 453–483, 1988.

82. MOGENSEN, C. E. Therapeutic interventions in nephropathy of IDDM. *Diabetes Care* 11: 10–15, 1988.

83. MOGENSEN, C. E. Prediction of clinical diabetic nephropathy in IDDM patients: alternatives to microalbuminuria? *Diabetes* 39: 761–767, 1990.

84. MOORE, H. K., RADLOFF, J. F., HULL, F. E., and SWEELEY, C. C. Incomplete fatty acid oxidation by ischemic heart: b-hydroxy fatty acid production. *Am. J. Physiol. (Heart Circ. Physiol.* 8): H257–H265, 1980.

85. MORITA, J., UEDA, K., NANJO, S., and KOMANO, T. Sequence specific damage of DNA induced by reducing sugars. *Nucleic Acids Res.* 13: 449–458, 1985.

86. MORRISON, A. D., CLEMENTS, R. S., JR., TRAVIS, S. B., OSKI, F., and WINEGRAD, A. I. Glucose utilization by the polyol pathway in human erythrocytes. *Biochem. Biophys. Res. Commun.* 1: 199, 1970.

87. NORTON, E. W. D., and GUTMAN, F. Diabetic retinopathy studied by fluorescein angiography. *Ophthalmologica* 150: 5–17, 1965.

88. OATES, P. J., ELLERY, C. A., and PUSTILNIK, L. R. Renal hyperperfusion in 30% galactose-fed rats is prevented by two structurally distinct aldose reductase inhibitors. *Diabetologia* 33: A65, 1990.

89. OHI, T., PODUSLO, J. F., and DYCK, P. J. Increased endoneurial albumin in diabetic polyneuropathy. *Neurology* 35: 1790–1791, 1985.

90. OKUMURA, K., AKIYAMA, N., HASHIMOTO, H., OGAWA, K., and SATAKE, T. Alteration of 1,2-diacylglycerol content in myocardium from diabetic rats. *Diabetes* 37: 1168–1172, 1988.

91. ORTOLA, F. V., BALLERMANN, B. J., ANDERSON, S., MENDEZ, R. E., and BRENNER, B. M. Elevated plasma arterial natriuretic peptide levels in diabetic rats. *J. Clin. Invest.* 80: 670–674, 1987.

92. OSTERBY, R., and GUNDERSEN, H. J. G. Glomerular basement membrane thickening in streptozotocin diabetic rats despite treatment with an aldose reductase inhibitor. *J. Diabetic Complications* 3: 149–153, 1989.

93. PARVING, H.-H., and ROSSING, N. Simultaneous determination of the transcapillary escape rate of albumin and IgG in normal and long-term juvenile diabetic subjects. *Scand. J. Clin. Lab. Invest.* 32: 239–244, 1973.

94. PARVING, H.-H. Increased microvascular permeability to plasma proteins in short- and long-term juvenile diabetics. *Diabetes* 25: 884–889, 1976.

95. PARVING, H.-H., VIBERTI, G. C., KEEN, H., CHRISTIANSEN, J. S., and LASSEN, N. A. Hemodynamic factors in the genesis of diabetic microangiopathy. *Metabolism* 32: 943–949, 1983.

96. PIRART, J. Diabetes mellitus and its degenerative complications: a prospective study of 4,400 patients observed between 1947 and 1973. *Diabetes Care* 1: 168–188, 1977.

97. POULSON, R., MIRRLEES, D. J., EARL, D. C. N., and HEATH, H. The effects of an aldose reductase inhibitor upon the sorbitol pathway, fructose-1-phosphate and lactate in the retina and nerve of streptozotocin-diabetic rats. *Exp. Eye Res.* 36: 751–760, 1983.

98. PUGLIESE, G., TILTON, R. G., SPEEDY, A., CHANG, K., SANTARELLI, E., PROVINCE, M. A., EADES, D., SHERMAN, W. R., and WILLIAMSON, J. R. Effects of very mild versus overt diabetes on vascular haemodynamics and barrier function in rats. *Diabetologia* 32: 845–857, 1989.

99. PUGLIESE, G., TILTON, R. G., SPEEDY, A., CHANG, K., PROVINCE, M. A., KILO, C., and WILLIAMSON, J. R. Vascular filtration function in galactose-fed versus diabetic rats: the role of polyol pathway activity. *Metabolism* 39: 690–697, 1990.

100. PUGLIESE, G. TILTON, R. G., SPEEDY, A., SANTARELLI, E., EADES, D. M., PROVINCE, M. A., KILO, C., SHERMAN, W. R., and WILLIAMSON, J. R. Modulation of hemodynamic and vascular filtration changes in diabetic rats by dietary *myo*-inositol. *Diabetes* 39: 312–322, 1990.

101. PUGLIESE, G., TILTON, R. G., CHANG, K., SPEEDY, A., PROVINCE, M., EADES, D. M., LACY, P. E., KILO, C., and WILLIAMSON, J. R. Effects of islet isografts on hemodynamic and vascular filtration changes in diabetic rats. *Diabetes* 39: 323–332, 1990.

102. RASKIN, P., and ROSENSTOCK, J. Blood glucose control and diabetic complications. *Ann. Intern. Med.* 105: 254–263, 1986.

103. ROBISON, W. G., JR., NAGATA, M., LAVER, N., HOHMAN, T. C., and KINOSHITA, J. H. Diabetic-like retinopathy in rats prevented with an aldose reductase inhibitor. *Invest. Ophthalmol. Vis. Sci.* 30: 2285–2292, 1989.

104. ROBISON, W. G., JR., TILLIS, T. N., LAVER, N. and KINOSHITA, J. H. Diabetes-related histopathologies of the rat retina prevented with an aldose reductase inhibitor. *Exp. Eye Res.* 50: 355–366, 1990.

105. RUDERMAN, N. B., SCHMAHL, F. W., and GOODMAN, M. N. Regulation of alanine formation and release in rat muscle in vivo: effect of starvation and diabetes. *Am. J. Physiol.* 233 (*Endocrinol. Metab. Gastrointest. Physiol.* 2): E109–E114, 1977.

106. RUDERMAN, N. B., and HAUDENSCHILD, C. Diabetes as an atherogenic factor. *Prog. Cardiovasc. Dis.* 26: 373–412, 1984.

107. RUNYAN, J. W., JR. Statement on hypertension in diabetes. *Diabetes Care* 10: 764–776, 1987.

108. SANDLER, S., WELSH, M., and ANDERSSON, A. Streptozotocin-induced impairment of islet B-cell metabolism and its prevention by a hydroxyl radical scavenger and inhibitors of polyol(ADP-ribose) synthetase. *Acta Pharmacol. Toxicol.* 53: 392–400, 1983.

109. SIMMONS, D. A., and WINEGRAD, A. I. Mechanism of glucose-induced (Na^+, K^+)-ATPase inhibition in aortic wall of rabbits. *Diabetologia* 32: 402–408, 1989.

110. SINCLAIR, S. H., GRUNWALD, J. E., RIVA, C. E., BRAUNSTEIN, S. N., NICHOLS, C. W., and SCHWARTZ, S. S. Retinal vascular autoregulation in diabetes mellitus. *Ophthalmology* 89: 748–750, 1982.

111. SIPERSTEIN, M. D., UNGER, R. H., and MADISON, L. L. Studies of muscle capillary basement membranes in normal subjects, diabetic, and prediabetic patients. *J. Clin. Invest.* 47: 1973–1999, 1969. -

112. SMALL, K. W., STEFANSSON, E., and HATCHELL, D. L. Retinal blood flow in normal and diabetic dogs. *Invest. Ophthalmol. Vis. Sci.* 28: 672–675, 1987.

113. SOELDNER, J. S., CHRISTACOPOULOS, P. D., and GLEASON, R. E. Mean retinal circulation time as determined by fluorescein angiography in normal, prediabetic, and chemical-diabetic subjects. *Diabetes* 25: 903, 1976 (abstract).

114. STEFFES, M. W., OSTERBY, R., CHAVERS, B., and MAUER, S. M. Mesangial expansion as a central mechanism for loss of kidney function in diabetic patients. *Diabetes* 38: 1077–1081, 1989.

115. STERKY, G., and WALL, S. Determinants of microangiopathy in growth-onset diabetes. *Acta Paediatr. Scand.* 5–45, 1986.

116. STEVENS, V. J., VLASSARA, H., ABATI, A., and CERAMI, A. Nonenzymatic glycosylation of hemoglobin. *J. Biol. Chem.* 252: 2998–3002, 1977.

117. SZWERGOLD, B. S., KAPPLER, F., and BROWN, T. R. Identification of fructose 3-phosphate in the lens of diabetic rats. *Science* 247: 451–454, 1990.

118. TILTON, R. G., CHANG, K., WEIGEL, C., KILO, C., and WILLIAMSON, J. R. Increased ocular blood flow and ^{125}I-albumin permeation in galactose-fed rats: inhibition by sorbinil. *Invest. Ophthalmol. Vis. Sci.* 29: 861–868, 1988.

119. TILTON, R. G., CHANG, K., PUGLIESE, G., EADES, D. M., PROVINCE, M. A., SHERMAN, W. R., KILO, C., and WILLIAMSON, J. R. Prevention of hemodynamic and vascular albumin filtration changes in diabetic rats by aldose reductase inhibitors. *Diabetes* 38: 1258–1270, 1989.

120. TILTON, R. G., CHANG, K., OSTROW, E., ALLISON, W., and WILLIAMSON, J. R. Aminoguanidine reduces increased ^{131}I-albumin permeation of retinal and uveal vessels in streptozotocin-diabetic rats. *Invest. Ophthalmol. Vis. Sci.* 31: 342, 1990.

121. TILTON, R. G., PUGLIESE, G., and WILLIAMSON, J. R. Diabetes-induced glomerular structural changes in rats are not prevented by sorbinil. *Diabetes* 38: 94A, 1989.

122. TOMLANOVICH, S., DEEN, W. M., JONES, H. W., III., SCHWARTZ, H. C., and MYERS, B. D. Functional nature of glomerular injury in progressive diabetic glomerulopathy. *Diabetes* 36: 556–565, 1987.

123. Travis, S. F., Morrison, A. D., Clements, R. S., Jr., Winegrad, A. I., and Oski, F. A. Metabolic alterations in the human erythrocyte produced by increases in glucose concentration: the role of the polyol pathway. *J. Clin. Invest.* 50: 2104–2112, 1971.

124. Trus, M., Warner, H., and Matschinsky, F. Effects of glucose on insulin release and on intermediary metabolism of isolated perfused pancreatic islets from fed and fasted rats. *Diabetes* 29: 1–14, 1980.

125. Tsubota, K., Krauss, J. M., Kenyon, K. R., Laing, R. A., Miglior, S., and Cheng, H.-M. Lens redox fluorometry: pyridine nucleotide fluorescence and analysis of diabetic lens. *Exp. Eye Res.* 49: 321–334, 1989.

126. Tucker, B. J. Early onset of increased transcapillary albumin escape in awake diabetic rats. *Diabetes* 39: 919–923, 1990.

127. Uchigata, Y., Yamamoto, H., Kawamura, A., and Okamoto, H. Protection by superoxide dismutase, catalase, and poly(ADP-ribose) synthetase inhibitors against alloxan- and streptozotocin-induced islet DNA strand breaks and against the inhibition of proinsulin synthesis. *J. Biol. Chem.* 257: 6084–6088, 1982.

128. Ward, J. D., Baker, R. W. R., and Davis, B. H. Effect of blood sugar control on the accumulation of sorbitol and fructose in nervous tissue. *Diabetes* 21: 1173–1178, 1972.

129. Williamson, D. H., Lund, P., and Krebs, H. A. The redox state of free nicotinamide-adenine dinucleotide in the cytoplasm and mitochondria of rat liver. *Biochem. J.* 103: 514–527, 1967.

130. Williamson, J. R., Rowold, E., Chang, K., Marvel, J., Tomlinson, M., Sherman, W. R., Ackermann, K. E., Berger, R. A., and Kilo, C. Sex steroid dependency of diabetes-induced changes in polyol metabolism, vascular permeability, and collagen cross-linking. *Diabetes* 35: 20–27, 1986.

131. Williamson, J. R., Chang, K., Tilton, R. G., Prater, C., Jeffrey, J. R., Weigel, C., Sherman, W. R., Eades, D. M., and Kilo, C. Increased vascular permeability in spontaneously diabetic BB/W rats and in rats with mild versus severe streptozotocin-induced diabetes: prevention by aldose reductase inhibitors and castration. *Diabetes* 36: 813–821, 1987.

132. Williamson, J. R., Tilton, R. G., Chang, K., and Kilo, C. Basement membrane abnormalities in diabetes mellitus: relationship to clinical microangiopathy. *Diabetes/Metab. Rev.* 4: 339–370, 1988.

133. Williamson, J. R., Chang, K., Ostrow, E., Allison, W., Harlow, J., and Kilo, C. Sorbitol-induced increases in vascular albumin clearance (VAC) are prevented by pyruvate but not *myo*-inositol. *Diabetes* 38: 94A, 1989.

134. Williamson, J. R., Chang, K., Kilo, C., Sherman, W. R., Montenero, M., and Arrigoni-Martelli, E. Prevention of glucose-induced vascular functional changes by acetyl-L-carnitine. *Diabetologia* 33: A175, 1990.

135. Williamson, J. R., Ostrow, E., Eades, D. M., Chang, K., Allison, W., Kilo, C., and Sherman, W. R. Glucose-induced microvascular functional changes in nondiabetic rats are stereospecific and are prevented by an aldose reductase inhibitor. *J. Clin. Invest.* 85: 1167–1172, 1990.

136. Williamson, J. R., Tilton, R. G., and Kilo, C. The polyol pathway and diabetic complications. In: *Diabetic Complications: Epidemiology and Pathogenetic Mechanisms,* edited by F. Conti. New York: Raven, 1990, pp. 45–58.

137. Williamson, J. R., Chang, K., Allison, W., and Ostrow, E. Glucose-induced vascular functional changes in granulation tissue are largely prevented by H1 and H2 receptor antagonists. *FASEB J* 4: A1276, 1990.

138. Winegrad, A. I. Does a common mechanism induce the diverse complications of diabetes? *Diabetes* 36: 396–406, 1987.

139. Wolf, B. A., Williamson, J. R., Easom, R. A., Chang, K., Sherman, W. R., and Turk, J. Diacylglycerol accumulation and microvascular abnormalities induced by elevated glucose levels. *J. Clin. Invest.* 87: 31–38, 1990.

140. Yeh, L.-A., Rafford, C. E., Goddu, K. J., Ashton, M. A., Beyer, T. A., and Hutson, N. J. Na$^+$-K$^+$-ATPase pumping activity is not directly linked to *myo*-inositol levels after sorbinil treatment in lenses of diabetic rats. *Diabetes* 36: 1414–1419, 1987.

141. Yorek, M. A., Dunlap, J. A., and Ginsberg, B. H. *Myo*-Inositol metabolism in 41A3 neuroblastoma cells: effects of high glucose and sorbitol levels. *J. Neurochem.* 48: 53–61, 1987.

142. Zatz, R., Dunn, B. R., Meyer, T. W., Anderson, S., Rennke, H. G., and Brenner, B. M. Prevention of diabetic glomerulopathy by pharmacological amelioration of glomerular capillary hypertension. *J. Clin. Invest.* 77: 1925–1930, 1986.

143. Zatz, R., and Brenner, B. M. Pathogenesis of diabetic microangiopathy: the hemodynamic view. *Am. J. Med.* 80: 443–453, 1987.

7

Mechanisms of Early Hyperglycemia-Induced Alterations in Vascular Metabolism and Autoregulation

ALBERT I. WINEGRAD AND DAVID A. SIMMONS

To develop a valid framework for efforts to explain the association between diabetes mellitus and vascular disease, we must first resolve the question of the cause of the association between diverse types of diabetes and a characteristic group of late complicating syndromes that do not have a common pathological basis. Diabetes mellitus is a heterogeneous group of chronic hyperglycemic disorders with differing genetic and etiologic origins. However, all types of diabetes convey risks for progressive disease (subclinical structural alterations) and late clinical complications in the same restricted group of susceptible organs and regions of the nervous and arterial systems. Hyperglycemia is now generally agreed to be the factor that conveys these risks, but not to be the sole determinant of the clinical outcome in any of the susceptible tissues. Why hyperglycemia induces risks for disease in a specific group of organs and systems has been unknown, but a potential answer has developed. Hyperglycemia has been found to cause its initial metabolic and functional effects in all of the organs and systems susceptible to a late complication of diabetes mellitus by activating a "common initiating mechanism." The common initiating mechanism can be activated by hyperglycemia only in cells in which a restrictive combination of requirements is met, and its early effects in most of the susceptible organs and systems have been linked to risks for inciting disease. In retina, kidney, and aorta (a model arterial wall) the common initiating mechanism causes early alterations in vascular metabolism, autoregulation, permeability, and responses to specific vasoactive hormones or neurotransmitters. To place the probable role of the common initiating mechanism in the pathogenesis of the late complications of diabetes in context, a brief review of some general features of this problem is required.

LATE CLINICAL COMPLICATIONS OF DIABETES MELLITUS

Each late complication of diabetes is a syndrome resulting from disease in an individual organ or system region that occurs more frequently in patients with chronic diabetes. These syndromes are truly complications rather than inexorable consequences of chronic diabetes, and there is marked variation in the development of individual complications among individual diabetics. The late complications of diabetes were once believed to be simply local manifestations either of atherosclerotic arterial disease or of "diabetic microangiopathy," a putatively unique, generalized, and uniform type of capillary disease whose pathognomonic feature was basement membrane thickening. This view is now untenable. Neither microvascular disease or atherosclerotic arterial disease is a primary or consistent contributing factor in the development of the most common form of diabetic neuropathy, diabetic polyneuropathy (5). The term *diabetic microangiopathy* was introduced before it was recognized that the patterns of the pathology in the retinal and glomerular microcirculations in diabetes are different, even different in nature and degree from the pathology in other microcirculations in the same organ, and that they are not unique to diabetes (24,25,29,33). Moreover, capillary basement membrane thickening does not define a specific type of capillary disease or one that is unique to genetically determined diabetes mellitus (15). Furthermore, the categorization of diabetic nephropathy as a "microangiopathic complication" ignores the potential importance of arteriolarsclerosis and interstitial nephritis in the development of clinical diabetic nephropathy (29). Atherosclerotic coronary artery disease and peripheral vascular disease in the lower extremities are the clinical syndromes resulting from occlusive arterial disease that are specifically associated with diabetes. The peripheral arterial lesions in diabetics are indistinguishable from those in nondiabetics, but their distribution in diabetics is characteristically different from that in nondiabetics and is much more frequently associated with focal medial calcification (Mönckeberg's sclerosis) in the same arterial segment (28).

Current evidence indicates that each late complication of diabetes arises at the end stage of a complex sequence of progressive structural alterations that is peculiar to an individual organ or system, even with regard to any critical component of microvascular disease, and is not unique to diabetes. This suggests that, aside from the common inciting role of hyperglycemia, the pathogenesis of each clinical complication of diabetes is probably an independent process whose nature is determined primarily by distinctive features of the biology and structure of the affected organ or system.

There is evidence that hyperglycemia is the governing factor in the earlier stages in the pathology in the kidney and retina. However, once the initial pattern of pathology in the kidney and retina progresses to a given stage, processes that are not governed by hyperglycemia determine whether progression to clinical manifestations occurs (24,29,33). Since a similar situation may obtain in the other commonly affected tissues, efforts to identify the mechanisms by which hyperglycemia directly contributes to risks for late complications of diabetes must logically focus on early events. Hyperglycemia could contribute by many mechanisms, including some that operate only in a single organ or system. However, during the era in which virtually all type I diabetics were treated in a manner that resulted in chronic persistent hyperglycemia, albeit of varying degrees, a majority of the few fortunate patients who survived for 40 or more years had no clinically significant complication of any type (32). These survivors appear to have been a self-selected group with an innate "immunity" to hyperglycemia-induced risks for disease in all of the usually susceptible organs and systems. This first suggested that hyperglycemia might make its major contribution to the risks for all of the common complications of diabetes through a common biochemical mechanism whose modification by a genetic variation could reduce the risks in all of the susceptible organs and systems.

EARLY FUNCTIONAL ALTERATIONS

Evidence for a common initiating mechanism developed from studies of the early subclinical alterations that are commonly demonstrable in the organs and systems susceptible to late complications of diabetes in patients with type I diabetes of short duration. These are termed *functional* alterations because at the outset they can be corrected by stringent control of hyperglycemia (19,20,24,29). Animals with experimental or spontaneous diabetes develop similar functional alterations, which become readily demonstrable in the individual tissues within 10 days to several weeks; this has facilitated their study (19,23,25,35,48,49). The functional alteration in the individual tissues varies markedly in nature (Table 7.1). However, all of the well studied early functional alterations are now known to be markers for early hyperglycemia-induced derangements in the tissue that result from activation of the common initiating mechanism in some tissue components and the inhibition of a specific Na^+K^+-ATPase regulatory system. This induces diverse secondary effects in the individual tissues, which can, in most instances, be linked to risks for inciting disease. It is of note that in a number of the affected tissues the common initiating mechanism induces alterations in vascular autoregulation or/ and permeability to which secondary alterations in the effects of specific vasoactive hormones and neurotransmitters contribute (Table 7.1). The early functional alteration in peripheral nerve is decreased nerve conduction velocity; this initially results from the effects of an abnormally high axonal $[Na^+]$ on the function of the voltage-gated Na^+-channels in the nodes of large myelinated axons. The common initiating mechanism also causes early changes

TABLE 7.1. Early Functional Alterations

Peripheral nerve conduction velocity ↓
   ↑ Axonal $[Na^+]$ affects voltage-gated Na^+-channels in myelinated fibers

Renal glomerular hyperfiltration
   Deranged regulation of glomerular hemodynamics; altered effects of angiotension II and adenosine

Retinal blood flow ↑, *deranged autoregulation, changes in blood–retinal barrier(s)*
   ↑ Albumin permeation corrected by histamine H_1 receptor antagonist
   ↓ R. pigmented epithelium transport functions, ↑ RPE $[Na^+]$

Blood pressure responses to norepinephrine and angiotension II ↑
Aortic contractile responses to above agonists ↑
   Aortic Na^+K^+-ATPase ↓ Impaired modulation of contraction

Plasma albumin permeation into aorta ↑
   Corrected by histamine H_1 receptor antagonist

---

in the number of intramembranous (proteinaceous) particles in the freeze-fracture surfaces of internodal myelin membrane and has been linked to the later development of axoglial dysjunction, which is postulated to be the first irreversible structural alteration in nerve (19,38).

The early functional alteration in kidney is glomerular hyperfiltration; this results from a derangement in the regulation in glomerular capillary hemodynamics at the afferent arteriole, to which secondary derangements in the normal effects of angiotensin II and adenosine contribute (17,23,29,34). Some nephrologists postulate that the resulting renal glomerular hypertension is the major factor in inciting the development of diabetic glomerulopathy (23). The emphasis they place on physical effects is open to question, but the derangements in metabolism and hemodynamic regulation induced in the glomerular microcirculation by the common initiating mechanism are generally agreed to play a role in inciting disease in the kidney in diabetes.

Type I diabetics and diabetic animals exhibit early increases in retinal blood flow that reflect a derangement in vascular autoregulation, which normally coordinates local blood flow with local energy utilization (25,35). The retinal capillary mural cells (pericytes) are thought to play a major role in retinal vascular autoregulation, and hyalinization of mural cells is one early structural alteration in retinal capillaries in diabetes (25). The retinal capillaries resemble brain capillaries in structure and permeability characteristics and are one component of the blood–retinal barrier. The other component, the retinal pigmented epithelium (RPE), lies between the choroid and the neuroretina. The composition of the retinal extracellular fluid (ECF) is normally regulated by active transport of ions and metabolites in the retinal capillary endothelial cell and RPE and by their roles as diffusion barriers (e.g. to albumin). In addition to causing early alterations in retinal vascular autoregulation, the common initiating mechanism causes early alterations in the blood–retinal barrier and in the transport functions of the RPE. In diabetic animals the initiating mechanism causes an abnormal increase in plasma albumin permeation into retina, which can be prevented by treating the animals with a histamine H_1 receptor antagonist [(35); Chapter 6].

Some workers have reported an early reversible alteration in the blood–retinal barrier to IV injected fluorescein in type I diabetics and in diabetic animals (25). In diabetic animals the RPE exhibits decreased Na^+K^+-ATPase activity, an abnormally elevated $[Na^+]$, impaired active transport of fluorescein out of retina, early ultrastructural changes, and an alteration in its contribution to the electroretinogram, which is also an effect of the common initiating mechanism (27). It is of note that alterations in retinal vascular autoregulation, in the blood–retinal barrier, and in the function of the RPE are factors implicated in the development of specific types of retinopathy in nondiabetics. Furthermore, the common initiating mechanism has been linked to the later development of retinal capillary basement membrane thickening in diabetic animals (7).

Normotensive type I diabetics exhibit increased pressor responses to norepinephrine and angiotensin II, and aortae from diabetic animals exhibit increased contractile responses to the same agonists (4,8,13,36). The common initiating mechanism induces decreased Na^+K^+-ATPase activity in aorta (41), which is a potential explanation for the increased contractile responses to these vasoactive agonists in aorta (and some resistance vessels). In addition, as will be noted later, it also has the potential of impairing adenosine modulation of vascular smooth muscle contraction in some blood vessels. Abnormal albumin accumulation in the walls of many arteries has been observed in patients with diabetes. In diabetic animals the common initiating mechanism causes an early abnormal increase in plasma albumin permeation into aorta, which presumably reflects some abnormality in the aortic endothelium (35); this effect can be prevented by treatment with a histamine H_1 receptor antagonist (Chapter 6).

EARLY FORMULATIONS OF THE COMMON INITIATING MECHANISM

It became apparent that hyperglycemia acts through a common mechanism in peripheral nerve, kidney, and retina to cause decreased Na^+K^+-ATPase activity and early functional alterations in some tissue components, when it was observed that these effects in the three tissues could be prevented in diabetic animals by the same distinctive panel of three independent types of treatment (48,19,10,35). They can be prevented by very stringent control of the hyperglycemia with insulin. They can also be prevented without insulin treatment or any decrease in the hyperglycemia, either by administering an aldose reductase inhibitor or by raising the otherwise normal micromolar plasma *myo*-inositol levels ~7-fold by increasing dietary *myo*-inositol content to a pharmacological level. Thus before the nature of the common initiating mechanism was clarified its identifying characteristics were known to be that it mediates a hyperglycemia-induced decrease in Na^+K^+-ATPase activity and induces functional alterations that can be prevented both by aldose reductase inhibitors and by raising normal plasma *myo*-inositol levels ~7-fold.

Virtually all of the earlier efforts to clarify the nature of the initiating mechanism were of the following nature. In tissues from normal animals and from diabetic animals that had been untreated or treated with insulin, an aldose reductase inhibitor, or by raising their plasma *myo*-inositol, investigators examined the affected functional parameter, Na^+K^+-ATPase activity (usually by assaying total ouabain-inhibitable ATPase activity in tissue homogenates), and the levels of specific metabolites. They attempted to relate the effects of the different treatments on Na^+K^+-ATPase activity and the functional parameter to their effects on the tissue levels of glucose, polyol pathway metabolites (sorbitol, fructose), and *myo*-inositol. In these studies tissues from the diabetic animals were almost invariably examined at an arbitrarily selected time point 2 to several weeks after the onset of diabetes. This resulted from the assumption that weeks of hyperglycemia were required to activate the common initiating mechanism and cause the decreased Na^+K^+-ATPase activity that induced the functional alteration. In interpreting the data it was tacitly assumed that the metabolite levels observed at the time point selected reflected those present when the effect of the initiating mechanism on Na^+K^+-ATPase activity first developed (10,19,48,49). Such studies provided some useful information, which is summarized below, but they also generated misinterpretations and controversy because of the limitations of the experimental approach and the assumptions employed in interpreting the data (49).

In general, the tissues in which the effects of the common initiating mechanism are observed are tissues in which insulin does not regulate glucose transport (or utilization), and in which hyperglycemia causes an increase in tissue glucose that reflects an increase in the free intracellular glucose level. In whole peripheral nerve (and isolated endoneurium), renal glomeruli, and retina, the increased glucose level in tissue from diabetic animals was associated with increased levels of polyol pathway metabolites. The polyol pathway involves the reduction of D-glucose to sorbitol by an aldose reductase and the subsequent oxidation of sorbitol to D-fructose by a NAD:polyol dehydrogenase. Contrary to a common misperception, the enzymes of the polyol pathway are widely distributed, and most mammalian tissues contain components in which this pathway is operative under physiological conditions, although in most tissues its normal function is unknown. Aldose reductases have high K_ms for glucose (~50 mM in human placenta), and in most tissues and cell types in which hyperglycemia increases the free intracellular glucose level, it induces increased polyol pathway activity, which fluctuates with the plasma glucose level. In a number of tissues and cell types (e.g. human erythrocytes) this increased polyol pathway activity does not have significant adverse effects in diabetics (49). However, in the tissues in which the common initiating mechanism causes decreased Na$^+$K$^+$-ATPase activity and induces early functional effects in diabetic animals, treatment with an aldose reductase inhibitor that prevented the increased levels of polyol metabolites prevented the effects of the initiating mechanism. In the same tissues the effects of the initiating mechanism were prevented without any decrease in the elevated levels of polyol pathway metabolites when the normal plasma *myo*-inositol levels in diabetic animals were raised ~7-fold. Increased polyol pathway activity was known to impair *myo*-inositol transport in a number of tissues and cell types, and it was found that this effect could be rapidly induced in normal peripheral nerve endoneurium by raising medium glucose from a normal to an elevated plasma glucose level to induce increased polyol pathway activity, and that the effect was prevented when an aldose reductase inhibitor was added (16). *Thus it was inferred that in the tissues in which the common initiating mechanism operates, hyperglycemia induces increased polyol pathway activity that impairs* myo-*inositol transport at a normal plasma (ECF)* myo-*inositol level, which leads to some secondary alteration in* myo-*inositol metabolism that causes decreased Na$^+$K$^+$-ATPase activity and induces the functional alteration* (19,48).

The controversy generated by these studies concerned the "*myo*-inositol depletion" hypothesis (19). It was found that diabetes of a specific number of weeks duration caused a 20%–30% decrease in the normal *myo*-inositol contents of peripheral nerve and renal glomeruli that was prevented in diabetic animals treated with an aldose reductase inhibitor or by raising their plasma *myo*-inositol (10,19). The *myo*-inositol depletion hypothesis postulated that the effect of the common initiating mechanism on Na$^+$K$^+$-ATPase activity required a slowly developing, significant decrease in the tissue's normal *myo*-inositol content (19). This hypothesis became untenable when it was observed that the decrease in Na$^+$K$^+$-ATPase activity in renal glomeruli is demonstrable weeks before there is any detectable decrease in the tissue's *myo*-inositol content (10). Current evidence indicates that activation of the initiating mechanism does not require a measurable decrease in the tissue's normal *myo*-inositol content, but that in some of the affected tissues there is a delayed secondary decrease in *myo*-inositol content, which can be transient (49,26). Thus these earlier studies left unexplained why, in specific tissues, a polyol pathway–induced impairment of *myo*-inositol transport causes decreased Na^+K^+-ATPase activity that occurs without a measurable decrease in the tissue's normal *myo*-inositol content. This problem was resolved by recent studies in which the common initiating mechanism was acutely activated and studied in vitro for the first time in normal rabbit aortic intima-media (AIM); this led to the recognition that the initiating mechanism decreases Na^+K^+-ATPase activity by inhibiting a novel adenosine-Na^+K^+-ATPase regulatory system that is critically dependent on ECF *myo*-inositol transport to maintain its normal operation, although *myo*-inositol transport is not required for the maintenance of the major *myo*-inositol pools in the tissue (41,42). Before considering this new information some aspects of the metabolism of *myo*-inositol and of phosphoinositides (*myo*-inositol-containing phospholipids) require comment.

myo-INOSITOL AND PHOSPHOINOSITIDE METABOLISM

myo-inositol, a cyclic hexitol, is a normal constituent of the diet and plasma, and it is present in all cells both as free *myo*-inositol and as a constituent of phosphoinositides. Plasma *myo*-inositol is regulated by the kidney in a manner that is specifically designed to maintain very low (micromolar) stable levels that are only minimally affected by normal variations in dietary *myo*-inositol intake (9). In contrast most tissues normally maintain high total *myo*-inositol contents (e.g. ~6 mmol/kg in normal rabbit aortic intima-media) that do not require dietary *myo*-inositol for their maintenance (9). The major mechanisms by which most tissues maintain their high *myo*-inositol contents are endogenous synthesis and the recovery of *myo*-inositol from the phosphorylated-*myo*-inositols released during the turnover (hydrolysis) of endogenous phosphoinositides (37). Active transport of ECF *myo*-inositol is demonstrable in most tissues, but it does not appear to be essential for the maintenance of the major *myo*-inositol pools in most tissues (37). However, tissue *myo*-inositol is comprised of heterogeneous cellular and subcellular pools, and some tissues appear to contain very small discrete *myo*-inositol pools that are peculiarly dependent on ECF *myo*-inositol transport for their maintenance. The major fate of *myo*-inositol in cells is its use for phosphatidylinositol synthesis. Phosphatidylinositol is a normal constituent of most cellular membranes and is the precursor from which the smaller quantities of the classic membrane polyphosphoinositides [phosphatidylinositol 4-phosphate (PIP) and phosphatidylinositol 4,5-biphosphate (PIP_2)] are derived by sequential phosphorylations of the *myo*-inositol-moiety of phosphatidylinositol. Phosphatidylinositol synthesis occurs primarily in endoplasmic reticulum, which characteristically contains a phosphatidylinositol synthetase that has a millimolar K_m for *myo*-inositol, but in some cells it also occurs in plasma membrane, where it is mediated by a phosphatidylinositol synthetase that has a very low (micromolar) K_m for *myo*-inositol.

Many hormones and neurotransmitters (e.g. angiotensin II, norepinephrine, histamine) act through receptors whose transduction mechanism is activation of phospholipase C hydrolysis of PIP_2 in a small, discrete plasma membrane pool (3,22). This initiates biological effects by releasing a specific phosphorylated *myo*-inositol (D-*myo*-inositol 1,4,5-P_3), which acutely increases cytosolic Ca^{2+} by stimulating its release from intracellular stores, and by releasing a *sn*-1,2-diacylglycerol (DAG), which can activate a protein kinase C at the membrane site where it is produced and transiently accumulates. When an agonist that acts through a receptor that stimulates phospholipase C hydrolysis of PIP_2 stimulates a resting tissue it evokes agonist-stimulated phosphoinositide turnover (ASPT), acute sequential increases in the isotopic turnover of discrete pools of PIP_2 and phosphatidylinositol (22). The increased phosphatidylinositol turnover in ASPT reflects, in part, a secondary (non-receptor-controlled) increase in phospholipase C hydrolysis of phosphatidylinositol in specific discrete phosphatidylinositol pools, which has effects that are attributed to a release of DAG (12,22). Stimulation of a resting tissue by an agonist that evokes ASPT commonly causes a secondary increase in a fraction of phosphatidylinositol synthesis that selectively replenishes the phosphatidylinositol and PIP_2 pools, in which the agonist stimulates hydrolysis (22). The biological effects of agonists that evoke ASPT and their secondary stimulation of phosphatidylinositol synthesis have been routinely demonstrated in isolated tissues and cells in medium lacking *myo*-inositol, i.e. under conditions in which *myo*-inositol transport is inhibited (3,6,21,22). Thus there is no intimation that the maintenance of the phosphoinositide pools required for the effects of agonists that evoke ASPT are critically dependent on *myo*-inositol transport. This made it unlikely that the common initiating mechanism causes decreased Na^+K^+-ATPase activity by inhibiting a Na^+K^+-ATPase regulatory mechanism that involved classic ASPT. This view was reinforced by the observation that diabetes does not impair PIP_2 synthesis or turnover in rat peripheral nerve (14). However, it was found that the decreased Na^+K^+-ATPase activity exhibited by resting intact peripheral nerve endoneurium from diabetic rabbits is acutely corrected by a synthetic DAG that can activate protein kinase(s) C in intact cells; this DAG did not stimulate Na^+K^+-ATPase activity in endoneurium from normal animals (18). This suggested that the common initiating mechanism decreases Na^+K^+-ATPase activity by inhibiting a regulatory system that uses phospholipase C hydrolysis of a phosphoinositide and a release of DAG as its effector arm. For the reasons previously cited it was unlikely that this regulatory system involved classic ASPT, and this view was reinforced by the fact that the common initiating mechanism causes a decrease in Na^+K^+-ATPase activity that is apparent in resting peripheral nerve endoneurium.

It had been known for decades that in a number of resting tissues a small phosphatidylinositol pool exhibits persistent rapid basal turnover, even when an antagonist of an agonist that evokes ASPT in the tissue is added (1,45). Because basal phosphatidylinositol turnover was distinct from ASPT, it was not believed to play a role in mediating hormonal effects. We speculated that some basal phosphatidylinositol turnover might reflect the transduction mechanism of an autacoid (local hormone) that normally operates in the resting isolated tissue.

CLARIFICATION OF THE COMMON INITIATING MECHANISM

Identification of an Adenosine-Na$^+$K$^+$-ATPase Regulatory System That Uses Basal Phosphatidylinositol Turnover as Its Effector Arm

The possibility that the tissues in which the common initiating mechanism operates contain a Na$^+$K$^+$-ATPase regulatory system that involves basal phosphatidylinositol turnover and requires *myo*-inositol transport at a normal ECF *myo*-inositol level to maintain its operation was initially examined in the following manner. Normal resting rabbit peripheral nerve endoneurium and aortic intima-media (AIM) were incubated with 5 mM glucose and the micromolar *myo*-inositol levels normally present in CSF and plasma (70 μM), respectively, and the effects of inhibiting *myo*-inositol transport by depriving these tissues of their normal ECF *myo*-inositol levels were examined (39,40). Endoneurium and AIM do not require their normal ECF *myo*-inositol levels to maintain their normal high *myo*-inositol contents during incubations, but depriving either tissue of its normal ECF *myo*-inositol level for 30 min selectively inhibits a major distinct component of its normal resting Na$^+$K$^+$-ATPase activity and a distinct fraction of its normal basal phosphatidylinositol synthesis. In AIM provided with medium *myo*-inositol in a normal plasma level, the addition of a competitive inhibitor of *myo*-inositol transport (scylloinositol) selectively and reversibly inhibits the same distinct components of normal resting Na$^+$K$^+$-ATPase activity and of basal phosphatidylinositol synthesis. Thus in both nerve and aortic wall *myo*-inositol transport is required to maintain distinct components of normal resting phosphatidylinositol synthesis and Na$^+$K$^+$-ATPase activity, but it is not required to maintain the major tissue *myo*-inositol pools or another major fraction of normal basal phosphatidylinositol synthesis. These observations were explained by an extension of these studies in AIM (40,41,42).

Aorta intima-media was found to contain a novel adenosine-Na$^+$K$^+$-ATPase regulatory system by which endogenously released adenosine normally stimulates and maintains a major distinct component of normal resting Na$^+$K$^+$-ATPase activity (42). [Adenosine is released by most tissues in a manner that varies with their activity and energy state. Extracellular adenosine functions as a local hormone and mediates diverse autoregulatory effects through receptors of several types (2,11,31,44). Most adenosine effects are mediated through receptors that inhibit (A$_1$) or stimulate (A$_2$) adenylate cyclase, but other types of receptors have been postulated (11,44).] The adenosine effect on Na$^+$K$^+$-ATPase activity in resting AIM is mediated through a novel type of adenosine receptor, whose transduction mechanism is stimulation of rapid basal phosphatidylinositol turnover (hydrolysis) in a small discrete phosphatidylinositol pool (Fig. 7.1). As will be discussed later in greater detail, the phosphatidylinositol pool that is required for the adenosine stimulation of a distinct component of Na$^+$K$^+$-ATPase activity is maintained by a distinct frac-

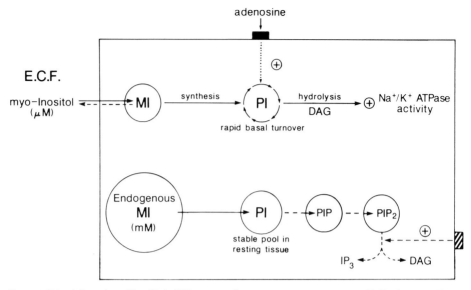

FIGURE 7.1. Adenosine-(Na$^+$K$^+$)-ATPase regulatory system in aortic wall. Endogenously released adenosine stimulates a distinct component of normal resting (Na$^+$K$^+$)-ATPase activity by stimulating basal phosphatidylinositol (PI) turnover (hydrolysis) in a discrete PI pool; this appears to act by releasing diacylglycerol (DAG) at specific membrane sites. The PI pool required for the operation of this system is maintained by a fraction of PI synthesis that is selectively dependent on *myo*-inositol (MI) transport at a normal E.C.F. (plasma) level. The common initiating mechanism causes decreased (Na$^+$K$^+$)-ATPase activity by inducing increased polyol pathway activity, which impairs MI transport at a normal plasma level, and inhibiting the replenishment of the "adenosine-sensitive" PI pool. The major tissue MI pools do not require MI transport for their maintenance; they support another major fraction of basal PI synthesis that is not dependent on MI transport, which provides PI that enters the PI pool but that does not turn over rapidly in resting tissue, but that is used to a very small extent for polyphosphoinositide (PIP and PIP$_2$) formation in resting tissue. MI transport is not required to maintain the PIP$_2$ pools used to initiate the effects of agonists that act through receptors that stimulate PIP$_2$ hydrolysis; and the common initiating mechanism does not inhibit the effects of these agonists.

tion of normal basal de novo phosphatidylinositol synthesis that selectively requires *myo*-inositol transport at a normal plasma *myo*-inositol level to prevent its inhibition. The rapid basal turnover of the adenosine-sensitive phosphatidylinositol pool is not attributable to its use for polyphosphoinositide formation and reflects basal phosphatidylinositol hydrolysis of some type (40). When the adenosine-stimulated component of normal resting Na$^+$K$^+$-ATPase activity is selectively inhibited by adding adenosine deaminase (ADA) to the medium to degrade endogenously released adenosine, it can be restored by adding a synthetic DAG, 1-oleoyl-2-acetylglycerol (OAG), which can activate protein kinase(s) C in intact cells. The synthetic OAG does not stimulate Na$^+$K$^+$-ATPase activity in AIM when the adenosine-stimulated component is operative (42). Thus endogenously released adenosine normally stimulates and maintains a major distinct component of normal resting Na$^+$K$^+$-ATPase activity in AIM through a receptor that stimulates rapid basal phosphatidylinositol hydrolysis in a discrete phosphatidylinositol pool, and this appears to be a phospholipase C hydrolysis of phosphatidylinositol that acts through a release of DAG at specific membrane sites to stimulate a distinct component of Na^+K^+-ATPase activity. Whether adenosine selectively stimulates the activity of a specific Na^+K^+-ATPase molecular isoform remains to be clarified, but this is suspected to be the case.

The continued normal operation of the adenosine-Na^+K^+-ATPase regulatory system in resting AIM is critically dependent on *myo*-inositol transport at its normal low ECF (plasma) concentration. In resting AIM incubated with 5 mM glucose, *myo*-inositol transport is not required to maintain the major fraction of the tissue's normal basal de novo phosphatidylinositol synthesis; this fraction remains constant when the tissue is deprived of medium *myo*-inositol in a normal plasma level or when a competitive inhibitor of *myo*-inositol transport is added (40,41). It forms glycerol and arachidonic acid-labeled phosphatidylinositol during a 15 or 30 min pulse that selectively labels phosphatidylinositol pools that exhibit no significant turnover during a 30 min chase, but have been shown to be the source of all of the very small quantities of newly synthesized glycerol and arachidonic acid–labeled phosphatidylinositol that are converted to classic PIP and PIP_2 in resting AIM [(40); Fig. 7.1]. The adenosine-sensitive phosphatidylinositol pool is replenished by another distinct fraction of normal basal de novo phosphatidylinositol synthesis and arachidonic acid incorporation into phosphatidylinositol, which is demonstrable only when medium *myo*-inositol in a normal plasma level is provided and is selectively inhibited when a competitive inhibitor of *myo*-inositol transport is added [(40,41); Fig. 7.1]. This fraction of basal phosphatidylinositol synthesis forms an additional component of labeled phosphatidylinositol during a 15 or 30 min pulse that completely disappears during a 30 min chase (40,41). The rapid basal turnover of this fraction of labeled phosphatidylinositol is completely inhibited when ADA is added to degrade endogenously released adenosine (42). The adenosine-sensitive phosphatidylinositol pool turns over completely within 30 min in resting AIM in response to endogenously released adenosine, and if the replenishment of this phosphatidylinositol pool is inhibited by omitting medium *myo*-inositol in a normal plasma level or by adding a competitive inhibitor of *myo*-inositol transport, then the adenosine-stimulated component of Na^+K^+-ATPase activity disappears within 30 min. Under these conditions it cannot be restored by adenosine analogues, but it is restored by a synthetic DAG, 1-oleoyl-2-acetylglycerol (42). Thus the continued normal operation of the adenosine-Na^+K^+-ATPase regulatory system is peculiarly dependent on *myo*-inositol transport at a normal plasma *myo*-inositol level, because the fraction of basal phosphatidylinositol synthesis that maintains the "adenosine-sensitive" phosphatidylinositol pool appears to be located in a specific cell type or subcellular site (plasma membrane?), where it requires a small *myo*-inositol pool that is peculiarly dependent on *myo*-inositol transport for its maintenance.

The Common Initiating Mechanism Inhibits the Adenosine Na^+K^+-ATPase Regulatory System

It was recently found that the common initiating mechanism can be acutely activated and studied in vitro in normal resting AIM, and that it selectively inhibits the component of Na^+K^+-ATPase activity that is normally maintained by the adenosine-Na$^+$K$^+$-ATPase regulatory system (41,42). In resting AIM incubated with normal plasma levels of glucose (5 mM) and *myo*-inositol (70 μM), raising the medium glucose to a threshold elevated plasma level (10 mM) for 40 min prior to and during a 20 min assessment of Na$^+$K$^+$-ATPase–mediated ^{86}Rb$^+$/K$^+$ uptake selectively and completely inhibits the adenosine-stimulated component of normal resting Na$^+$K$^+$-ATPase activity. Raising the medium glucose to 20 or 30 mM causes no greater decrease in the tissue's Na$^+$K$^+$-ATPase activity. The inhibition of Na$^+$K$^+$-ATPase activity caused by exposing AIM to medium glucose in an elevated plasma level (30 mM) can be prevented by adding an aldose reductase inhibitor (both 10 μM sorbinil and 1 μM tolrestat are effective) or by raising the medium *myo*-inositol from a normal plasma level to one ~7-fold higher (500 μM). (Adding an aldose reductase inhibitor or raising the medium *myo*-inositol has no effect on Na$^+$K$^+$-ATPase activity in AIM incubated with 5 mM glucose.) Thus exposing AIM to medium glucose at an elevated plasma level causes an inhibition of Na$^+$K$^+$-ATPase activity that has the identifying characteristics of the common initiating mechanism. Raising the medium glucose induces increased polyol pathway activity in AIM (30), which makes *myo*-inositol transport at a normal plasma level inadequate to prevent the selective inhibition of the fraction of phosphatidylinositol synthesis that replenishes the "adenosine-sensitive" phosphatidylinositol pool [(41); Fig. 7.1]. This fraction of phosphatidylinositol synthesis is restored when the medium *myo*-inositol is raised ~7-fold or when an aldose reductase inhibitor is added. It is of note that exposing AIM to medium glucose in an elevated plasma glucose level causes no measureable decrease in its normal total *myo*-inositol content (30,41). *Thus in tissues in which the common initiating mechanism operates, hyperglycemia induces increased polyol pathway activity that impairs* myo-*inositol transport at a normal ECF* myo-*inositol level, which causes decreased Na$^+$K$^+$-ATPase activity because the affected tissue components contain a novel adenosine-Na$^+$K$^+$-ATPase regulatory system that is critically dependent on* myo-*inositol transport to maintain its normal operation (Fig. 7.1).*

IMPLICATIONS OF THE NATURE OF THE COMMON INITIATING MECHANISM

A number of the features of the common initiating mechanism provide potential explanations for aspects of the association between diabetes mellitus and risks for disease and late clinical complications in a restricted group of susceptible organs and systems. It is now clear that hyperglycemia can activate the initiating mechanism only in tissues that contain cells in which a restrictive combination of requirements are met. Hyperglycemia must induce an increase in free intracellular glucose in these cells and induce increased polyol pathway activity. The later must impair *myo*-inositol transport at the cells' normal ECF *myo*-inositol level. The cells must contain the adenosine-Na$^+$K$^+$-ATPase regulatory system that requires *myo*-inositol transport to maintain its operation. This restrictive combination of requirements for the activation of the common initiating mechanism could explain why a specific group of organs and systems is peculiarly susceptible to hyperglycemia-induced risks for disease.

The nature of the common initiating mechanism is such that it has the potential to be the major mechanism by which hyperglycemia directly affects the organs and systems in which it incites risks for disease. It can also explain why diabetes of short duration induces alterations in vascular autoregulation and permeability to which secondary alterations in the effects of specific vasoactive hormones and neurotransmitters may contribute. It was previously assumed that the adverse effects of activating the common initiating mechanism in components of a tissue were restricted to the numerous potential consequences of inducing a persistent inappropriately low level of Na^+K^+-ATPase activity in them. These well-recognized potential consequences include alterations in intracellular $[Na^+]$; the Na^+ and K^+ gradients across the plasma membrane; the function of voltage-gated Na^+-channels and voltage-gated Ca^{2+}-channels; the active transport of metabolites that are co-transported with Na^+ (e.g. amino acids, creatine); the regulation of cell volume, pH, and cytosolic Ca^{2+}; and, the effects of hormones and neurotransmitters whose effects might be augmented by a secondary impairment of the Na^+/Ca^{2+}-exchange mechanism (e.g. angiotensin II, norepinephrine, histamine). Many of the early functional alterations and early metabolic derangements observed in tissues in which the common initiating mechanism operates are attributable to potential effects of a chronic, inappropriately low level of Na^+K^+-ATPase activity in some component cells. Moreover, the nature of these potential effects is such that the prolonged survival of the affected cells might be expected to require significant cellular adaptations. However, in addition to these effects, the initiating mechanism has the potential of causing adverse effects by inhibiting some acute autoregulatory effects that may normally be mediated through the adenosine-Na^+K^+-ATPase regulatory system.

Adenosine release by most tissues increases with biological activity and in response to acute imbalances in ATP utilization and production (11,31). Extracellular adenosine mediates acute autoregulatory effects on local tissue metabolism, local microcirculatory hemodynamics, arterial tone, and local tissue responses to specific hormones and neurotransmitters (2,11,31). It has been suggested that the pattern of adenosine's effects is designed to help maintain normal energy balance, as exemplified by adenosine's role in coordinating the regulation of local microcirculatory blood flow with local tissue biological activity and energy utilization (2). Most adenosine effects are mediated through receptors that inhibit or stimulate adenylate cyclase (11,44), and it was not previously known that in specific tissues adenosine can also act through a different type of receptor to stimulate Na^+K^+-ATPase activity. Our studies of the adenosine-Na^+K^+-ATPase regulatory system have been restricted to studies in resting tissue, because this facilitated the establishment of a distinction between the mechanism of the adenosine effect on Na^+K^+-ATPase activity and classic ASPT. There is, however, a strong probability that one of the normal functions of this system is to mediate some of adenosine's acute autoregulatory effects in stimulated peripheral nerve and vascular smooth muscle (VSM) through acute increases in electrogenic Na^+K^+-ATPase activity. Na^+K^+-ATPase activity is electrogenic because it translocates Na^+ and K^+ across the plasma membrane in a ratio of 3:2, and it makes a significant contribution to the membrane potential in peripheral nerve and VSM under some physiological conditions. In these excitable tissues an acute stimulation of Na^+K^+-ATPase activity that induces hyperpolarization is known to mediate specific acute autoregulatory effects, such as post-tetanic hyperpolarization (50) and modulation of VSM contraction by an endogenously released vasodilator, "hyperpolarizing factor" (46). The stimulus for the acute increase in Na^+K^+-ATPase activity that abruptly occurs after cessation of repetitive nerve stimulation and the chemical nature of "hyperpolarizing factor" are still unknown. It is of interest that peripheral nerve stimulation increases adenosine release (31) and that adenosine is known to be one of the vasodilator factors released by arteries and resistence vessels in response to specific vasoconstrictive stimuli (46). Inhibition of the adenosine-Na^+K^+-ATPase regulatory system by the common initiating mechanism and the loss of specific normal adenosine-mediated acute autoregulatory effects is a likely explanation for the early initiating-mechanism–induced alterations in vascular autoregulation in retina and glomeruli in human and experimental diabetes and may contribute to the increased contractile responses to norepinephrine and angiotensin II in aortae from diabetic animals. It is of note that it has recently been found that the normal effect of adenosine on glomerular filtration rate (a decrease) is lost in diabetic animals and is restored when they are treated with an aldose reductase inhibitor (34).

The common initiating mechanism also has the potential to explain hyperglycemia-induced risks for disease in the tissues in which it operates that are not a simple and predictable function of the usual absolute level of hyperglycemia in a patient with diabetes. This is apparent from the previously discussed evidence that secondary alterations in the effects of specific vasoactive hormones significantly contribute to the effects of the mechanism in a number of the tissues susceptible to late complications. In addition, the observation that in normal aortic wall exposure for only 60 min to a relatively modest threshold level of "hyperglycemia" (180 mg/dl) is adequate to activate the initiating mechanism and induce its maximal initial effect on Na^+K^+-ATPase activity, clearly indicates that there can be no simple relationship between the usual absolute degree of hyperglycemia and the effects of the mechanism in the individual organs and systems susceptible to late complications of diabetes. This observation also explains why the demonstration of an effect of insulin treatment on the early initiating-mechanism–induced functional alterations in type I diabetics and diabetic animals generally requires a period of persistent, very stringent restriction of their hyperglycemia.

THE COMMON INITIATING MECHANISM AND RISKS FOR VASCULAR DISEASE IN DIABETICS

It is now clear that in diabetic states hyperglycemia acts through the common initiating mechanism to cause its initial metabolic and functional effects in the retinal and glomerular microcirculations (which are not necessarily restricted to effects on capillaries or capillary endothelium) and in arterial wall. This suggests that in efforts to understand how hyperglycemia incites risks for disease in these tissues, the logical starting point is to develop a detailed understanding of the sequential consequences of continual activation of the initiating mechanism in them. There are already grounds to believe that the mechanism probably plays a major role in mediating the hyperglycemia-induced risks for disease in the retinal and glomerular microcirculations in diabetes. However, the specific manner in which the components of these two very different microcirculations are affected by continual activation of the mechanism over an extended period must be clarified before the critical factors in inciting risks for progressive structural alterations in them can be identified. It is already apparent that even at an early stage the in vivo effects of activating the common initiating mechanism in these microcirculations include effects resulting from secondary alterations in the release or response to specific vasoactive hormones, which may be difficult to reproduce in in vitro systems, such as cultured vascular cell types. This is a problem, but it also presents an opportunity since it is possible that some alterations in the effects of vasoactive hormones will prove to be critical in inciting risks for disease, and lead to new pharmacological approaches to reducing the risks for specific late complications.

Whether the common initiating mechanism contributes to the risks for the atherosclerotic late complications of diabetes mellitus remains a matter of conjecture. The prevailing view is that hyperglycemia-induced alterations in the arterial wall per se do not contribute to these risks. This view may prove to be correct, but even the early effects of the initiating mechanism in aorta (a model arterial wall) are such that one cannot summarily dismiss the possibility that the mechanism makes some contribution to the increased risks for atherosclerotic arterial disease in diabetes. The common initiating mechanism causes an alteration in aortic endothelium that results in an abnormal increase in plasma albumin (and presumably albumin-bound free fatty acids, a large fraction of which is unsaturated FFA) into the aortic wall. It also deranges Na^+K^+-ATPase regulation and has the potential to inhibit specific adenosine-mediated autoregulatory effects, which can explain the increased contractile responses of some arteries (and some resistance vessels) to angiotensin II and norepinephrine in diabetic states. There are possible links between these effects and current views of the pathogenesis of atherosclerosis (43) that require evaluation before a role for the common initiating mechanism can be excluded. The alteration in arterial endothelium induced by the mechanism (an alteration to which histamine contributes) might convey a predisposition to local endothelial injury or alter interactions of the endothelium with blood platelets or macrophages. The increased plasma albumin free fatty acid permeation into arterial wall might tax the capacity of the local antioxidants and increase the peroxidation of the polyunsaturated fatty acid components of any low-density lipoprotein (LDL) that enters the arterial wall and increase its atherogenic potential (43). Finally, whether the effects of the common initiating mechanism in arterial wall can alter the proliferative response of locally subjacent VSM to focal endothelial injury merits evaluation. A separate, but not inconsequential, consideration is whether an initiating-mechanism–induced derangement in Na^+K^+-ATPase regulation in some resistance vessels contributes to the risks for hypertension in diabetes.

REFERENCES

1. AGRANOFF, B., and BLEASDALE, J. E. The acetylcholine phospholipid effect: What has it told us? In: *Cylitols and Phosphoinositides,* edited by W. W. Wells and F. Eisenberg, Jr. New York: Academic Press, 1978, pp. 105–120.
2. BERNE, R. M., KNABB, R. M., ELY, R. W., and RUBIO, R. Adenosine in the local regulation of blood flow; a brief overview. *Federation Proc.* 42: 3136–3142, 1983.
3. BERRIDGE, M. J. Inositol triphosphate and diacylglycerol: two interacting second messengers. *Annu. Rev. Biochem.* 56: 159–193, 1987.
4. BORDY, M. D., and DIXON, R. L. Vascular reactivity in experimental diabetes. *Circ. Res.* 14: 494–501, 1964.
5. BRADLEY, J., THOMAS, P. K., KING, R. H. M., LIEWELYN, J. G., MUDDLE, J. R., and WATKINS, P. J. Morphometry of endoneurial capillaries in diabetic sensory and autonomic neuropathy. *Diabetologia* 33: 611–618, 1990.
6. CAMPBELLS, M. D., DETH, R. C., PAYNE, R. A., and HONEYMAN, T. W. Phosphoinositide hydrolysis is correlated with agonist-induced calcium influx and contraction in rabbit aorta. *Eur. J. Pharmacol.* 116: 129–136, 1985.
7. CHANDLER, M. I., SABON, W. A., and DeSANTIS, L. Prevention of retinal capillary basement membrane thickening in diabetic rats by aldose reductase inhibitors. *Invest. Ophthalmol. Vis. Sci.* 25(Suppl.): 159, 1984.
8. CHRISTLIEB, A. R. Vascular reactivity to angiotensin II and norepinephrine in diabetic subjects. *Diabetes* 25: 269–274, 1976.
9. CLEMENTS, R. S., and DIETHHELM, A. G. The metabolism of *myo*-inositol by human kidney. *J. Lab. Clin. Med.* 93: 210–219, 1979.
10. COHEN, M. P. Aldose reductase, glomerular metabolism and diabetic nephropathy. *Metabolism* 35(Suppl 1): 55–59, 1986.
11. DALY, J. W. Adenosine receptors: targets for future drugs. *J. Med. Chem.* 25: 197–207, 1982.
12. DIXON, J. F., and HOKIN, L. E. Kinetic analysis of the formation of inositol 1:2 cyclic phosphate in carbochol-stimulated pancreatic minilobules. *J. Biol. Chem.* 264: 11721–11724, 1989.
13. DRURY, P. L., SMITH, G. M., and FERRISS, J. B. Increased vasopressor responsiveness to angiotensin II in type 1 (insulin-dependent) diabetic patients without complications. *Diabetologia* 27: 174–179, 1984.
14. EICHBERG, J., BERTI-MATTERA, K., BELL, M. E., and PETERSON, R. G. Changes in peripheral nerve polyphosphoinositide metabolism in experimental diabetes; nature and significance. In: *Inositol and Phosphoinositides: metabolism and regulation,* edited by J. E. Bleasdale, J. Eichberg, and G. Hauser. Clifton, NJ: Humana Press, 1985, pp. 583–599.
15. FEINGOLD, K. R., LEE, T. H., CHUNG, N. Y., and SIPERSTEIN, M. D. Muscle capillary basement membrane thickening in patients with Vacor-induced diabetes mellitus. *J. Clin. Invest.* 78: 102–107, 1986.
16. GILLON, K. R. W., and HAWTHORNE, J. N. Transport of MI into endoneurial preparations of sciatic nerve from normal and STZ-diabetic rats. *Biochem. J.* 210: 775–781, 1983.
17. GOLDFARB, S., SIMMONS, D. A., and KERN, E. F. O. Amelioration of glomerular hyperfiltration in acute experimental diabetes by dietary *myo*-inositol supplementation and aldose reductase inhibition. *Trans. Assoc. Am. Physicians* 99: 67–72, 1986.
18. GREENE, D. A., and LATTIMER, S. A. Protein kinase C agonists acutely normalize decreased ouabain-inhibitable respiration in diabetic nerve: implications for (Na$^+$,K$^+$)-ATPase regulation and diabetic complications. *Diabetes* 35: 242–245, 1986.
19. GREENE, D. A., LATTIMER, S. A., and SIMA, A. A. F. Biochemical alterations in peripheral nerve in animal diabetes. In: *Frontiers in Diabetes Research,* edited by E. Shaffrir and A. E. Renold. London: John Libbey & Co., 1988, pp. 463–470.
20. GREGERSON, G. Diabetic neuropathy: influence of age, sex, metabolic control and duration of diabetes on motor conduction velocity. *Neurology* 17: 972–980, 1967.
21. GRIENDLING, K. K., BERK, B. C., GANZ, P., GIMBRONE, M. A., JR., and ALEXANDER, R. W. Angiotensin II stimulation of vascular smooth muscle phosphoinositide metabolism. State of the art lecture. *Hypertension* 9(Suppl III): 181–185, 1987.
22. HOKIN, L. E. Receptors and phosphoinositide-generated second messengers. *Annu. Rev. Biochem.* 54: 205–235, 1985.
23. HOSTETTER, T. H., RENNKE, H. G., and BRENNER, B. M. The case for intrarenal hypertension in the initiation and progression of diabetic and other glomerulopathies. *Am. J. Med.* 72: 375–380, 1982.

24. KOHNER, E. M., McLOED, D., and MARSHALL, J. Diabetic eye disease. In: *Complications of Diabetes*, edited by H. Keen and J. Jarrett. London: Edward Arnold, 1982, pp. 99–108.

25. KOHNER, E. M. Microangiopathy: diabetic retinopathy. In: *Diabetic Complications*, edited by M. James and C. Crabbe. London: Churchill Livingstone, 1987, pp. 41–65.

26. KUSUMA, H., and STEWART, M. A. Levels of *myo*-inositol in normal and degenerating peripheral nerve. *J. Neurochem.* 14: 1057–1066, 1970.

27. MACGREGOR, L. C., and MATSCHINSKY, F. M. Treatment with aldose reductase inhibitors or with *myo*-inositol arrests deterioration of the electroretinogram of diabetic rats. *J. Clin. Invest.* 76: 887–889, 1985.

28. McMILLAN, D. E. The role of blood flow in diabetic vascular disease. In: *Diabetes Mellitus,* edited by H. Rifkin and D. Porte. New York: Elsevier Science, 1990, pp. 234–248.

29. MOGENSEN, E. E., and OSTERBY, R. Structural and functional alterations in the diabetic kidney. *Front Diabetes* 8: 67–81, 1987.

30. MORRISON, A. D., ORCI, L., PERRELET, A., and WINEGRAD, A. I. Studies of the effects of an elevated glucose concentration on the ultrastructure and composite metabolism of the intact aortic intima-media preparation. *Diabetes* 28: 720–723, 1979.

31. NEWBY, A. C. Adenosine and the concept of retaliatory metabolites. *Trends Biol. Sci.* 9: 42–44, 1984.

32. OAKLEY, W. G., PYKE, D. A., TATTERSALL, R. B., and WATKINS, P. J. Long-term diabetes. A clinical study of 92 patients after 40 years. *Q. J. Med.* 43: 145–146, 1974.

33. OSTERBY, R., GUNDERSEN, H. J. G., NYBERG, G., and AURELL, M. Advanced diabetic glomerulopathy. Quantitative structural characterization of nonoccluded glomeruli. *Diabetes* 36: 612–619, 1987.

34. PERMUTTER, J., JACOBS, J., ZIYADEH, F., SENESKY, D., SIMMONS, D. A., KERN, E. F. O., and GOLDFARB, S. Reduced renal vasoconstrictive response to adenosine and reversal by aldose reductase inhibition in acute experimental diabetes. *Clin. Res.* 37: 583A, 1989.

35. PUGLIESE, G., TILTON, R. G., SANTARELLI, E., EADES, D. M., PROVINCE, M. A., KILO, C., SHERMAN, W. R., and WILLIAMSON, J. R. Modulation of hemodynamic and vascular filtration changes in diabetic rats by dietary *myo*-inositol. *Diabetes* 39: 312–322, 1990.

36. SCARBOROUGH, N. L., and CARRIER, G. O. Increased alpha-2 adrenoreceptor mediated contraction in diabetic rats. *J. Auton. Pharmacol.* 3: 177–183, 1983.

37. SHERMAN, W. R., MUNSELL, L. Y., GISH, B. G., and HONCHAR, M. P. Effects of systemically administered lithium on phosphoinositide metabolism in rat brain, kidney, and testes. *J. Neurochem.* 44: 798–807, 1985.

38. SIMA, A. A. F., YAGIHASHI, S., and GREENE, D. A. Morphological features of human and animal diabetic nerve. In: *Diabetic Neuropathy,* edited by J. Ward and Y. Goto. Chichester: John Wiley & Sons, 1990, pp. 17–28.

39. SIMMONS, D. A., WINEGRAD, A. I., and MARTIN, D. B. Significance of tissue *myo*-inositol concentrations in metabolic regulation in nerve. *Science* 217: 848–851, 1982.

40. SIMMONS, D. A., KERN, E. F. O., WINEGRAD, A. I., and MARTIN, D. B. Basal phosphatidylinositol turnover controls aortic (Na$^+$,K$^+$)-ATPase activity. *J. Clin. Invest.* 77: 503–513, 1986.

41. SIMMONS, D. A., and WINEGRAD, A. I. Mechanism of glucose-induced (Na$^+$,K$^+$)-ATPase inhibition in aortic wall of rabbits. *Diabetologia* 32: 402–408, 1989.

42. SIMMONS, D. A., and WINEGRAD, A. I. Elevated extracellular glucose inhibits an adenosine-(Na$^+$,K$^+$)-ATPase regulatory system in rabbit aortic wall. *Diabetologia* 34: 157–163, 1991.

43. STEINBERG, D., PARTHASARATHY, S., CAREW, T. E., KHOO, J. C., and WITZUM, J. L. Beyond cholesterol: modifications of low density lipoprotein that increases it atherogenicity. *N. Engl. J. Med.* 320: 915–924, 1989.

44. STILES, G. L. Adenosine receptors: structure, function, and regulation. *Trends Physiol. Sci.* 7: 486–490, 1986.

45. TAKHAR, A. P. S., and KIRK, C. J. Stimulation of inorganic phosphate incorporation into phosphatidylinositol in rat thoracic aorta mediated through V$_1$-vasopressin receptors. *Biochem. J.* 194: 167–172, 1981.

46. VANHOUTTE, P. M. The endothelium-modulator of vascular smooth muscle tone. *N. Engl. J. Med.* 319: 512–513, 1988.

47. WEBB, R. C., LOCKETTE, W. E., VANHOUTTE, P. M., and BOHR, D. F. Sodium potassium-adenosine triphosphatase and vasodilation. In: *Vasodilation,* edited by P. M. Vanhoutte and I. Leusen. New York: Raven, 1981, pp. 319–330.

48. WINEGRAD, A. I. Does a common mechanism induce the diverse complications of diabetes? *Diabetes* 36: 396–406, 1987.

49. WINEGRAD, A. I., and SIMMONS, D. A. Common initiating mechanism for diabetic compli-
    cations. In: *Frontiers in Diabetes Research,* edited by E. Shaffrir and A. E. Renold.
    London: John Libbet & Co., 1988, pp. 455–462.
50. YAROWSKY, P. J., and INGVAR, D. H. Neuronal activity and energy metabolism. *Federation
    Proc.* 40: 2362–2362, 1981.

8

Dissociation of Retinopathy and Nephropathy in Animal Models of Diabetes: Diabetes vs Galactosemia

RONALD L. ENGERMAN AND TIMOTHY S. KERN

Microvascular disease in the retina and kidney accounts for much of the morbidity and mortality associated with diabetes mellitus. Retinopathy is seen in 98% of insulin-dependent patients at 15 yr of diabetes, and the risk of blindness in diabetes is reportedly 25 times greater than in the general population (16,23). Diabetic nephropathy is the major cause of all new cases of end-stage renal disease, becoming clinically apparent in 35% of diabetic patients (27,33).

The relationship of the microvascular disease to the metabolic disorders of diabetes, and to hyperglycemia in particular, has been difficult to determine in human subjects, and has remained a subject of continuing controversy. Much needed perspective on the question has been gained, however, in recent years from study of models of the retinopathy and nephropathy in laboratory animals. Many retinal and renal abnormalities of interest may develop in diabetic rats and other small animals, but such animals have yet to be shown to develop in a consistent fashion the saccular capillary aneurysms, pericyte loss, and mesangial expansion that are characteristic of diabetes mellitus in humans. Anatomic features of the retinopathy and nephropathy are more closely reproduced by diabetes in dogs, and studies in our laboratory have accordingly focused on that animal model.

RETINOPATHY IN THE DIABETIC DOG

Retinal lesions comparable to those of diabetic humans develop in dogs in which diabetes has appeared spontaneously or has been induced experimentally by any of several means (9). The lesions characteristic of early diabetic retinopathy in both humans and dogs include microaneurysms, acellular and nonperfused capillaries, varicose dilated capillaries (IRMAs; intra-retinal microvascular abnormalities), and dot and blot hemorrhages. The capillary aneurysms, which are typically saccular and at inception thin-walled, usually do not appear in the dog until after 2 or more years following the induction of diabetes. By that time, some subtle loss of capillary pericytes and closure of capillaries may be found.

151

With progression of the retinopathy, increasing numbers of retinal capillaries come to possess endothelial cells but few or no pericytes. The disappearance of pericytes may be evident from an increasing prevalence of pericyte "ghosts" on capillaries having endothelial cells, the ghost being an outline of the missing pericyte in the basement membrane. A change in the ratio of endothelial cells and pericytes may be attributed to a loss of pericytes, but may also be a consequence of a more rapid regeneration of endothelial cells than of pericytes after degeneration of both cell types. Endothelial cells do disappear from retinal vessels in diabetes, and under some circumstances they show proliferation as well.

Capillary nonperfusion seems to begin with occlusion and atrophy of individual capillaries at scattered places within the vasculature but, at later stages of retinopathy, may involve clusters of atrophic capillaries associated with sclerosed arterioles. Nonperfused capillaries in diabetic retinopathy commonly lack endothelial cells or pericytes, and thus they appear to be acellular. These vessels, which are nearly normal in caliber, are not truly acellular, and upon electron microscopy may be seen to be filled with cytoplasmic processes of neuroglia. Whether the invasion of retinal capillaries by glia in diabetes is secondary to nonperfusion, or whether it contributes to vessel occlusion is not known.

The microaneurysms, vaso-obliteration, and associated lesions are especially important because they appear early in retinopathy, and they seem to represent disease processes that are responsible for such late complications as retinal neovascularization and recurrent vitreous hemorrhage. In diabetic dogs, when retinopathy is severe and large patches of the capillary network have become hypocellular or acellular, newly formed vessels do commonly appear in the retina. Such newly formed vessels have not been observed in the vitreous, and therefore diabetic dogs may be of limited value as a model for treatment of the preretinal neovascularization that can occur in humans. As a model for investigating the pathogenesis and early stages of retinal neovascularization, the proliferative lesions in dogs with diabetes or galactosemia are unique.

Role of Glycemic Control

In alloxan-diabetic dogs, the development of retinopathy was found many years ago to be inhibited by strict glycemic control (8), provided control was established shortly after the onset of diabetes. That report has been confirmed by a more recent study in our laboratory (11). Dogs were made diabetic with alloxan and randomly assigned to either of two prospectively identified levels of glycemic control: poor control or good control.

In the poor control group, hyperglycemia was severe, as intended, and persisted through all hours of the day (Table 8.1). In animals assigned prospectively to good control, intensified treatment with insulin reduced the blood glucose level to the range of normal for much of the day, lowered HbA$_1$ to normal, and greatly reduced the severity of glycosuria.

The animals were killed for histologic study when they had been diabetic for 5 years. As shown in Table 8.1, poor control resulted in significantly greater

TABLE 8.1. Inhibition of retinopathy in alloxan-diabetic dogs (mean ± SEM)

| | Diabetes | | Normal |
	Poor control (n = 8)	Good control (n = 7)	Normal (n = 14)
Plasma glucose (mmol/liter)			
8:00 AM	21 ± 0.7	5.9 ± 0.5	4.4 ± 0.1
8:00 PM	21 ± 0.9	3.9 ± 0.3	4.3 ± 0.2
Glycosuria (g/day)	104 ± 8	<2	0
Sugar-free days (%)	0	65	100
Hemoglobin A_1 (%)	11.1 ± 0.4	6.6 ± 0.3	6.5 ± 0.2
Retinopathy			
Aneurysms/eye	42 ± 10	2 ± 1.3	1 ± 0.2
Capillary atrophy[a]	264 ± 25	80 ± 20	39 ± 6
Pericyte loss	+ + +	0 to +	0
Hemorrhage	+ +	0	0
Capillary basement membrane width (nm)	319 ± 34	186 ± 14	168 ± 8

[a]Acellular capillaries per 11 mm^2 of trypsin digest. *Source:* Engerman and Kern, *Diabetes* 36: 808–12, 1987.

than normal numbers of aneurysms and acellular capillaries, and in severe losses of pericytes. Retinal hemorrhages were identified in seven of the eight animals of the group. The development of retinopathy was significantly inhibited by good glycemic control, aneurysms and acellular capillaries were significantly reduced in number, and retinal hemorrhages and varicose vessels were entirely absent. The aneurysm count in this group, two aneurysms/eye, did not differ significantly from that in the normal group of animals. It is noteworthy that in the retinas of nondiabetic dogs, as well as in retinas of seemingly normal human subjects, one may encounter an occasional capillary aneurysm, acellular capillary, or pericyte ghost. Such abnormalities tend to be few compared to their prevalence in diabetic retinopathy, but failure to quantitate their frequency may preclude valid evaluation of the effect of therapy on retinopathy, especially in the early stages of the retinopathy.

The effect of improved glycemic control on the development or progression of retinopathy in human diabetics remains less clear. Randomized controlled clinical trials have not reproducibly found good control to inhibit diabetic retinopathy, and have even found the retinopathy to be initially worsened upon improvement of glycemic control. A multi-center, randomized, controlled clinical trial now under way (Diabetic Complications Clinical Trial) is expected to help clarify the ability of improved glycemic control to inhibit the progression of diabetic retinopathy in humans. An assumption that existing retinopathy can be arrested (as opposed to prevented) is inherent in the design of most clinical trials, due in part to the enormous cost and time necessary to investigate prevention of retinopathy in patients from the onset of diabetes. Studies in diabetic dogs suggest this assumption may be faulty (11), and may lead to underestimating a treatment's potential efficacy in a test for primary prevention. In dogs, like patients, an interval of months or years of poor glycemic control may pass before retinopathy becomes apparent. When diabetic dogs in poor glycemic control for 30 months (and having no visible retinopathy) were brought into good glycemic control, the retinopathy did not cease to progress. In fact, severe retinopathy ensued although the degree of control maintained is known to inhibit the onset of retinopathy when such control is initiated early in the course of the disease.

Correction of hyperglycemia with insulin is associated with a coincidental correction of other metabolic consequences of deficient insulin activity, such as disorders of lipid and amino acid metabolism. Therefore, the finding that good control serves to inhibit retinopathy in dogs does not warrant the conclusion that the microvascular disease of diabetes is due to hyperglycemia rather than some other consequence of insulin deficiency.

Sequelae of Hyperglycemia

New light on the importance of hyperglycemia itself has been provided by studies of nondiabetic animals in which hyperglycemia was induced by elevating the blood level of galactose rather than glucose. Normal dogs whose blood hexose was elevated experimentally by a diet containing 30% D-galactose develop a retinopathy indistinguishable from that of diabetic humans and dogs (10). The early stages of galactose-induced retinopathy are marked by excessive prevalence of microaneurysms, pericyte ghosts, acellular capillaries, occasional varicose vessels, and dot and blot hemorrhages. The experimental retinopathy is progressive as the periods of galactosemia are lengthened. Microaneurysms are absent during the first 2 + yr of galactosemia, a long latent period equivalent to that observed in experimental diabetic dogs.

Retinopathy develops in galactosemic dogs in the absence of a number of metabolic and pathophysiologic disorders characteristic of diabetes. Blood glucose is not elevated in the galactosemic dog, but the blood aldohexose concentration is excessive due to galactose, and sequelae of "hyperglycemia" therefore are characteristic of the two animal models, as well as of diabetic humans. No less significant is the fact that the galactosemic dog does not show the abnormal blood levels of insulin, free fatty acids, branched chain amino acids, fibrinogen, and various other defects often associated with diabetes. Thus the data suggest that hyperglycemia per se is sufficient to account for the development of retinopathy.

The mechanism by which hyperglycemia causes retinopathy remains to be identified, but comparison of the physiological and biochemical abnormalities that characterize the diabetic and galactosemic dog models offers a valuable perspective on the etiology of the retinal disease. Metabolic and pathophysiologic abnormalities not shared by the two dog models and diabetic humans seem unlikely to be critical to the pathogenesis of the retinopathy (Table 8.2). It is of interest, for example, that retinopathy develops in galactosemic dogs despite an absence of the abnormal blood filterability seen with diabetes (18). Moreover, neither diabetic dogs nor galactosemic dogs exhibit the abnormal platelet aggregation and plasma aggregation–enhancing factor that have been described in diabetic humans (17).

In recent years, the potential role of excessive polyol production and accumulation in the pathogenesis of diabetic microvascular complications has

TABLE 8.2. Comparison of diabetic dogs to experimental galactosemic dogs

	Diabetic dog	Galactosemic dog
Blood chemistry		
Glucose	↑	Normal
Aldohexose	↑	↑
Glycated hemoglobin	↑	↑
Glycated plasma protein	↑	↑
RBC polyol	↑	↑
Insulin	↓	Normal
Free fatty acids	↑	Normal
Branched-chain amino acids	↑	Normal
Fibrinogen	↑	Normal
Platelet aggregation	Normal	Normal
Blood filterability	↓	Normal
Blood viscosity	↑	↑
Heart weight (blood pressure)	Normal	Normal

attracted much attention. Pharmacologic inhibition of aldose reductase has been reported to inhibit a variety of anatomic and pathophysiologic abnormalities in experimentally galactosemic or diabetic rodents. Inhibition of aldose reductase has been reported to inhibit thickening of capillary basement membrane in the retina of galactosemic or diabetic rats (5,13,28), but apparently it has no such effect in the glomerulus of affected animals (7,24–26,32).

A postulated role of excessive polyol production in the pathogenesis of retinopathy is being investigated in our laboratory in galactosemic dogs and in diabetic dogs receiving the aldose reductase inhibitor sorbinil. Preliminary results of the experiment involving galactose-fed dogs are reported in Table 8.3. Normal young adult dogs were randomly assigned to a diet of 30% galactose and subdivided into a sorbinil-treated group and a placebo-treated group, each containing ten dogs. The drug and placebo are given orally each morning and evening at a daily dose of usually 60–80 mg/kg. The severity of hyperglycemia (that is to say, galactosemia) is judged chiefly from nonenzymatically glycated hemoglobin (HbA$_1$) and the plasma level of nonenzymatically glycated protein. The efficacy of the aldose reductase inhibitor is judged chiefly from the erythrocyte polyol concentration. Eyes and other tissues are being studied histologically at the time of autopsy after 60 months of galactosemia, and retinopathy is being evaluated histologically at 42 months of galactosemia in an eye obtained surgically from each of the animals.

Retinas have been obtained from each of the 20 dogs after 42 months of galactosemia, and also from half of the same animals when autopsied after 60 months of galactosemia. The severity of galactosemia seems to be comparable in the animals given sorbinil and those given the placebo, as judged from measurement of HbA$_1$ and nonenzymatically glycated plasma protein; in the sorbinil group, the values shown for HbA$_1$ are slightly and significantly greater than in the placebo group, whereas the plasma concentrations of nonenzymatically glycated protein are significantly lower than in the placebo group.

TABLE 8.3. Retinopathy in dogs receiving sorbinil (mean ± SD)

	Galactose + placebo		Galactose + sorbinil		Normal
	(n = 10)	(n = 5)	(n = 10)	(n = 5)	(n = 7)
Duration (months)	42	60	42	60	42–60
Nonenzymatic glycated					
Hemoglobin (%; HbA1)	6.4 ± 0.3	6.2 ± 0.3	6.7 ± 0.4	6.6 ± 0.3	5.7 ± 0.2
Plasma protein (nmol/g)	69 ± 6	69 ± 5	64 ± 4	60 ± 5	56 ± 5
Hexitol					
Erythrocyte (nmol/g Hb)	1454 ± 535	1465 ± 583	135 ± 32	127 ± 49	42 ± 9
Muscle (nmol/mg prot)	222 ± 148[a]		25 ± 9[a]		ND[b]
Retinopathy					
Aneurysms/eye	25 ± 41	41 ± 28	28 ± 39	84 ± 64	1 ± 1[c]
Pericyte ghosts/1,000 cells	15 ± 13	34 ± 17	16 ± 19	37 ± 19	2 ± 2[c]
Capillary basement membrane width (nm)	145 ± 28	210 ± 25	164 ± 70	245 ± 76	133 ± 28[c]

[a]Biopsied at 42 mo; n = 5.
[b]ND, not detected; n = 2.
[c]n = 3; duration 60 mo.

Treatment with the aldose reductase inhibitor effectively inhibited tissue polyol accumulation. The placebo group showed a 30- to 40-fold increase in polyol concentration in reds cells and skeletal muscle, and treatment with sorbinil was found to inhibit about 93% of that large increase.

In contrast to the clear inhibition of polyol path activity by sorbinil, histologic studies have revealed no similar inhibitory effect of the drug on retinopathy. Unmistakable retinopathy has appeared in the placebo group, and lesions no less severe are occurring in animals given sorbinil. By 60 mo, capillary basement membrane in the retina is significantly thicker than normal in both groups of galactosemic animals, and no inhibition by sorbinil is apparent in the animals that have been killed to date. Our present observations suggest that the development of retinopathy is not especially dependent on excessive polyol path activity, but this finding has yet to be confirmed by study of the entire group of 20 galactosemic dogs for the full 60 months. Moreover, data will soon become available for comparison of the results with those from a similar study in our laboratory of alloxan-diabetic dogs given the aldose reductase inhibitor for 60 months, and for comparison of animal experiments with a recently completed clinical trial of sorbinil in diabetic patients with retinopathy.

Recent reports by others have claimed that retinopathy has been inhibited by administration of an aldose reductase inhibitor (15,29). These studies, however, are difficult to interpret inasmuch as each has neglected to show whether the hyperglycemia (galactosemia or diabetes), which presumably is responsible for the retinopathy, was as severe in the inhibitor-treated animals as in the controls. Moreover, in each case, the retinopathy was described as being inhibited by an aldose reductase inhibitor, but the severity of the vascular pathology was not quantitatively compared. The retinopathy that has been reported recently in rats fed 50% galactose (29) seems promising, if confirmed, but at present it is of questionable significance; retinal lesions not typical of diabetes (such as retinal folds) also are produced in rats by diets having very high concentrations of galactose (34).

NEPHROPATHY IN DIABETIC DOGS

Satisfactory treatment of diabetes in patients will require the prevention or arrest not only of the ocular complications but also of such life-threatening complications as nephropathy. The development of retinopathy in alloxan-diabetic dogs is associated with the development of renal lesions that are also characteristic of diabetes in humans.

The renal lesions that are characteristic of insulin-deficient diabetes in humans and dogs include nephromegaly, glomerular sclerosis, occasional exudative deposits, and mesangial nodules (4,19). Excretion of protein and albumin tends to become greater than normal in many but not all dogs kept insulin-deficient for 5 yr (20). Obliterated glomeruli become relatively numerous, the glomerular and mesangial volumes and capillary filtering surface area become greater than normal, and the basement membrane of glomerular capillaries becomes thickened [Table 8.4; (12)]. Mesangial expansion is evident re-

TABLE 8.4. Glomerular structure in diabetic dogs and galactosemic dogs killed at 5 years (mean ± SD)

| | Normal (n = 9) | Diabetes | | | Galactose (n = 5) |
		Poor control (n = 7)	Good control (n = 6)		
Kidney weight (g/kg)	2.2 ± 0.3	4.0 ± 0.6	2.5 ± 0.6		2.2 ± 0.2
Glomerular volume (10^6 μm^3)	2.0 ± 0.6	5.1 ± 1.0	2.5 ± 0.9		1.9 ± 0.4
Mesangial volume (10^6 μm^3)	0.31 ± 0.2	1.08 ± 0.4	0.43 ± 0.2		0.24 ± 0.1
% of glomerulus	14 ± 6	25 ± 10	18 ± 3		11 ± 4
Obliterated glomeruli (%)	0.6 ± 0.8	11 ± 10	1.0 ± 0.3		0.3 ± 0.5
Capillary basement membrane width (nm)	361 ± 76	644 ± 79	416 ± 34		472 ± 90

Mean ± SD.
Source: Engerman and Kern, Kidney Int. 36: 41–45, 1988.

158

gardless of whether mesangial volume is expressed in absolute units or relative to the total volume of the glomerulus. Mesangial expansion and a subsequent reduction in glomerular capillary filtering surface area are believed to play an important role in the development of renal dysfunction in diabetes (30).

Strict glycemic control significantly inhibits development of the lesions in the kidney of the diabetic dog, similar to effects of strict control on the retina (4,12). As shown in Table 8.4, animals randomly assigned to good glycemic control are found to differ significantly from those in poor glycemic control, and not from normal animals, with respect to kidney weight, glomerular and mesangial volumes, frequency of glomerular obliteration, and basement membrane thickness. Therefore, although the renal lesions appear to be a result of deficient insulin activity, the possible role of hyperglycemia in renal disease is less clear than is the case with retinopathy.

In contrast to the marked nephropathy observed in insulin-deficient diabetic dogs, kidneys from the galactosemic dogs have been found to remain relatively normal (12,19). Galactosemia sufficient to produce diabetic-like retinopathy has failed to produce the mesangial expansion, glomerular obliteration, and renal hypertrophy typical of diabetes in humans and dogs. Capillary basement membrane in the glomerulus, like that in the retina, nonetheless, has become significantly thickened in both diabetes and galactosemia. Mesangial matrix, a basement membrane-like component of the glomerulus, has shown no sign of enlargement in the galactosemic dogs. Interestingly, glomerular filtration rate was found to be significantly greater than normal in both diabetic dogs and galactosemic dogs (21), a finding that seems inconsistent with a postulated role of hyperfiltration in the pathogenesis of diabetic nephropathy (1).

As in other tissues, polyol concentration in the renal cortex of galactosemic dogs (6.0 ± 1.2 nmol/mg protein, SD) was significantly greater than in normal dogs (0.23 ± 0.05) and diabetic dogs [0.43 ± 0.08; (12)]. The high polyol concentration in kidneys of long-term galactosemic dogs who develop so little nephropathy suggests that the development of the nephropathy may not be a result of excessive polyol production and accumulation. This conclusion is consistent with recent reports that the thickening of glomerular basement membrane in diabetic or galactosemic animals is not influenced by administration of aldose reductase inhibitors (7,24–26,32). Moreover, aldose reductase inhibitors have been found not to inhibit the elevation of glomerular filtration rate by diabetes or galactosemia in dogs (22). Whether aldose reductase inhibitors are able to inhibit the elevation of glomerular filtration rate by diabetes or galactosemia in the rat is controversial (2,3,6,14,31).

SUMMARY

The observed dissociation of retinopathy from glomerulopathy in experimental galactosemia raises the possibility that these complications differ appreciably in their pathogenesis. Diabetic glomerulopathy in the dog appears to be initiated as a result of sequelae of deficient insulin activity that are not simulated by galactosemia and its associated elevation of tissue polyol production and glomerular filtration rate. Animal experimentation has provided clear evidence, nevertheless, that the development of diabetic complications in a number of tissues, including retina, kidney, and nerve, may be significantly inhibited as a result of strict glycemic control.

REFERENCES

1. ANDERSON, S., and BRENNER, B. Pathogenesis of diabetic nephropathy: hemodynamic considerations. *Diabetes/Metab. Rev.* 4: 163–177, 1988.
2. BANK, N., COCO, M., and AYNEDJIAN, H. S. Galactose feeding causes glomerular hyperperfusion: prevention by aldose reductase inhibition. *Am. J. Physiol.* 256 (*Renal Fluid Electrolyte Physiol.*): F994–999, 1989.
3. BANK, N., MOWER, P., AYNEDJIAN, H. S., WILKES, B. M., and SILVERMAN, S. Sorbinil prevents glomerular hyperperfusion in diabetic rats. *Am. J. Physiol.* 256 (*Renal Fluid Electrolyte Physiol.*): F1000–1006, 1989.
4. BLOODWORTH, J. M. B., JR., and ENGERMAN, R. L. Experimental diabetic glomerulosclerosis. In: *Secondary Diabetes: The Spectrum of the Diabetic Syndromes*, edited by S. Podolsky and M. Viswanathan. New York: Raven, 1980, pp. 521–540.
5. CHAKRABARTI, S., and SIMA, A. A. F. Effect of aldose reductase inhibition and insulin treatment on retinal capillary basement membrane thickening in BB rats. *Diabetes* 38: 1181–1186, 1989.
6. DANIELS, B. S., and HOSTETTER, T. H. Aldose reductase inhibition and glomerular abnormalities in diabetic rats. *Diabetes* 38: 981–986, 1989.
7. DAS, A., FRANK, R. N., ZHANG, N. L., TURCZYN, T., and SAMADANI, E. Glomerular basement membrane thickening in galactosemic rats and role of polyol pathway. *Diabetes* 38(Suppl 2): 109, 1989 (abstr).
8. ENGERMAN, R. L., BLOODWORTH, J. M. B., JR., and NELSON, S. Relationship of microvascular disease to metabolic control. *Diabetes* 26: 760–769, 1977.
9. ENGERMAN, R. L., FINKELSTEIN, D., AGUIRRE, G., DIDDIE, K. R., FOX, R. R., FRANK, R. N., and VARMA, S. D. Ocular complications. *Diabetes* 31: 82–88, 1982.
10. ENGERMAN, R. L., and KERN, T. S. Experimental galactosemia produces diabetic-like retinopathy. *Diabetes* 33: 97–100, 1984.
11. ENGERMAN, R. L., and KERN, T. S. Progression of incipient diabetic retinopathy during good glycemic control. *Diabetes* 36: 808–812, 1987.
12. ENGERMAN, R. L., and KERN, T. S. Hyperglycemia and development of glomerular pathology: diabetes compared with galactosemia. *Kidney Int.* 36: 41–45, 1988.
13. FRANK, R. N., KEIRN, R. J., KENNEDY, A., and FRANK, K. W. Galactose-induced retinal capillary basement membrane thickening: prevention by sorbinil. *Invest. Ophthalmol. Vis. Sci.* 24: 1519–1524, 1983.
14. GOLDFARB, S., SIMMONS, D. A., and KERN, E. F. O. Amelioration of glomerular hyperfiltration in acute experimental diabetes mellitus by dietary *myo*-inositol supplementation and aldose reductase inhibition. *Trans. Assoc. Am. Physicians* 99: 67–72, 1986.
15. KADOR, P. F., AKAGI, Y., TERUBAYASHI, H., WYMAN, M., and KINOSHITA, J. H. Prevention of pericyte ghost formation in retinal capillaries of galactose-fed dogs by aldose reductase inhibitors. *Arch. Ophthalmol.* 106: 1099–1102, 1988.
16. KAHN, H. A., and HILLER, R. Blindness caused by diabetic retinopathy. *Am. J. Ophthalmol.* 78: 58–67, 1974.
17. KERN, T. S., and ENGERMAN, R. L. Platelet aggregation in experimental diabetes and experimental galactosemia. *Diabetes* 33: 846–850, 1984.
18. KERN, T. S., ROMANG, T. C., and ENGERMAN, R. L. Erythrocyte filterability in alloxan-diabetes and in experimental galactosemia. *Clin. Hemorheology* 6: 395–404, 1986.
19. KERN, T. S., and ENGERMAN, R. L. Kidney morphology in experimental hyperglycemia. *Diabetes* 36: 244–249, 1987.
20. KERN, T. S., and ENGERMAN, R. L. Urinary protein excretion rates in experimentally diabetic dogs and experimentally galactosemic dogs. *Diabetologia* 31: 928–932, 1988.
21. KERN, T. S., and ENGERMAN, R. L. Renal hemodynamics in dogs with diabetes and galactosemia. *Diabetes* 38(Suppl.2): 93A, 1989 (abstr).
22. KERN, T. S., and ENGERMAN, R. L. Renal hemodynamics in experimentally galactosemic dogs and diabetic dogs. *Metabolism* 40: 450–454, 1991.
23. KLEIN, R., KLEIN, B. E., MOSS, S. E., DAVIS, M. D., and DEMETS, D. L. The Wisconsin

Epidemiologic Study of Diabetic Retinopathy. II. Prevalence and risk of diabetic retinopathy when age at diagnosis is less than 30 years. *Arch. Ophthalmol.* 102: 520–526, 1984.

24. MAUER, S. M., STEFFES, M. W., AZAR, S., and BROWN, D. M. Effects of sorbinil on glomerular structure and function in long-term diabetic rats. *Diabetes* 38: 839–846, 1989.

25. MCCALEB, M. L., SREDY, J., MILLEN, J., ACKERMAN, D. M., and DVORNIK, D. Prevention of urinary albumin excretion in 6 month streptozotocin-diabetic rats with the aldose reductase inhibitor Tolrestat. *J. Diabetic Complications* 2: 16–18, 1988.

26. OSTERBY, R., and GUNDERSEN, H. J. G. Glomerular basement membrane thickening in streptozotocin diabetic rats despite treatment with an aldose reductase inhibitor. *J. Diabetic Complications* 3: 149–153, 1989.

27. RAO, T. K. S., and FRIEDMAN, E. A. Diabetic nephropathy in Brooklyn. In: *Diabetic Renal-Retinal Syndrome,* Vol. 2, edited by E. Friedman and F. A. L'Esperance. New York: Grune & Stratton, 1981, p. 3.

28. ROBISON, W. G., JR., KADOR, P. F., AKAGI, Y., KINOSHITA, J. H., GONZALEZ, R., and DVORNIK, D. Prevention of basement membrane thickening in retinal capillaries by a novel inhibitor of aldose reductase, Tolrestat. *Diabetes* 35: 295–299, 1986.

29. ROBISON, W. G., JR., NAGATA, M., LAVER, N., HOHMAN, T. C., and KINOSHITA, J. H. Diabetic-like retinopathy in rats prevented with an aldose reductase inhibitor. *Invest. Ophthalmol. Vis. Sci.* 30: 2285–2292, 1989.

30. STEFFES, M. W., OSTERBY, R., CHAVERS, B., and MAUER, S. M. Mesangial expansion as a central mechanism for loss of kidney function in diabetic patients. *Diabetes* 38: 1077–1081, 1989.

31. TILTON, R. G., CHANG, K., PUGLIESE, G., EADES, D. M., PROVINCE, M. A., SHERMAN, W. R., KILO, C., and WILLIAMSON, J. R. Prevention of hemodynamic and vascular albumin filtration changes in diabetic rats by aldose reductase inhibitors. *Diabetes* 37: 1258–1270, 1989.

32. TILTON, R. G., PUGLIESE, G., and WILLIAMSON, J. R. Diabetes-induced glomerular structural changes in rats are not prevented by sorbinil. *Diabetes* 38(Suppl 2): 374, 1989 (abstr).

33. VIBERTI, G. C., and WALKER, J. D. Diabetic nephropathy: etiology and prevention. *Diabetes/Metab. Rev.* 4: 147–162, 1988.

34. VINORES, S. A., and CAMPOCHIARO, P. A. Prevention or moderation of some ultrastructural changes in the RPE and retina of galactosemic rats by aldose reductase inhibition. *Exp. Eye Res.* 49: 495–510, 1989.

9

Cell Culture Model for the Study of Vascular Complications of Diabetes: The Effect of High Glucose Levels on Metabolism and Growth of Vascular Cells

GEORGE L. KING, TERUO SHIBA, EDWARD P. FEENER, AND RAMESH NAYAK

Vascular complications affect all diabetic patients to some extent and involve both microvessels and macrovessels. In this chapter we discuss studies that show the effects of elevated glucose levels on the metabolism of retinal and aortic vascular cells in culture.

There are many advantages to using cultured vascular cells for the study of diabetic retinopathy and vascular complications of diabetes in general. One clear advantage is the ability to control variables so as to allow the investigator to determine the effects of a single parameter. Another advantage is that cultured cells can be used to dissect out biochemical and molecular mechanisms rapidly. In contrast, animal models of diabetic complications may not be available, may be expensive, and may require years to produce the right histopathologies (17–19,49). There are many potential pitfalls as well in interpreting and extrapolating data derived from cultured cells to in vivo conditions. The most serious is that cultured cells do not retain many of their *in vivo* properties. In addition, cells in vivo exist and communicate with many other types of cells, whereas in vitro pure cultures of a single cell type are studied. These are important concerns that we have tried to address in our studies to understand diabetic retinopathy.

RETINAL VASCULAR CELL CHANGES IN DIABETES

The sequence of cellular changes that result in the development of diabetic retinopathy are beginning to be clarified as described in Figure 9.1. Most of the retinal abnormalities in diabetic patients or animal models are located in the retinal microvessels involving the pericyte, endothelial cells, and basement membranes (17,18,34,49). One of the earliest histopathological findings is the loss of pericytes in the retinal capillaries. The number of endothelial cells is relatively unaffected, and as a result the endothelial cell/pericyte ratio is 1:1 to 9:1 after a few years of diabetes (11,16,17,29,35,49). After the loss of pericytes, the capillaries demonstrate an increased diameter, thickening of base-

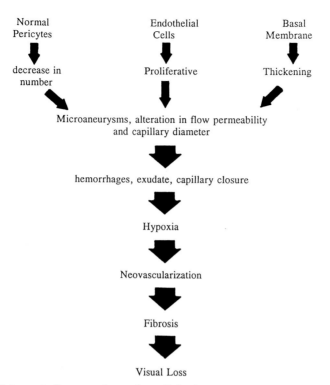

FIGURE 9.1. Schematic diagram of vascular cellular histopathology of diabetic retinopathy.

ment membrane, and formation of microaneurysms. Microaneurysms are composed of a cluster of endothelial cells and are the result of cellular proliferation or aggregation. Associated with these cellular changes are functional alterations such as abnormalities in blood flow and vascular permeability (10,15,23,33,34,48). These early vascular functional changes are followed by more obvious retinal pathologies such as hemorrhages, exudates, and regions of nonperfusion due to capillary closures (9,10,34,48). The late changes of diabetic background retinopathy probably set up regions of hypoxia, which is a potent inducer of neovascularization (2,20,56). The onset of neovascularization defines the beginning of proliferative retinopathy, which, if left untreated, leads to retinal hemorrhage and fibrosis that will cause a majority of patients to lose vision (10,34,48).

These pathological changes are usually separated into background and proliferative retinopathy. The pathologies found in the early stages of background diabetic retinopathy are very specific to the disease, whereas the later, proliferative findings, which are common to many diseases, are probably due to tissue reactions to hypoxia, inflammation, and injury (34). Studies in animals and humans with diabetes in which euglycemia was effectively maintained by intensive insulin therapy or a pancreatic transplant have shown that the restoration of euglycemia, by itself, does not reverse the late histopathologies of diabetic retinopathy (47). Presumably, this therapeutic intervention needs to be initiated early in the course of the disease to prevent the adverse effects of hyperglycemia. The importance of early glycemic intervention has been amply characterized by Engerman et al., who used dogs with chemically-induced diabetes, and is discussed in Chapter 8 (17).

CHARACTERIZATION OF RETINAL MICROVASCULAR CELLS IN CULTURE

As already stated, if it can be ascertained that cultured retinal vascular cells retain in vivo properties, they could be a useful tool for examining the mechanism by which elevated glucose levels can produce dysfunction in vascular cells. To determine whether the cultured retinal capillary cells retain their in vivo properties, they have been characterized by morphological and antigenic properties. Retinal capillary endothelial cells in culture exhibited cuboidal, monolayer morphology which is typical of these cells in vivo (28,30,42). In addition, they express factor VIII antigen and are able to incorporate acetylated-LDL, typical properties of endothelial cells in vivo. In contrast to endothelial cells, retinal pericytes grow in an overlapping manner and are negative to an-

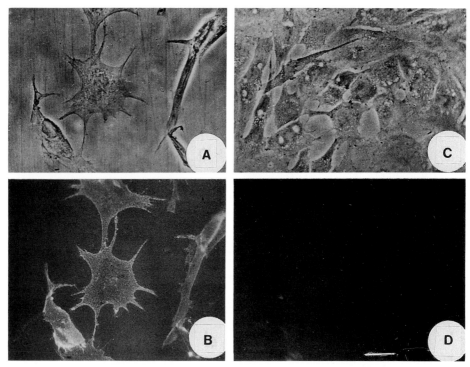

FIGURE 9.2. Immunofluorescent stain of vascular cells in vitro. *A*. Phase contrast micrograph of bovine retinal pericytes; *B*. mAb 3G5 staining of the same field shown in *A*.; *C*. Phase contrast micrograph of retinal endothelial cells; *D*. mAb 3G5 staining of the same field shown in *C*. Reproduced with permission of the Rockefeller University Press, from: Nayak, R.C., Berman, A. B., George, K. L., Eisenbarth, G. S., King, G. L. A monoclonal antibody (3G5)-defined ganglioside antigen is expressed on the cell surface of microvascular pericytes. *J. Exp. Med.* 1988, 167: 1003–1015.

tibody made against factor VIII (28,30,42). Since these are nonspecific properties, we have characterized a pericyte-specific monoclonal antibody, 3G5,
which is made against a glycolipid in the plasma membrane (Fig. 9.2). Recently, we have shown that 3G5 stains specifically retinal pericytes and is negative against retinal endothelial cells, smooth muscle and retinal pigmented
epithelial cells. Pericytes in vivo also express the antigen for 3G5 (42). Interestingly, renal glomerular epithelial cells and islet cells are also positive for
3G5 antigens. Thus, cultured retinal capillary cells exhibited many of the same
morphological and antigenic properties with those in vivo, which suggests that
they could be useful for metabolic or functional studies.

The effects of an elevated glucose level on the growth of retinal endothelial
cells and pericytes in culture have also been found to mirror its histology in
vivo. When pericytes are grown in a medium containing 400 mg/dl of glucose,
they attain a steady-state cell density level 2–3-fold less than in the presence
of 100 mg/dl glucose [Fig. 9.3; (32,38)]. The effect of glucose can be partially
reversed by the addition of insulin but not by the addition of an aldose reductase inhibitor like sorbinil. In addition, pericytes are very responsive to insulin, even in the presence of plasma, as shown in Figure 9.4. This is unlike most
other types of cultured cells, which require an insulin concentration of $10^{-8} M$
and $10^{-7} M$ before growth effects are observed (4,30). This dose-response curve
of insulin suggests that the growth effect of insulin is mediated via the insulin
receptor rather than the insulin-like growth factor (IGF-1) receptors. Both of
these receptors have been reported to be present on retinal pericytes (28,30).

In contrast to pericytes, the proliferation of bovine aortic retinal endothelial cells in culture is not affected significantly by exposure to 400 mg/dl glucose as compared with 100 mg/dl (Fig. 9.5). Similar results have been observed
with endothelial cells from bovine aorta and microvessels from rat epididymal

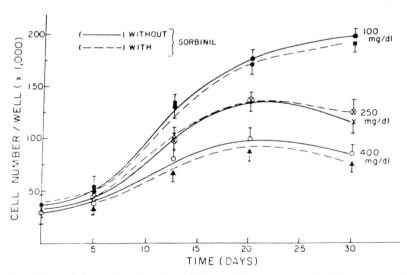

FIGURE 9.3. Effect of glucose levels and sorbinil, an aldose reductase inhibitor, on retinal pericyte growth.

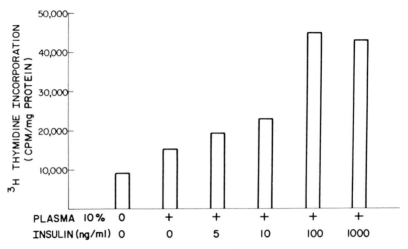

FIGURE 9.4. Effect of insulin and plasma on DNA synthesis in retinal pericytes.

fat pads. Thus, these in vitro studies of retinal capillary cell growth suggested that the loss of pericytes, in vivo, which leads to an increase in the ratio of endothelial cells to pericytes, is due to the elevated glucose levels and the relative lack of insulin in the diabetic state.

Besides pericyte loss, exposure of human umbilical vein endothelial cells to elevated glucose levels has been reported to increase the expression of such basement membrane components as type IV collagen, fibronectin, and laminin (12). Since these components of the membrane have been shown to be in-

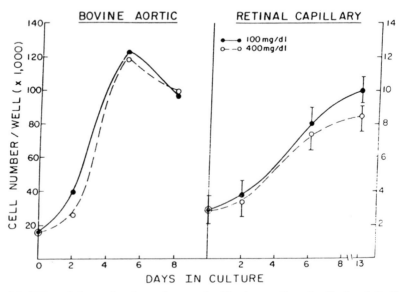

FIGURE 9.5. Effect of glucose levels on the growth of bovine aortic and retinal endothelial cells in culture.

creased in the renal glomeruli, these reports postulated that the thickening of basement membrane is due to the effects of glucose on increasing the synthesis of these proteins. More recently, Yamauchi et al. demonstrated that the production of endothelin-1 (ET-1), a vasoactive hormone, by aortic endothelial cells is enhanced at high concentrations of glucose (59), suggesting that hyperglycemia could be a factor in causing hypertension in diabetic patients. Interestingly, these effects of glucose are not mimicked by mannitol or inhibited by aldose reductase inhibitors.

The data presented so far support the validity of using cultured vascular cells for proving the mechanisms of the adverse effects of glucose on vascular metabolism, functions, and growth. Several theories have been postulated to explain these adverse effects of glucose (8,22,32,58). Many are described in other chapters; here we focus on the effects of an elevated glucose level on phospholipid metabolism and protein kinase C (PKC) activities.

CHANGES IN PHOSPHOLIPID AND PROTEIN KINASE C BY ELEVATED GLUCOSE LEVELS

We concentrated on the effect of elevated glucose levels on cellular phosphoinositols (PIs) and PKC activities for several reasons. Most important is that numerous reports have suggested that PI metabolites and the activation of PKC can affect vascular cell growth, metabolism, and functions. For example, the activation of PKC activities has been reported to increase vascular permeability (39,58), enhance contraction (55), alter basement membrane synthesis, and stimulate cellular proliferation (40). Since all of these vascular parameters have been shown to be abnormal in diabetic patients and animals, it seemed logical to characterize the effect of glucose on PKC activities.

Since retinal endothelial cells in culture express the antigens in vivo and respond to high glucose concentrations, we first characterized the effect of a high glucose level on PI levels and PKC activities. Exposure of bovine retinal endothelial cells in culture to glucose levels of 400 mg/dl for greater than five days will increase the PKC activities found in the membrane pool, whereas no significant changes were noted in the cytosolic pool (Fig. 9.6). This finding suggests that hyperglycemia can cause an activation of PKC, probably by its translocation from cytosol to the membrane. This action of glucose is time-dependent, since incubating retinal endothelial cells with 400 mg/dl glucose for a period less than 24 h, did not cause a similar change in membrane PKC activities. The activation of PKC found in the retinal endothelial cells can be generalized to other cultured vascular cells; a similar alteration of PKC activities was observed in aortic smooth muscle cells exposed to high glucose concentrations (Table 9.1).

Since the expression and regulation of enzymes in cultured cells may differ from that of the same cell type in vivo, we also measured PKC activities in various tissues from rats with chemically induced diabetes. In whole retinas isolated from rats with streptozotocin-induced diabetes, an increase of PKC activities in the membrane pool was observed. Similar increases were also found in the aorta from diabetic rats. Craven et al. recently reported that renal

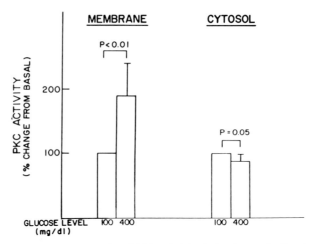

FIGURE 9.6. Effect of glucose level on PKC activities in bovine retinal endothelial cells.

glomeruli from diabetic rats have an increase in the PKC activities of the membrane pool with a corresponding decrease in the cytosol, suggesting that the diabetic state causes an activation of PKC by translocation of the enzyme from the cytosol to the membrane (13,14). These investigators also reported that incubating isolated glomeruli from nondiabetic animals with glucose concentrations of 400 mg/dl increases membranous PKC activities within a few minutes when compared to glomeruli exposed to 100 mg/dl of glucose (13,14), indicating that hyperglycemia is the major offending metabolic factor.

So far the data have shown that PKC activities appear to be increased in multiple types of vascular cells in culture and in various vascular tissues from rats with both chemically and genetically induced diabetes. However, PKC activities are not always increased in all tissues derived from diabetic animals. We examined brain PKC activities from streptozotocin-treated diabetic rats and found it to be comparable with those from nondiabetic animals, both in the membrane compartment and the cytosol compartment. Others have reported that PKC activities may actually be decreased in the liver of diabetic rats (46). Thus, these findings suggest that diabetes or the effect of elevated glucose on PKC activities can vary, depending on the source of tissue. In addition, the mechanisms that regulate PKC activities by glucose appear to be similar in most vascular tissues, but they differ from the mechanisms that regulate PKC activities in nonvascular tissues.

To investigate the mechanisms by which the PKC activities are altered when the vascular cells are exposed to hyperglycemia in vivo, or to elevated glucose levels in a cultured medium, we characterized some of the metabolites that have been demonstrated to regulate PKC activities under physiological conditions. In the cell, PKC activities are activated when they are bound to the diacylglycerol (DAG) level in the membranes (6,43). Thus, the activation of PKC in response to a high glucose level in the vascular tissues could be due to increases in the DAG level, suggesting an increase of PKC in the membrane. It is also possible that PKC activities can be enhanced by increases in total

TABLE 9.1. Summary of PKC activity and DAG changes in various cells in culture

In vitro	PKC activity	DAG (total)
Retinal endothelial cells	↑	↑
Aortic endothelial cells	↑	↑
Aortic smooth muscle cells	↑	↑
Tissues		
Retina (diabetic rats)	↑	↑
Heart (diabetic rats)	?	↑
Aorta (diabetic rats)	↑	↑
Renal glomeruli (diabetic rats)	↑	↑
Brain (diabetic rats)	↔	↔
Granulation tissue (exposed to glucose level)	?	↑

cellular amount of enzymes where both cytosol and membrane pool are increased. Recent preliminary data have indicated that both of these possibilities might be occurring. In cultured retinal endothelial cells, high glucose levels increased only membranous PKC without altering cytosol activities. This would indicate possible activities by translocation. In the retina of diabetic rats, we have found increases in both cytosol and membrane pools. These findings suggest that the total amount of PKC could be increased in vivo, in addition to translocation. In cultured endothelial cells PKC activation could be due to increased DAG. We therefore investigated DAG level to determine whether it can be altered by varying glucose levels.

The DAG level was measured in several ways, since DAG can be derived by multiple pathways (6,44,58). The first mechanism of DAG formation studied was the conversion of phosphoinositol (PIP_2) to DAG and inositol triphosphate (IP_3) by phospholipase C (6,44,58). Previous reports suggested that a pool PI turnover may be decreased in cells exposed to elevated levels of glucose and in diabetes. The reduction in PIP_2 is due to a lack of precursors in cellular concentrations of *myo*-inositol, which is inhibited in its uptake by elevated glucose and intracellular sorbitol levels (22). Since most of these data were derived from studying peripheral nerve we have characterized these parameters in vascular cells in culture.

As shown in Figure 9.7, sorbitol levels were increased in all vascular cells from bovine aorta and retinal microvessels studied when exposed to glucose levels of 400 mg/dl vs 100 mg/dl. Since the increase in sorbitol level was diminished in the presence of the aldose reductase inhibitor, sorbinil, these findings suggest that all the cells contain a significant amount of aldose reductase. Unlike sorbitol, the cellular *myo*-inositol levels did not change in most of the vascular cells, whereas the pericytes showed a significant decrease (Table 9.2). These findings are consistent with previous reports of Sussman et al., who used pericyte cultures from the brain microvessel cells and others on the aortic

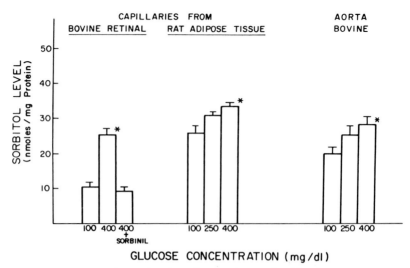

FIGURE 9.7. Effect of glucose levels and sorbinil on sorbitol levels in vascular cells.

cells (38,53). Those investigators showed that the *myo*-inositol level was not changed in endothelial cells exposed to elevated levels of glucose. In contrast, the myoinositol level was decreased in pericytes (53).

In studies using pancreatic islet cells, Wollheim et al. found that the elevation of glucose levels in the medium will increase the concentration of DAG, in part by de novo synthesis pathways (45). That is, an increase in glycolytic flux by the elevation of glucose level will lead to an increased level of glyceraldehyde 3-phosphate, which is a precursor for the synthesis of phosphotidic acid [PA; (see Figure 9.8)], which can then be converted to DAG. In turn, the increase in DAG level can activate PKC. Recent publications by Rasmussen et al. have shown that glucose level regulated mainly the α-isoform of PKC (21). This hypothesis is feasible for the endothelial cells if it can be shown that the elevation of glucose levels from 5.5 mM to 20 mM of glucose in the external media of endothelial cells will increase glucose flux through glycolysis. To test this hypothesis, we compared the amount of ^{3}H$_2$O glucose formation from [^{3}H]glucose over 2 hours, which is a reflection of glucose uptake and estimation of glycolytic rate in endothelial cells. Endothelial cells from both retinal microvessels and aorta were studied. Elevation of glucose level increased the glycolytic rate, suggesting that endothelial and islet cells may share similar regu-

TABLE 9.2. Effect of elevated glucose level

	Sorbitol	Myoinositol levels
Bovine aortic endothelial cells	↑	↔
Bovine aortic smooth muscle cells	↑	↔
Bovine retinal endothelial cells and pericytes	↑	↓
Rat capillary endothelial cells	↑	↔

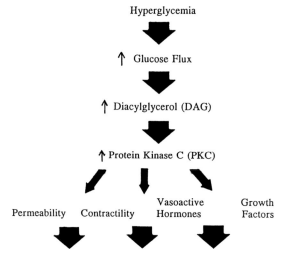

Hyperglycemia

↑ Glucose Flux

↑ Diacylglycerol (DAG)

↑ Protein Kinase C (PKC)

Permeability   Contractility   Vasoactive   Growth
                                 Hormones   Factors

Retinopathy , Hypertension , Flow Changes , Proliferative Changes

FIGURE 9.8. Schematic drawing of the DAG-PKC hypothesis.

lation in the uptake and metabolism of glucose. It is unclear which step in glucose transport or glycolysis is limiting glucolytic flux in endothelial cells when glucose levels are fluctuating between 5 and 20 mM. It is unlikely that the limiting step is glucose phosphorylation since most hexokinases generally have a K_m of 0.3 mM or lower, except for the specific glucokinase located in the liver or pancreatic islets, which have a high K_m hexokinases (56). There is no evidence, however, that this enzyme is found in significant quantity in endothelial cells. Another possibility is that glucose transport could be limiting. Research on the regulation of glucose transport and transporters in endothelial cells is beginning to be reported, and more information is critically needed to resolve these issues.

So far our findings suggest that PKC activities in cultured vascular endothelial cells are increased in the membrane pool when exposed to elevated glucose concentrations. This could be due to an increase in the activity or protein of PKC in vascular cells or tissue. The question of whether there are protein changes comparable to PKC activity increase is an important one since there are several members in the PKC family of proteins and they may be regulated differently (25,43,44). The distribution of the isoforms for PKC is different in various tissues and may even be located at different subcellular sites (25). These differences have given rise to the suggestion that various PKC isoforms may have unique functions within the cells. The PKC enzyme family is separated into α, β_1, β_2, γ, ε, d, and z isoforms, with the latter three having less sensitivity to Ca^{2+} (25,43,44). The brain contains all seven isoforms, but our initial analysis of vascular tissue in culture using anti-peptide antibodies has revealed only isoforms α and β_2. In Figure 9.9, these PKC isoforms are shown by immunoblotting. Both isoforms can be shown to be activated by phorbol ester, as is evident from translocation of the cytosol to the membrane pool in the presence of PMA, a DAG analog. In addition, both PKC isoforms can be

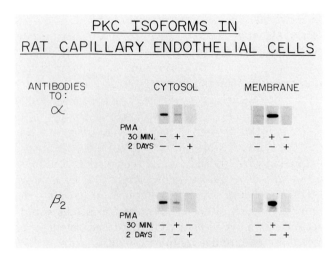

FIGURE 9.9. Identification of PKC isoforms in vascular cells in culture.

downregulated by prolonged exposure to the phorbol ester, PMA, with loss of both activities and proteins.

A survey of multiple types of vascular cells from microvessels and macrovessels showed that only α and β₂ PKC isoforms are expressed. Since the effect of a high glucose level on PKC activities is probably due to an increase of DAG concentrations, both of these PKC isoforms presumably will be increased in the membrane pool by glucose levels. Initial studies on vascular tissue seem to support this postulate.

From the perspective of the pathogenesis of diabetic retinopathy, the finding of PKC activation is interesting, but it would be even more meaningful if its physiological significances were understood. This is so because glucose is used by numerous biochemical pathways; therefore, the finding of a metabolic parameter being altered in the diabetic state or when cells are exposed to elevated glucose levels is not surprising. It would be much more significant, however, if the changes could be linked to physiological dysfunctions.

POSSIBLE CONSEQUENCES OF PKC CHANGES

To characterize the effect of PKC activation in the vascular cells, we and others have begun to evaluate the changes in insulin receptor processing, type IV collagen synthesis, vasoactive hormone production, and vascular flow and permeability when cells are exposed to high glucose concentrations. As described previously, all of these parameters have been reported to be abnormal in vascular tissue from diabetic animals and humans (40,41,55,58). I will describe them each briefly.

Insulin receptors have been found in all vascular cells from both the macrovasculature and microvasculature of a variety of species, including the human, bovine, and rat, among others (27–29,30,36). Interestingly, there is a differential responsiveness to insulin between endothelial cells of macrovessels and microvessels, although no difference in binding affinity or receptor number has been found (28,30). Capillary endothelial cells isolated from normal rats are responsive to insulin for both metabolic and growth effects (36). In contrast, the same cells isolated from capillaries of diabetic rats have been reported to have a decreased number of insulin receptors and actions, as measured by receptor autophosphorylation and glucose incorporation into glycogen (36). The mRNA and the protein structure of the insulin receptors from the endothelial cells of diabetic and control rats did not demonstrate any differences as determined by Northern blot and trypsin digest analysis, respectively. It is possible that the decreased number of insulin receptor in cells from diabetic rats may be due to alterations in receptor processing or degradation (Fig. 9.10). We believe that such alterations in the processing could be due to PKC activation, because we have shown that increased serine phosphorylation of the insulin receptor can enhance its internalization rate in the endothelial cell (3,7,24). Serine phosphorylation of the insulin receptor could be due to PKC. In this context we have found that PMA, an activator of PKC, could induce insulin receptor internalization and phosphorylation, whereas an inactive phorbol ester, 4α, was without effect. Thus, it is possible that the changes in PKC activities in endothelial cells, when exposed to elevated glucose levels, could alter insulin receptor processing and lead to a decrease in insulin effect. In other cell types, an increase of serine phosphorylation of the insulin receptor has been reported to inhibit insulin receptor tyrosine kinase activity, which is postulated to be essential for insulin action (54).

In addition to insulin's classical actions, we have shown that the insulin receptor participates in transcytosis, the process of transporting insulin across the endothelial cell barrier without degradation (3,27,31). In endothelial cells from diabetic rats, we have shown that the transcytosis process is also de-

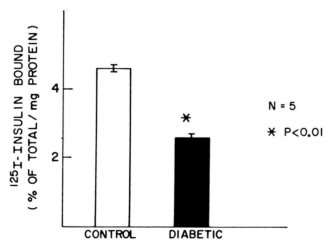

FIGURE 9.10. Characterization of insulin receptors on capillary endothelial cells from control and diabetic rats.

creased. Recent in vivo studies have provided supporting evidence that the transcytosis pathway is important in the physiological action of insulin and responsible for some of the insulin resistance observed in diabetes (5). Interestingly, hypoglycemic agents such as sulfonyluria have been reported to increase insulin binding on endothelial cells. Metformin, another hypoglycemic agent, did not affect insulin receptor but appears to increase the transport of insulin across endothelial cells from diabetic rats without affecting those from normal rats.

It is possible that other growth factor receptors may also be altered in vascular tissue of diabetic animals and patients. The processing for a number of these growth factor receptors, including epidermal growth factor (EGF), insulin-like growth factor (IGF), and, possibly, platelet-derived growth factor (PDGF) are regulated by PKC (3). This may therefore be a major way by which PKC activation interferes with cellular junctions in diabetes.

Another vascular function that could be modulated by PKC- and phospholipid-derived signals is the regulation of blood flow and vascular permeability (40,59). In the diabetic state, abnormalities involving both increases and decreases in blood flow have been reported (1,51,52,58). In the kidney, hyperperfusion has been demonstrated to occur in both diabetic animals and patients in the early stages of the disease (1). This mechanism is less clear for the retina, where decreased perfusion may be present in early stages of disease, but hyperperfusion may occur in later stages (51,52). Besides flow changes, increased vascular permeability has been noted in tissues with continuous capillaries, such as in the retina (15). Activation of PKC activities has been shown to affect junctional complexes between endothelial cells and to enhance vascular smooth muscle contractions (40,58). Preliminary studies on control and diabetic rats in our laboratory, have shown that there is a decrease in retinal blood flow, paralleled by an increase in PKC activities in the diabetic rat (51). In support of the retinal PKC changes responsible for this alteration of retinal blood flow, we have shown that the activation of retinal PKC with a phorbol ester will slow retinal blood flow in a similar manner. Further studies using PKC inhibitors in diabetic animals are necessary to confirm this hypothesis.

Another possible effect of elevated glucose concentration that could be attributed to altered PKC activity in the vascular endothelial cells is an abnormality in the expression of vasoactive hormones such as endothelin and angiotensin. Endothelin is a recently discovered vasoactive hormone of 21 amino acids, among which there are three different but very homologous polypeptides located on three different genes (26). In vascular tissues, endothelin is a very potent vasoconstrictor that can be synthesized by endothelium, and that stimulates contraction of smooth muscle cells or pericytes (60). Yamauchi et al. have reported that elevating the glucose levels in the medium enhances the production of endothelin-1 (ET-1) by bovine aortic endothelial cells (59). This effect of glucose is not related to sorbitol formation since it was not affected by an aldose reductase inhibitor. Because activation of PKC by phorbol ester is known to enhance the expression of ET-1, it is reasonable to suggest that this represents another example of a hyperglycemic effect mediated via PKC activation (37). It is tempting to speculate that abnormalities in ET production and effect in the vascular cells could be significant causal factors in the development of the abnormal hemodynamics and the hypertension found in the diabetic population (50).

We have presented evidence to demonstrate the feasibility of using cultured vascular cells as models to determine the metabolic and functional alterations caused by hyperglycemia. Studies using a combination of cultured cells and animal models have shown that PKC activities are generally increased in vascular tissue in hyperglycemic and diabetic states, and they also indicate that the mechanism of activation appears to be related to an increased production of DAG, de novo, secondary to an increase in glycolytic flux. The effects of PKC activation are multiple and could involve alterations of growth factor receptor processing, hemodynamics, vasoactive hormone expression, and basement membrane synthesis (Fig. 9.8). Further studies in these areas will clarify the roles of phospholipids and PKC in regulating vascular metabolism and functions during physiological and pathophysiological conditions.

ACKNOWLEDGMENTS

The authors wish to acknowledge their appreciation for the secretarial assistance of Leslie Balmat and Terri-Lyn Bellman. The studies in this report were supported in part by Joslin's Diabetes and Endocrinology Research Center grant (NIH DK 36836), NIH grants EY 05110, DK 39783, DK 36433, and the Lion's research grant.

REFERENCES

1. ANDERSON, S., and BRENNER, B. M. Pathogenesis of diabetic glomerulopathy: hemodynamic considerations. *Diabetes/Metab. Rev.* 4: 163–177, 1988.
2. ASHTON, N. Oxygen and the growth and development of retinal vessels. In vivo and in vitro studies. In: *Vascular Complications of Diabetes Mellitus,* edited by S. J. Kimura and W. M. Caggill. St. Louis: Mosby, 1967.
3. BACKER, J. M., and KING, G. L. Regulation of receptor-mediated endocytosis by phorbol esters. *Biochem. Pharmacol.* 41: 1267–1277, 1991.
4. BANSKOTA, N. K., TAUB, R., ZELLNER, K., and KING, G. L. Insulin, insulin-like growth factor I and platelet-derived growth factor interact additively in the induction of the protooncogene c-*myc* and cellular proliferation in cultured bovine aortic smooth muscle cells. *Mol. Endocrinol.* 3: 1183–1190, 1989.
5. BERGMAN, R. N. Toward physiological understanding of glucose tolerance. *Diabetes* 38: 1512–1527, 1989.
6. BERRIDGE, M. J. Inositol triphosphate and diacylglycerol: two interacting second messengers. *Annu. Rev. Biochem.* 56: 159–193, 1987.
7. BOTTARO, D. P., BONNER-WEIR, S., and KING, G. L. Insulin receptor recycling in vascular endothelial cells. *J. Biol. Chem.* 264: 5916–1923, 1989.
8. BROWNLEE, M., CERAMI, A., and VALASSARA, H. Advanced glycosylation end products in tissue and the biochemical basis of diabetic complications. *N. Engl. J. Med.* 318: 1315–1321, 1988.
9. BURDITT, A. F., CAIRD, F. I., and PROPER, G. J. The natural history of diabetic retinopathy. *Q. J. Med.* 371: 303–317, 1968.
10. CAIRD, F. I., BURDITT, A. F., and DRAPER, G. J. Diabetic retinopathy, a further study of prognosis for vision. *Diabetes* 17: 121–128, 1968.
11. COGAN, D. G., and KUWABARA, T. Capillary shunts in the pathogenesis of diabetic retinopathy. *Diabetes* 12: 293–300, 1983.
12. COGLIERO, E., MAIELLO, M., BOERI, D., ROY, S., and LORENZI, M. Increased expression of basement membrane components in human endothelial cells cultured in high glucose. *J. Clin. Invest.* 82: 735–738 1988.
13. CRAVEN, P. A., DAVIDSON, C. M., and DERUBERTIS, F. R. Increase in diacylglycerol mass in isolated glomeruli by glucose from de novo synthesis of glycerolipids. *Diabetes* 39: 667–674, 1990.

14. CRAVEN, P. A., DAVIDSON, C. M., and DERUBERTIS, F. R. Increase in diacylglycerol mass in isolated glomeruli by glucose from de novo synthesis of glycerolipids. *Diabetes* 39: 667–674, 1990.
15. CUNDA-VAZ, J., DEABREW, J. R. F., and CAMPOS, A. J. Early breakdown of the blood retinal barrier in diabetes. *Br. J. Ophthalmol.* 59: 649–656, 1975.
16. DEOLIVEIRA, F. Pericytes in diabetic retinopathy. *Br. J. Ophthalmol.* 50: 134–143, 1966.
17. ENGERMAN, R. L., and KERN, T. S. Progression of incipient diabetic retinopathy during glycemic control. *Diabetes* 36: 808–812, 1987.
18. ENGERMAN, R. L. Pathogenesis of diabetic retinopathy. *Diabetes* 38: 1203–1206, 1989.
19. ENGERMAN, R. L., and KERN, T. S. Hyperglycemia and development of glomerular pathology: diabetes compared with galactosemia. *Kidney Int.* 36: 41–45, 1989.
20. FOLKMAN, J., and KLAGSBRUN, M. Angiogenic factors. *Science* 235: 442–447, 1987.
21. GANESAN, S., CALLE, R., ZAWALICK, K., SMALLWOOD, J. I., ZAWALICH, W., and RASMUSSEN, H. Glucose-induced translocation of protein kinase C in rat pancreatic islets. *Proc. Natl. Acad. Sci. USA* 87: 9893–9897, 1990.
22. GREEN, D. A., LATTIMER, S. A., and SIMA, A. A. F. Sorbitol, phosphoinositides and sodium-potassium ATPase in the pathogenesis of diabetic complications. *N. Engl. J. Med.* 316: 599–606, 1987.
23. GRUNWALD, J. E., BRUCKER, A. J., SCHWARTZ, S. S., BRAUNSTEIN, S. N., BAKER, L., PETRIG, B. L., and RIVA, C. E. Diabetic glycemic control and retinal blood flow. *Diabetes* 39: 602–607, 1990.
24. HACHIYA, H. L., TAKAYAMA, S., WHITE, M. F., and KING, G. L. Regulation of insulin receptor internalization in vascular endothelial cells by insulin and phorbol ester. *J. Biol. Chem.* 262: 6417–6424, 1987.
25. HOCEVAR, B. A., and FIELD, A. P. Selective translocation of BII-protein kinase C to the nucleus of human promyelocytic (HL60) leukemia cells. *J. Biol. Chem.* 266: 38–33, 1991.
26. INOUE, A., YANAGISAWA, M., KIMURA, S., KASUYA, Y., MIYAUCHI, T., GOTO, K., and MASAKI, T. The human endothelin family: three structurally and pharmacologically distinct isopeptides predicted by three separate genes. *Proc. Natl. Acad. Sci. USA* 86: 2863–2867, 1989.
27. JIALAL, I., KING, G. L., BUCHWALD, S., KAHN, C. R., and CRETTAZ, M. Processing of insulin by bovine endothelial cells in culture. *Diabetes* 33: 794–800, 1984.
28. KING, G. L., BUZNEY, S. M., KAHN, C. R., HETA, N., BUCHWALD, S., MacDONALD, S. G., and RAND, L. I. Differential responsiveness to insulin of endothelial and support cells from micro and macrovessels. *J. Clin. Invest.* 71: 974–979, 1983.
29. KING. G. L. Cell biology as an approach to the study of vascular complications of diabetes. *Metabolism* 34 (Suppl. 1) 34: 17–24, 1985.
30. KING, G. L., GOODMAN, A. D., BUZNEY, S. M., MOSES, A., and KAHN, C. R. Receptors and growth-promoting effects of insulin and insulin-like growth factors on cells from bovine retinal capillaries and aorta. *J. Clin. Invest.* 75: 1028–1036, 1985.
31. KING, G. L., and JOHNSON, S. Receptor-mediated transport of insulin across endothelial cells. *Science* 227: 1583–1586, 1985.
32. KING, G. L., JOHNSON, S., and WU, G. Possible growth modulators involved in the pathogenesis of diabetic proliferative retinopathy. In: *Growth Factors in Health and Disease,* edited by B. Westermark, C. Betsholtz, and B. Hokfelt. Netherlands: Elsevier Science, 1990, pp. 303–317.
33. KOHNER, E. M. The problems of retinal blood flow in diabetes. *Diabetes* 25 (Suppl. 2): 839–844, 1976.
34. KOHNER, E. M., McLEOD, D., and MARSHALL, J. Diabetic retinopathy. In: *Complications of Diabetes,* edited by H. Keen and J. Jarrett. London: Edward Arnold, 1982, pp. 19–121.
35. KUWABARA, T., and COGAN, G. Studies on the retinal vascular pattern. I. Normal architecture. *AMA Arch. Ophthalmol.* 64: 904–916, 1960.
36. KWOK, C. F., GOLDSTEIN, B. J., MULLER-WIELAND, D., LEE, T.-S., KAHN, C. R., and KING, G. L. Identification of persistent defects in insulin receptor structure and function in capillary endothelial cells from diabetic rats. *J. Clin. Invest.* 83: 127–136, 1989.
37. LEE, M.-E., BLOCK, K. D., CLIFFORD, J. A., and QUERTERMOUS, T. Functional analysis of the endothelin-1 gene promoter. *J. Biol. Chem.* 265: 10446–10450, 1990.
38. LI, W., SHEN, S., KHATAMI, M., and ROCKEY, J. H. Stimulation of retinal pericytes, protein and collagen synthesis in culture by high glucose concentration. *Diabetes* 33: 785–789, 1984.
39. LOY, A., LURIE, K. G., GHOSH, A., WILSON, J. M., MacGREGOR, L. C., and MATSCHINSKY, F. M. Diabetes and the myoinositol paradox. *Diabetes* 39: 1305–1312, 1990.

40. LYNCH, J. L., FERRO, T. J., BLUMENSTOCK, F. A., BROCKENAUER, A. M., and MALIK, A. B. Increased endothelial albumin permeability mediated by protein kinase C activation. *J. Clin. Invest.* 85: 1991–1998, 1990.

41. MONTESANO, R., and ORCI, L. Tumor-promoting esters induce angiogenesis in vitro. *Cell* 42: 469–477, 1985.

42. NAYAK, R. C., BERMAN, A. B., GEORGE, K. L., EISENBARTH, G. S., and KING, G. L. A monoclonal antibody (3G5)-defined ganglioside antigen is expressed on the cell surface of microvascular pericytes. *J. Exp. Med.* 167: 1003–1015, 1988.

43. NISHIZUKA, Y. The family of protein kinase C for signal transduction. *JAMA* 262: 1826–1833, 1989.

44. ONO, Y., FUJII, T., OGITA, K., KIKKAWA, U., IGARASHI, K., and NISHIZUKA, Y. Protein kinase C subspecies from rat brain: its structure, expression, and properties. *Proc. Natl. Acad. Sci. USA* 86: 3099–3103, 1989.

45. PETER-RIESCH, B., FAHTI, M., SCHLEGEL, W., and WOLLHEIM, C. B. Glucose and carbachol generate 1,2-diacylglycerols by different mechanisms in pancreatic islets. *J. Clin. Invest.* 81: 1154–1161, 1988.

46. PUGAZHENTHI, S., MANTHA, S. V., and KHANDELWOL, R. L. Decrease of liver protein kinase C in streptozotocin-induced diabetic rats and restoration by vanadate treatment. *Biochem. Int.* 21: 651–657, 1990.

47. RAMSAY, R. C., GOETZ, F. C., SUTHERLAND, D. E. R., MAUER, S. M., ROBISON, L. L., CANTRILL, H. L., KNOBLOCH, W. H., and NAJARIAN, J. S. Progression of diabetic retinopathy after pancreatic transplantation for insulin dependent diabetic mellitus. *N. Engl. J. Med.* 318: 208–214, 1988.

48. RAND, L. I. Recent advances in diabetic retinopathy. *Am. J. Med.* 70: 595–602, 1981.

49. ROBISON, W. G., TILLIS, T. N., LAVER, N., and KINOSHITA, J. Diabetes-related histopathologies of rat retina prevented with an aldose reductase inhibitor. *Exp. Eye Res.* 50: 355, 1970.

50. SAAD, M. F., LILLIOJA, S., NYOMBA, B. L., CASTILLO, C., FERRARO, R., GREGORIO, M. D., RAVUSSEN, E., KNOWLER, W. C., BENNETT, P. H., HOWARD, B. V., and BOGARDUS, C. Racial differences in the relation between blood pressure and insulin resistance. *N. Engl. J. Med.* 324: 733–739, 1991.

51. SHIBA, T., BURSELL, S.-E., CLERMONT, A., SPORTSMAN, R., HEATH, W., and KING, G. L. Protein kinase C activation is a causal factor for the alteration of retinal blood flow in diabetes of short duration. *Invest. Ophthalmol. Vis. Sci. USA* 32: 785, 1991.

52. SMALL, K. W., STEFANSSON, E., and HATCHELL, D. C. Retinal blood flow in normal and diabetic dogs. *Invest. Ophthalmol. Vis. Sci.* 28: 672–675, 1987.

53. SUSSMAN, I., CARSON, M. P., SCHULTZ, V., WU, V. P., MCCALL, A. L., RUDERMAN, N. B., and TORNHEIM, K. Chronic exposure to high glucose decreases myo-inositol in cultured cerebral microvascular pericytes but not in endothelium. *Diabetologia* 31: 771–775, 1988.

54. TAKAYAMA, S., WHITE, M. F., LAURIS, V., and KAHN, C. R. Phorbol esters modulate insulin receptor phosphorylation and insulin in cultured hepatoma cells. *Proc. Natl. Acad. Sci. USA* 81: 7797–7801, 1984.

55. TESFAMARIAN, B., BROWN, M. L., and COHEN, R. A. Elevated glucose impairs endothelium-dependent relaxation by activation protein kinase C. *J. Clin. Invest.* 87: 1643–1648, 1991.

56. TRUS, M. D., ZAWALICH, W. S., BURCH, P. T., BERNER, D. K., WEILL, V. A., and MATSHINSKY, F. M. Regulation of glucose metabolism in pancreatic islets. *Diabetes* 30: 911–922, 1981.

57. WISE, G. N. Retinal neovascularization. *Trans. Am. Ophthalmol. Soc.* 54: 729–826, 1956.

58. WOLF, B. A., WILLIAMSON, J. R., EASOM, R. A., CHANG, K., SHERMAN, W. R., and TURK, J. Diacylglycerol accumulation and microvascular abnormalities induced by elevated glucose levels. *J. Clin. Invest.* 87: 31–38, 1991.

59. YAMAUCHI, T., KEIZO, O., TAKAYANAGI, R., UMEDA, F., and NAWATA, H. Enhanced secretion of endothlin-1 by elevated glucose levels from cultured bovine aortic endothelial cells. *FEBS Lett.* 267: 16–18, 1990.

60. YANAGISAWA, M., KURIHARA, H., KIMURA, S., TOMOBE, Y., KOBAYASHI, M., MITSUI, Y., YAZAKI, Y., GOTO, K., and MASAKI, T. A novel potent vasoconstrictor peptide produced by vascular endothelial cells. *Nature* 332: 411–415, 1988.

10

Mobilization of Arachidonic Acid from Diacyl and Ether Phospholipids in Cultured Endothelial Cells

MICHAEL L. BROWN

Cultured endothelial cells are invaluable tools in studying the effect of diabetes and its vast symptomology on the metabolism of the vasculature. The culture of endothelial cells provides an important tissue model, pure in cell type and easily manipulated. Although tissue culture offers slight possibilities of mimicking the total diabetic milieu, specific conditions that arise in the course of diabetes can be reproduced in a controlled and isolated manner. In this chapter, the discussion focuses on studies undertaken to examine arachidonic acid metabolism in endothelial cells and the influence upon it by elevated glucose levels similar to those found in patients with diabetes.

ARACHIDONIC ACID METABOLISM AND DIABETES

Arachidonic acid (AA; eicosatetraenoic acid; 20:4n-6; 20:4 delta [5,8,11,14]) is the parent compound for a variety of biologically active compounds known as *eicosanoids*. Eicosanoids are ubiquitously produced by the action of cyclooxygenases, lipoxygenases, and cytochrome P-450 monooxygenases on AA [(10,27,36); see Fig. 10.1]. The effects of the end product eicosanoids are many and are usually autacoid in nature. A single compound may have extremely varied effects, depending on the species, cell type, or location. In endothelial cells, prostacyclin (PGI_2) is generally the major eicosanoid produced. In most vascular systems its actions are vasodilatory with potent antiaggregatory capabilities. Such actions directly oppose those of the major platelet eicosanoid, thromboxane A_2, a vasoconstrictor and proaggregatory agent. Vascular occlusion and increased thrombosis could result if the balance of these metabolites is disturbed. Thus, it was the alteration of the metabolism and release of these two compounds that were originally implicated in the pathophysiology of diabetic vascular disease. Indeed, platelet thromboxane A_2 production in diabetes and diabetic models has been intensely studied and reviewed elsewhere (13,14). It is generally agreed that diabetes leads to a more pronounced release of thromboxane A_2, and thus more rapid aggregation times, decreased bleeding times, and increased number of vascular occlusions due to thrombi.

The production and release of prostacyclin by blood vessels of diabetic pa-

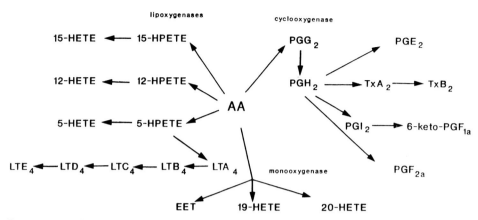

FIGURE 10.1. Abbreviated, generalized pathway of eicosanoid production. Arachidonic acid can be metabolized to a variety of eicosanoids. Production is species, tissue, and cell specific. Cyclooxygenase activity results in thromboxane (Tx) and prostaglandin (PG) synthesis. Lipogenase activity results in hydroperoxy- (HPETE) and hydroxy- (HETE) derivatives of AA and the leukotrienes (LT). Cytochrome P 450 monooxygenase activity can result in epoxy- (EET) and hydroxy- (HETE) metabolites.

tients (1,38,40), animal models (19,31,42,46,52), and from cells cultured in conditions to mimic diabetes (5,18,27,51) is less well studied. Although not conclusive, the release of prostacyclin in most cases has been found to be diminished compared to matched controls. In our laboratories, the production of 6-keto-PGF$_{1a}$, the stable metabolite of prostacyclin, by isolated cerebral microvessels from streptozotocin-induced diabetic rats was diminished only if the vessels were challenged with exogenous free AA (52). In endothelial cells in culture, glucose elevation alone did not affect 6-keto-PGF$_{1a}$ release (5).

ARACHIDONIC ACID METABOLISM IN ENDOTHELIAL CELLS

It is of interest to establish how AA is mobilized and redistributed in endothelial cells and how elevated glucose concentration influences these and other processes in the cultured endothelial cell.

Arachidonic acid is one of the essential fatty acids that must be obtained dietetically as AA or as one of its less desaturated or elongated precursors such as linoleic acid or dihomo-gamma-linolenic acid. Endothelial cells in culture lack the demonstrable delta-6 desaturase activity necessary for this conversion (32,41). As a result they must be supplied with AA through supplementations, such as with fetal calf serum, or by the addition of AA/bovine serum albumin complexes in serum-free systems. Once taken up by the cell, AA is distributed throughout phospholipid classes and the various neutral lipid subclasses. Arachidonic acid is esterified almost exclusively to the *sn*-2 position of phospholipids (Fig. 10.2). It is liberated by Ca^{2+}-dependent phospholipases. For example, phospholipase A$_2$ action would yield free AA and a 2-lyso-phospholipid. Phospholipase C action would yield 1-radyl,2-arachidonoyl-glycerol

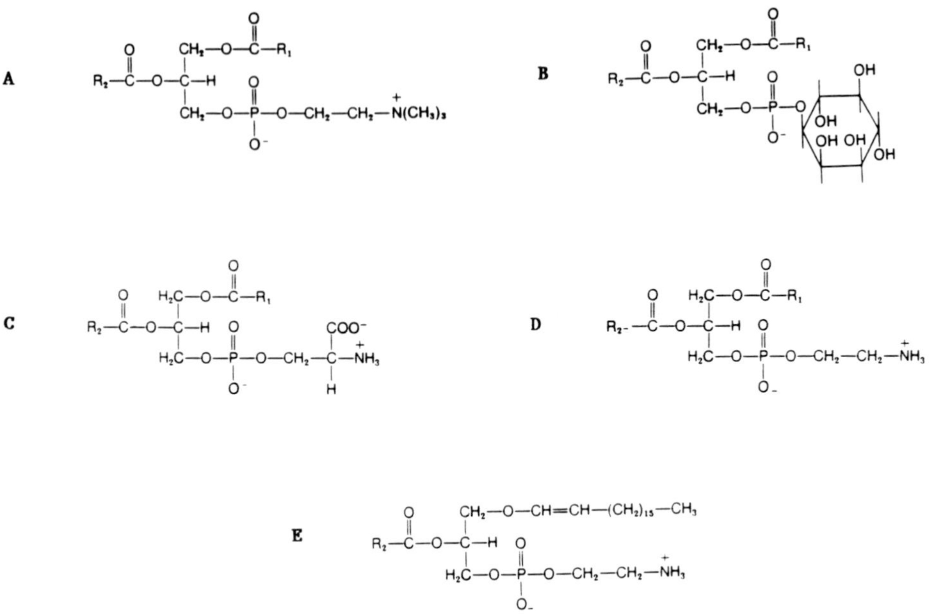

FIGURE 10.2. Phospholipid structure. The structure of the common endothelial phospholipids is illustrated. *A:* phosphatidylcholine, *B:* phosphatidylinositol; *C:* phosphatidylserine; *D:* phosphatidylethanolamine; *E:* alkenyl phosphatidylethanolamine. *A–D:* diacyl forms; *E:* alkenylacyl form. R_2COOH is the near-exclusive position of AA and other polyunsaturated fatty acids.

and a phosphobase. Further action of a diglyceride lipase would yield free AA. Once free, AA can be oxygenated by cyclooxygenase, lipoxygenase, or mono-oxygenase with the release of the corresponding products. Arachidonic acid can be released free into the medium and may have bioactive properties of its own (28). Free AA can be reesterified to recently formed lyso-compounds by the action of acyltransferases (15), or it can enter the neutral lipid pool and form triglycerides (9) or intermediates of de novo phospholipid synthesis. Phospholipase A_2, by forming a lysophospholipid, may also initiate a transfer of AA by the action of transacylases (11,20,21,30).

GENERATION OF SPECIFIC CYCLOOXYGENASE AND LIPOXYGENASE
PRODUCTS FROM SELECT POOLS OF PHOSPHOLIPIDS

Earlier Investigations

It is a frequently propagated notion that, once released from phospholipids, AA enters a miscible pool and can enter any of the above oxygenating pathways for conversion to product. There is evidence that select pools may exist for the conversion of AA to prostaglandins and lipoxygenase products.

In an early attempt to examine this question, Thomas et al. (47) prelabeled human umbilical vein endothelial cells (HUVEC) with [³H]AA for 24 h, then examined the loss of radiolabel from phospholipids upon stimulation with 5 μM calcium ionophore A23187. The only significant net loss of AA was from phosphatidylcholine. This loss occurred while prostacyclin and free AA was being released into the medium. The low total release of radiolabel (<6% of the total incorporated) and the lack of a detailed time course of release detract from the clarity of their conclusions. Selection of a single time point also does not allow one to monitor the pattern of release nor the potential of rapid reacylation of labeled AA into a specific pool especially in the absence of albumin in the incubation medium. A larger magnitude of mobilization would unmask subtle changes in the AA release or redistribution.

Hong and Deykin (17) prelabeled primary porcine aortic endothelial cells with both [^{14}C]stearic acid and [^{3}H]AA. As anticipated, the [^{14}C]stearic acid esterified primarily to the sn-1 position of phospholipids and the [^{3}H]AA almost exclusively to the sn-2 position. Following the application of bradykinin, the net change in radioactivity for both isotopes as well as the ratio of ^{14}C:^{3}H was measured in individual phospholipid, lysophospholipid and neutral lipid classes. It was determined that bradykinin induced the synthesis of diacylglycerol and the release of prostacyclin. The ^{14}C:^{3}H ratio of diacylglycerol was very similar to phosphatidylinositol, suggesting specific action of phospholipase C. During the 4 min experiment lysophosphatidylinositol, lysophosphatidylethanolamine, and lysophosphatidylcholine were also generated, suggesting the action of phospholipase A$_2$, and that these phospholipids contributed AA for prostacyclin synthesis. The release of other eicosanoids was not detailed in this study, and the shortness of the time course study may have limited their elaboration.

In later studies Thomas et al. (48) reevaluated the phospholipid origin of AA in HUVEC using thrombin as an agonist. In the basic experimental designs, cultures were prelabeled with [^{3}H]AA for 24 h, rinsed with buffer, and stimulated with thrombin, after which medium and cell lipids were extracted and analyzed. As in a previous report by these investigators, prostacyclin was the major eicosanoid released along with free AA. They reported that the major net loss occurred at the expense of phosphatidylcholine AA content, with lesser net loss in phosphatidylinositol. A rise in intracellular free AA led to the conclusion that the major arachidonic liberating enzyme was phospholipase A$_2$.

In the hands of Thomas et al. (48), the labeling of endothelial cultures with radioactive AA over 24 h resulted in pools of phospholipid arachidonate of nearly equivalent specific activities. However, Wey et al. (53), using bovine aortic endothelial cells (BAEC), noticed a dramatic shift in the amount of AA entering phosphatidylcholine over an extended time course. Uptake of radiolabeled AA into phosphatidylcholine was near linear for 8 h. After this time, a decrease in phosphatidylcholine-arachidonate was noticed, while phosphatidylethanolamine continued to increase. A more careful examination of this observation was allowed by a 2 h pulse-labeling study. The BAEC were incubated for 2 h with [^{14}C]AA/bovine serum albumin complex, after which the cultures were rinsed and the medium containing 10% fetal calf serum was added. The [^{14}C]AA content of cellular lipids was monitored for an additional 24 h. From an original distribution (following 2 hr exposure to [^{14}C]AA) of 53.0% phosphatidylcholine, 14.9% phosphatidylethanolamine, 28.9% phosphatidylinositol, and 1.7% phosphatidylserine, the AA was redistributed after a 24 h "chase" with 10% fetal calf serum to 27.6% phosphatidylcholine, 41.0% phosphatidylethanolamine, 28.5% phosphatidylinositol, and 1.7% phosphatidylserine. Phosphatidylcholine lost 25.4% of its radiolabel while an equivalent level of 26.1% was gained by phosphatidylethanolamine. Analysis of acyl and ether subclasses of these two phospholipids demonstrated that the loss came from diacyl phosphatidylcholine and that the gain was equally distributed in diacyl- and alkenyl phosphatidylethanolamine. We can conclude from this study that the extent and conditions of labeling with AA can enrich phospholipid fractions beyond the homogeneity of specific activities previously observed.

Ragab-Thomas and colleagues (29) continued their studies tracing the source of agonist-induced AA release by labeling HUVEC with [U-^{14}C]AA for 20 h. Application of the calcium ionophore A23187 or thrombin promoted the release of free AA and prostaglandins into the medium. Addition of A23187 resulted in a rapid loss of radioactivity from phosphatidylcholine and a minor decrease from phosphatidylethanolamine. Phosphatidylinositol displayed a minor decrease in radioactivity followed by resynthesis to baseline levels at 10 min. The investigators' observations concerning thrombin stimulated HUVEC were confirmed with the additional observation of thrombin-induced triacylglycerol hydrolysis. In the same report, this group prelabeled HUVEC with both [^{14}C]AA acid and [^{3}H]palmitic acid. They determined that the ^{14}C/^{3}H ratio of the diacylglycerol fraction generated compared with the ratio that would result from phospholipase C action on phosphatidylcholine and not phosphatidylinositol.

STUDIES IN PORCINE AORTIC ENDOTHELIAL CELLS

Research in our laboratory has centered on the use of porcine aortic endothelial cells [PAEC; (3,4,5)] because these cells in culture are highly responsive to agonists, especially A23187 and bradykinin. In our initial studies (4), we prelabeled PAEC with [^{14}C]AA for times up to 24 h and found that the uptake of AA was essentially complete at 8 h (Fig. 10.3). The pattern of uptake into the various phospholipid and neutral lipid fractions closely paralleled that of Wey et al. (53) using BAEC. For the first 8 h the most avid uptake was into phosphatidylcholine; after 8 h the absolute amount of radiolabel in phosphatidylcholine diminished, and the predominant labeled fraction became phosphatidylethanolamine. Analysis of the subclasses of phosphatidylcholine and phosphatidylethanolamine throughout the uptake curve revealed that the AA lost from phosphatidylcholine was from the diacyl fraction while alkenyl phosphatidylethanolamine, and to a lesser extent diacyl phosphatidylethanolamine, gained radioactivity. The distribution of [^{14}C]AA after 24 h and the distribution of lipid phosphorus of PAEC is shown in Table 10.1. These results demonstrate that differences in specific activities of phospholipid classes is feasible with careful labeling and culture conditions. Such labeling permits tracking of AA in the alkenyl as well as diacyl subclasses. Further, if there is a singular or dominant source of AA resulting from agonist stimulation, then the specific activity of the released AA and eicosanoids should be reflective of that source.

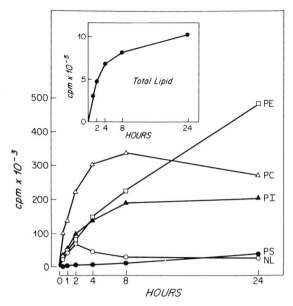

FIGURE 10.3. Incorporation of [¹⁴C]AA into PAEC. PAEC were incubated for times up to 24 h with 1 μM [¹⁴C]AA (0.55 μCi). Lipids were resolved by HPLC and the radioactivity assayed. Data represent the mean of three experiments performed in duplicate. [From (4); used with permission.]

After 24 h of prelabeling, the PAEC were incubated with 1 μM A23187 for times up to 30 min (Fig. 10.4). Up to 24% of the incorporated AA was recovered as released radioactivity in the medium (Table 10.2). Release of prostaglandins (50% of which was prostacyclin) was complete within 5 min. Release of lipoxygenase products (mostly 15-hydroxyeicosatetraenoic acid; 15-HETE) was slow in the first 5 min and more rapid thereafter. Release of free AA, the major eicosanoid released, proceeded in a biphasic manner—a rapid linear release in the first 10 min followed by a secondary near-linear and less rapid release

TABLE 10.1. Distribution of lipid phosphorus and [¹⁴C] arachidonic acid in PAEC[a]

Phospholipid[b]	Subclass	% Total [¹⁴C]AA	% Phospholipid mass
PC	Diacyl	16.8	44.2
	Alkyl	2.9	7.8
	Alkenyl	1.1	1.3
PE	Diacyl	15.7	12.4
	Alkyl	4.3	1.5
	Alkenyl	27.9	11.7
PI		22.4	5.5
PS		1.5	4.0

[a]Confluent cultures of PAEC (approximately 6.5×10^6 cells/100 mm dish) were prelabeled with 1 μM [¹⁴C]AA for 24 h (1.201 dpm $\times 10^{-6}$ total radioactivity associated with cell lipid. Lipids separated by HPLC and assayed for radioactivity and lipid phosphorus.

[b]PC, phosphatidylcholine; PE, phosphatidylethanolamine; PI, phosphatidylinositol; PS, phosphatidylserine.

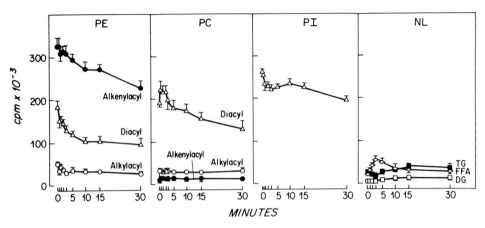

FIGURE 10.4. Changes in [^{14}C]AA content of individual lipid fractions of PAEC in response to ionophore A23187. Data represent the mean ± SE of six experiments performed in duplicate. [From (4); used with permission.]

thereafter. Early, from 30 s to 5 min, substantial losses of [^{14}C]AA from diacyl phosphatidylethanolamine and phosphatidylinositol were observed. These losses coincided with the release of cyclooxygenase products, mainly prostacyclin into the medium. After 5 min, we observed a progressive and sustained loss of [^{14}C]AA from alkenyl phosphatidylethanolamine and from diacyl phosphatidylcholine. These late changes coincided with the elaboration of ^{14}C-lipoxygenase products. Although unequivocal assignments could not be made, the data suggest that specific pools of AA provide precursors for individual classes of eicosanoids. Since the net changes of many phospholipid classes exceeded those of the eicosanoids in the medium, any single or combined fraction of phospholipids could have provided AA for eicosanoid production. The patterns of release from phospholipids and the appearance of radiolabel in the medium are striking enough to suggest specific sources of AA from individual classes of eicosanoids (Fig. 10.5). The coincident loss of AA from phosphatidylinositol and diacyl phosphatidylethanolamine with the appearance of cyclooxygenase products in the medium suggest one relationship. While the loss AA from alkenyl phosphatidylethanolamine and diacyl phosphatidylcholine and the finding that this correlates with the appearance of lipoxygenase, but not cyclooxygenase, products suggests another relationship. This study was the first to demonstrate the role of alkenyl phosphatidylethanolamine as a source of AA release for eicosanoid synthesis in endothelial cells.

FURTHER CONSIDERATION OF THE MODEL

Our model provides an excellent starting point for studying precursor–product relationships. It has a few potential weaknesses that we are working to overcome. One possible problem when one assigns products to precursors based on temporal relationships may be the coincidental activation/deactivation of AA metabolizing enzymes. We know that the activation of phospholipases is rapid

TABLE 10.2. A23187-induced release of ^{14}C-labeled eicosanoids from prelabeled PAEC[a]

Time (min)	Polar front	6-Keto-prostaglandin F_{1a}	Other CO products	Leuko-trienes	5-HETE	15-HETE	Arachidonic acid	Total	6-Keto-prostaglandin F_{1a}[b]
0	0.5 ± 0.4	0.9 ± 0.4	0.2 ± 0.1	0	0.2 ± 0.1	0.2 ± 0.1	1.8 ± 0.4	5.2 ± 1.3	2.1 ± 2.1
0.5	0.6 ± 0.2	0.9 ± 0.4	0.6 ± 0.3	trace	0.2 ± 0.3	1.0 ± 0.3	4.3 ± 0.4	9.0 ± 1.2	2.6 ± 0.2
1	0.8 ± 0.1	2.5 ± 0.4	1.7 ± 0.1	0.9 ± 0.4	1.0 ± 0.3	1.3 ± 0.4	12.0 ± 2.4	20.7 ± 2.3	6.2 ± 0.2
2	0.7 ± 0.2	5.5 ± 1.2	5.5 ± 1.5	1.1 ± 0.4	0.7 ± 0.1	1.3 ± 0.2	18.4 ± 2.8	38.4 ± 5.9	18.8 ± 0.5
3	3.1 ± 0.7	10.7 ± 1.5	9.3 ± 1.2	2.0 ± 0.6	0.9 ± 0.2	1.1 ± 0.2	36.8 ± 2.4	63.9 ± 1.3	90.0 ± 4.3
5	4.9 ± 0.8	19.8 ± 4.4	14.1 ± 2.9	1.9 ± 0.4	2.1 ± 0.7	3.9 ± 1.4	63.4 ± 8.6	120 ± 7.7	153 ± 3.2
10	4.8 ± 1.1	21.1 ± 5.1	11.8 ± 1.2	2.4 ± 0.7	1.8 ± 0.3	4.2 ± 0.4	79.5 ± 10.2	133 ± 11.0	201 ± 9.8
15	5.5 ± 1.7	21.6 ± 4.5	15.2 ± 1.4	3.8 ± 1.1	3.9 ± 0.9	6.1 ± 1.5	114 ± 11.1	182 ± 5.4	208 ± 10.5
30	10.3 ± 3.4	27.8 ± 3.8	16.7 ± 3.0	3.9 ± 0.8	5.8 ± 1.8	11.2 ± 3.4	193 ± 31.9	281 ± 2.7	215 ± 9.9

[a]PAEC prelabeled with [^{14}C]AA for 24 h were subsequently stimulated with 1 μM A23187 for times up to 30 min. The medium was aspirated, acidified, extracted, and the eicosanoids resolved by reverse-phase HPLC as previously described (4). Data are expressed as the mean ± SE of six experiments performed in duplicate. Values are cpm × 10^{-3}, except the far column of 6-keto-PGF$_{1a}$ is expressed as ng/plate.

[b]Parallel experiments using 1 μM unlabeled arachidonic acid were also performed, and 6-ketoprostaglandin F$_{1a}$ mass was determined by radioimmunoassay.

185

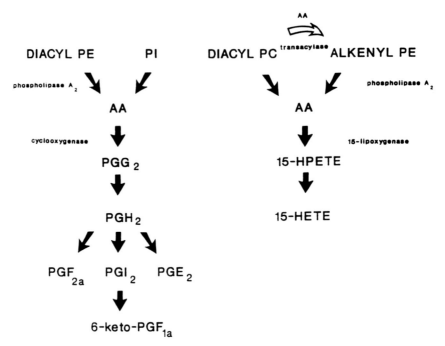

FIGURE 10.5. Hypothetical model of ionophore A23187-induced eicosanoid metabolism in endothelial cells.

following an increase in intracellular Ca^{2+}. Also, after a burst of activity, the cyclooxygenase is self-deactivated by the endoperoxide byproducts (2). For this reason, in endothelial cells, cyclooxygenase activation is often limited to 10 min. This secondary inactivation of cyclooxygenase hypothetically would allow lipoxygenase activity to continue without competition for substrate. In this context, lipoxygenase products exert many local effects on AA metabolism, including feedback inhibition of cyclooxygenase (12,16,38) and phospholipase (6).

Measurement of loss of radioactivity from a specific phospholipid pool provides information only on the net mobilization of that AA. Surely, lysophospholipids generated by phospholipase A_2 action are reacylated with fatty acids available at the time. In order to maintain an ordered system, it is not unreasonable to think that AA itself would be the preferred reacylation compound. With this in mind, our system greatly underestimates the mobilization of AA, and excludes estimates of transfer prior to release. Colard et al. (8), working with platelets prelabeled with [^{14}C]AA and stimulated with thrombin, reported that the AA could not come directly from diacyl phosphatidylcholine, but that two other phospholipids were the direct precursors following transfer from diacyl phosphatidylcholine. These phospholipids were alkyl phosphatidylcholine and diacyl phosphatidylethanolamine. These data were gathered by separation of diradylglycerobenzoate derivatives of phospholipids allowing direct, on-line measurement of mass by HPLC and thus measurement of specific activity of phospholipid class, subclass, and molecular species. Such techniques have been successfully applied to endothelial cells (44). We are actively using such techniques to assess simultaneous transfer and reacylation and to examine specific activities of labeled phospholipids and products. By combining mass measurements with metabolic perturbations (conditions that alter eicosanoid ratios), we hope to establish firmer specific phospholipid–eicosanoid relationships. Among the metabolic perturbations we have studied are the use of elevated glucose in the culture medium, the passage state of the cultured cells, and the use of different agonists to elicit eicosanoid production.

EFFECT OF ELEVATED GLUCOSE ON RELEASE OF EICOSANOIDS

PAEC were conditioned through two passages (5) for 6 days, (third passage at beginning of treatment) in glucose levels that mimic euglycemia (100 mg/dl; 5.2 mM; GN cells) or hyperglycemia (300 mg/dl; 15.6 mM; GE cells). The elevation of glucose in the culture medium did not affect cell growth, doubling times, morphology, or protein levels. More extreme levels of glucose, however, have been shown to be toxic to cultured endothelial cells (24,43). The cultures were labeled for 24 h with [^{14}C]AA as described above and stimulated with calcium ionophore A23187 for times up to 30 min. The high levels of glucose (GE group) did not affect the net uptake of [^{14}C]AA or its distribution in phospholipid classes at 24 h. However, it did influence the release of radioactivity into the medium and the profile of products found in the medium (Fig. 10.6). Release was identical for the GN and GE groups during the first 10 min but diverged thereafter. GN cells continued to release radiolabeled eicosanoids such that 33% of the incorporated radiolabel was recovered in the medium at

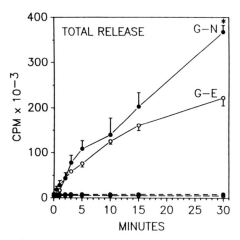

FIGURE 10.6. Ionophore-induced release of radioactivity from PAEC conditioned in normal (GN) and elevated (GE) glucose and prelabeled with [^{14}C]AA. PAEC conditioned through two passages with normal and elevated glucose levels were prelabeled for 24 h with 1 μM [^{14}C]AA, rinsed, and stimulated with 1 μM ionophore A23187. Data represent mean ± SE of three experiements performed in duplicate. *Dashed lines* represent exposure to the ionophore A23187 vehicle (dimethyl sulfoxide) alone. [From (5); used with permission.]

30 min. GE cells, however, continued to release only 20% of the incorporated total at 30 min. The specificity of this effect was examined using other sugars. Cells were cultured in GN levels of D-glucose, with additions of mannose, mannitol, sucrose, or L-glucose in amounts sufficient to achieve the same medium osmolarity as the GE group. In the presence of all of these compounds, release of ^{14}C-radioactivity was similar to that of GN cells and not the GE group. These findings indicate that the effect of elevated glucose was not due to increased osmolarity, but probably to an alteration of glucose metabolism caused by the increase in its concentration (see chapters 6, 7, and 9). The mechanism of diminished release of radiolabel remains unclear, although a role for altered phospholipase activity has been suggested. Early studies (39) indicated that the phospholipase A_2 from liver of streptozotocin-diabetic rats is greatly diminished as is the phospholipase A_2 activity in platelets of diabetic patients (45). However, Laychock (23) found that crudely purified phospholipase A_2 from pancreatic islet cells was directly stimulated by glucose.

As illustrated in Figure 10.7, closer examination of the eicosanoids released into the medium in our studies with PAEC revealed several interesting observations. The major product released into the medium upon stimulation with calcium ionophore A23187 was free [^{14}C]AA. GN cultures released up to 3 times the amount of [^{14}C]AA as GE cultures after 10 min of incubation with the calcium ionophore A23187. [^{14}C]cyclooxygenase products, considered as individual species or as a group, were released in equivalent amounts throughout the time course. This was confirmed in parallel experiments in which we measured immunoreactive 6-keto-PGF$_{1a}$. In contrast, the release of [^{14}C]lipoxygenase products was consistently elevated in GE cultures to as much as 3 times the rate observed in GN cultures. Of the lipoxygenase products released, [^{14}C]5-HETE was elevated in GE conditions but not to a significant degree. The major lipoxygenase product measured was [^{14}C]15-HETE, which accounted for half of the total lipoxygenase products. Beyond 10 min of agonist exposure the release of this metabolite was significantly increased. Parallel studies with unlabeled cultures incubated with the calcium ionophore A23187, bradykinin, or thrombin, both confirmed that elevated glucose increases 15-HETE release by cultured PAEC and demonstrated that this effect is independent of the agonist used. The role of glucose as a weak, but concentrated, free-radical scavenger has been suggested as augmenting lipoxygenase product release (33).

The importance of this 15-HETE or its parent compound 15-HPETE in diabetic vascular disease is as yet unclear. These compounds display many activities of potential importance in AA metabolism, vascular reactivity, and signal transduction. For instance, 15-HPETE has been shown to inhibit prostacyclin formation (16), and 15-HETE inhibits phospholipase A_2 activity in platelets and neutrophils (6). Furthermore, 15-HETE both stimulates and inhibits different steps in leukotriene synthesis by leukocytes (49,50), and it inhibits 5-HETE and 12-HETE formation in human leukocytes and platelets (34). 15-HETE has also been shown to block stimulation of guanylate cyclase activity in lymphocytes (7) and receptor-mediated cGMP formation in N1E-115 murine neuroblastoma cells (25). Finally, 15-HETE has been reported to be an endothelial cell mitogen (36,37).

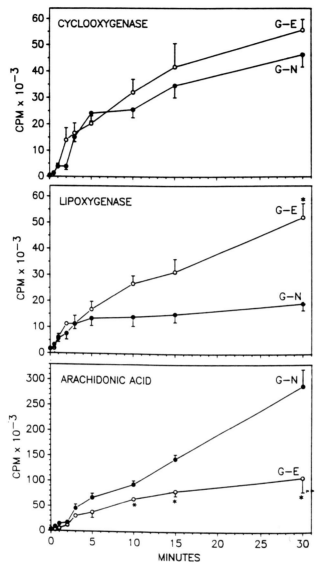

FIGURE 10.7. Effect of elevated glucose on ionophore A23187–induced release of eicosanoids from PAEC. PAEC were conditioned, labeled, and stimulated as in Figure 10.6. Classes of eicosanoids released into the medium were resolved by reverse-phase HPLC as in Table 10.2. (Mean ± SE, three experiments, performed in duplicate). [From (5); used with permission.]

EFFECT OF PASSAGE STATE ON EICOSANOID RELEASE

We have examined the effect of passage state on eicosanoid release in response to ionophore A23187 and AA levels in PAEC cultured through four passages from primary cultures (3). The content of AA in phosphatidylinositol and diacyl phosphatidylethanolamine remained constant at passage 1 but declined at passage 2 by 29% and at passage 4 by 59% (Fig. 10.8). The release of 6-keto-

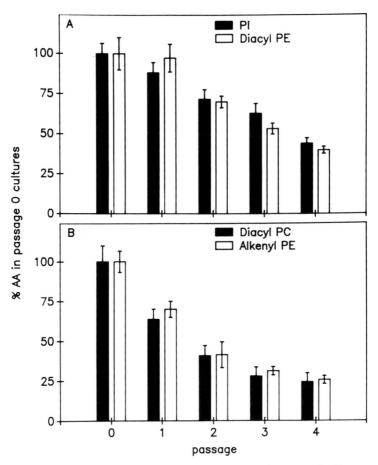

FIGURE 10.8. AA content of major phospholipid fractions as a function of cell passage. PAEC were cultured from primary cultures (passage 0) through four passages. Upon reaching confluence, the lipids were extracted, the classes separated, (passages 3,4), and the AA content measured by quantitative gas chromatography (mean ± SE; n = 5). [From (3); used with permission.]

PGF_{1a} in response A23187 (Fig. 10.9) was also unchanged at passage 1 but decreased by 60% at passage 2 and by 82% of its original value by passage 4. In contrast, the AA content of diacyl phosphatidylcholine and of alkenyl phosphatidylethanolamine declined with each passage—34% at passage 1, 59% at passage 2, 71% at passage 3 and 76% at passage 4 (Fig. 10.8). The release of 15-HETE decreased by 82% at passage 1, and diminished to a 97% decrement from the original value by passage 4 (Fig. 10.9). These data indicate that passage state strongly and nonuniformly affects both AA content in individual phospholipid classes and the release of eicosanoids in response to agonist stimulation. A relationship between the loss of AA from the phosphatidylinositol and diacyl phosphatidylethanolamine pools and the diminished release of 6-keto-PGF_{1a} is implied. Likewise a relationship between diacyl phosphatidylcholine and alkenyl phosphatidylethanolamine pools and 15-HETE release is suggested.

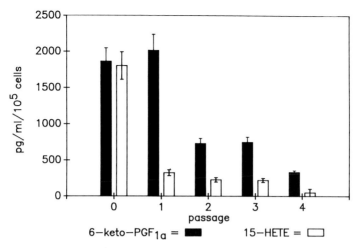

FIGURE 10.9. Effect of passage on ionophore A23187-induced release of 6-keto-PGF$_{1\alpha}$ and 15-HETE from PAEC. Cells were cultured from primary (passage 0) through four passages. At confluence the cultures were stimulated with 1 μM A23187 and the metabolites were measured by radioimmunoassay (mean ± SE; n = 8 separate determinations). [From (3); used with permission.]

A valuable result of these studies is that it becomes possible to use passage state as a tool to alter eicosanoid ratios. The ratios of metabolites released vary from a nearly equivalent level of A23187-induced release of 6-keto-PGF$_{1a}$ (1866 pg/ml/10,000 cells) and 15-HETE (1803 pg/ml/10,000 cells) at passage 0 to a ratio of 6:1 at passage 1 (2016 vs 325, respectively). If indeed specific pools of AA are linked to individual oxygenating enzyme systems then one would expect that relationship to be pronounced upon comparing the two passage states.

SUMMARY

In summary, agonist-induced release of AA is dependent on many factors, and assaying the specific pathways is often technically difficult and demanding. Pools of radiolabeled AA can be manipulated beyond homogeneous specific activities, enabling the investigator greater ease in assigning precursor–product relationships. Methods and agents that assist actual mass measurements and movement of AA-containing or AA-derived compounds such as immunoassays or metabolites, quantitative gas chromatography, and on-line quantitation of phospholipids and their molecular species will prove invaluable. Time course studies, though limited in capability when used alone, are of the utmost importance to such studies and should not be abandoned in favor of singular timepoint studies. Different medium supplementation and cell culture conditions (here we elevate glucose and exploit passage state) will become increasingly important tools in unraveling the pathways of AA release, its metabolism, and its redistribution. Each finding is and will be directly applicable to describing the dysfunction of AA metabolism in diabetes and potentially lead to therapeutic interventions. That AA metabolism is involved in diabetic vascular disease has been established; how it is involved remains unresolved. A ratio of TxA$_2$:PGI$_2$ in diabetes, favoring thrombosis and vascular occlusion is strongly suggested. The production and release of monohydroxylated AA metabolites such as 15-HETE resulting from hyperglycemic conditions can also be implicated in contributing to diabetic vascular disease through many possible pathways. The development of agents that block the TxA$_2$ receptor or modulate 15-lipoxygenase production should provide promising insight into future therapies for diabetic angiopathies.

ACKNOWLEDGMENTS

This work is supported by the Veterans Administration Medical Research Service and a grant from the National Institutes of Health (DK 39624).

REFERENCES

1. AANDERUD, S., KRANE, S. A., and NORDOY, A. Influence of glucose, insulin, and sera of diabetic patients on prostacyclin synthesis in vitro in cultured human endothelial cells. *Diabetologia* 28: 641–644, 1985.

2. ADAMS-BROTHERTON, A. F., and HOAK, J. C. Prostacyclin biosynthesis in cultured vascular endothelium is limited by deactivation of cyclooxygenase. *J. Clin. Invest.* 72: 1255–1261, 1983.

3. BROWN, M. L., and DEYKIN, D. Passage state affects arachidonic acid content and eicosanoid release in porcine aortic endothelial cells. *Arteriosclerosis* 11: 167–173, 1991.

4. BROWN, M. L., JAKUBOWSKI, J. A., LEVENTIS, L. L., and DEYKIN, D. Ionophore-induced metabolism of phospholipids and eicosanoid production in porcine aortic endothelial cells: selective release of arachidonic acid from diacyl and ether phospholipids. *Biochim. Biophys. Acta* 921: 159–166, 1987.

5. BROWN, M. L., JAKUBOWSKI, J. A., LEVENTIS, L. L., and DEYKIN, D. Elevated glucose alters eicosanoid release from porcine aortic endothelial cells. *J. Clin. Invest.* 82: 2136–2141, 1988.

6. CHANG, J., BLAZEK, E., KREFT, A. F., and LEWIS, A. J. Inhibition of platelet and neutrophil phospholipase A$_2$ by hydroxyeicosatetraenoic acids (HETEs). A novel pharmacological mechanism for regulating free fatty acid release. *Biochem. Pharmacol.* 34: 1571–1575, 1985.

7. COFFEY, R. G., and HADDEN, J. W. Phorbol myristate acetate stimulation of lymphocyte guanylate cyclase and cyclic guanosine 3′:5′-monophosphate phosphodiesterase and reduction of adenylate cyclase. *Cancer Res.* 43: 150–158, 1983.

8. COLARD, O., BRETON, M., PEPIN, D., CHEVY, F., BEREZIAT, G., and POLONOVSKI, J. Arachidonate cannot be released directly from diacyl-*sn*-glycero-3-phosphocholine in thrombin-stimulated platelets. *Biochem. J.* 259: 333–339, 1989.

9. DENNING, G. M., FIGARD, P. H., KADUCE, T. L., and SPECTOR, A. A. Role of triglycerides in endothelial cell arachidonic acid metabolism. *J. Lipid Res.* 24: 993–1001, 1983.

10. FITZPATRICK, F. A., and MURPHY, R. C. Cytochrome P-450 metabolism of arachidonic acid: formation and biological actions of "epoxygenase"-derived eicosanoids. *Pharmacol. Rev.* 40: 229–241, 1989.

11. GROSS, R. W., and SOBEL, B. E. Lysophosphatidylcholine metabolism in the rabbit heart. Characterization of metabolic pathways and partial purification of myocardial lysophospholipase-transacylase. *J. Biol. Chem.* 257: 6702–6708, 1982.

12. HADJIAGAPIOU, C., and SPECTOR, A. A. 12-Hydroxyeicosatetraenoic acid reduces prostacyclin production by endothelial cells. *Prostaglandins* 31: 1135–1144, 1986.

13. HALUSHKA, P. V., MAYFIELD, R., and COLWELL, J. A. Insulin and arachidonic acid metabolism in diabetes mellitus. *Metabolism* 34: 32–36, 1985.

14. HENDRA, T., and BETTERIDGE, D. J. Platelet function, platelet prostanoids and vascular prostacyclin in diabetes mellitus. *Prostaglandins, Leukotrienes and Essential Fatty Acids: Reviews* 35: 197–212, 1989.

15. HILL, E. E., and LANDS, W. E. M. Phospholipid Metabolism. In *Lipid Metabolism,* edited by S. J. Wakil. New York: Academic Press, 1970, pp. 185–279.

16. HONG, S. L., CARTY, T., and DEYKIN, D. Tranylcypromine and 15-hydroperoxyarachidonate affect arachidonic acid release in addition to inhibition of prostacyclin synthesis in calf aortic endothelial cells. *J. Biol. Chem.* 255: 9538–9540, 1980.

17. HONG, S. L., and DEYKIN, D. Activation of phospholipases A_2 and C in pig aortic endothelial cells synthesizing prostacyclin. *J. Biol. Chem.* 257: 7151–7154, 1982.

18. JEREMY, J. Y., MIKHAILIDIS, D. P., and DANDONA, P. Simulating the diabetic environment modifies in vitro prostacyclin synthesis. *Diabetes* 32: 217–221, 1983.

19. JEREMY, J. Y., THOMPSON, C. S., MIKHAILIDIS, D. P., and DANDONA, P. Experimental diabetes mellitus inhibits prostacyclin synthesis by the rat penis: pathological implications. *Diabetologia* 28: 365–368, 1985.

20. KRAMER, R. M., and DEYKIN, D. Arachidonoyl transacylase in human platelets. Coenzyme A-independent transfer of arachidonate from phosphatidylcholine to lysoplasmenylethanolamine. *J. Biol. Chem.* 258: 13806–13811, 1983.

21. KRAMER, R. M., PRITZKER, C. R., and DEYKIN, D. Coenzyme A–mediated arachidonic acid transacylation in human platelets. *J. Biol. Chem.* 259: 2403–2406, 1984.

22. KURACHI, Y., ITO, H., SUGIMOTO, T., SHIMIZU, T., MIKI, I., and UI, M. Arachidonic acid metabolites as intracellular modulators of the G protein-gated cardiac K^+ channel. *Nature* 337: 555–557, 1989.

23. LAYCHOCK, S. G. Phospholipase A_2 activity in pancreatic islets is calcium dependent and stimulated by glucose. *Cell Calcium* 3: 43–54, 1982.

24. LORENZI, M., CAGLIERO, E., and TOLEDO, S. Glucose toxicity for human endothelial cells in culture. Delayed replication, disturbed cell cycle, and accelerated death. *Diabetes* 34: 621–627, 1985.

25. MCKINNEY, M. Blockade of receptor-mediated cyclic GMP formation by hydroxyeicosatetraenoic acid. *J. Neurochem.* 49: 331–341, 1987.

26. NEEDLEMAN, P., TURK, J., JAKSCHIK, B. A., MORRISON, A. R., and LEFKOWITH, J. B. Arachidonic acid metabolism. *Ann. Rev. Biochem.* 55: 69–102, 1986.

27. ONO, H., UMEDA, F., INOGUCHI, T., and IBAYASHI, H. Glucose inhibits prostacyclin production by cultured aortic endothelial cells. *Thromb. Haemostas.* 60: 174–177, 1988.

28. ORDWAY, R. W., WALSH, J. V., JR., and SINGER, J. J. Arachidonic acid and other fatty acids directly activate potassium channels in smooth muscle cells. *Science* 244: 1176–1179, 1989.

29. RAGAB-THOMAS, J. M. F., HULLIN, F., CHAP, H., and DOUSTE-BLAZY, L. Pathways of arachidonic acid liberation in thrombin and calcium ionophore A23187-stimulated human endothelial cells: respective roles of phospholipids and triacylglycerol and evidence for diacylglycerol generation from phosphatidylcholine. *Biochim. Biophys. Acta* 917: 388–397, 1987.

30. ROBINSON, M., BLANK, M. L., and SNYDER, F. Acylation of lysophospholipids by rabbit alveolar macrophages. Specificities of CoA-dependent and CoA-independent reactions. *J. Biol. Chem.* 260: 7889–7895, 1985.

31. ROSEN, P., and SCHROR, K. Increased prostacyclin release from perfused hearts of acutely diabetic rats. *Diabetologia* 18: 391–394, 1980.

32. ROSENTHAL, M. D., and WHITEHURST, M. C. Fatty acyl delta[6]-desaturation activity of cultured human endothelial cells. Modulation by fetal bovine serum. *Biochim. Biophys. Acta* 750: 490–496, 1983.

33. SAGONE, A. L., JR., GREENWALD, J., KRAUT, E. H., BIANCHINE, J., and SINGH, D. Glucose: a role as a free radical scavenger in biological systems. *J. Lab. Clin. Med.* 101: 97–104, 1983.

34. SALARI, H., BRAQUET, P., and BORGEAT, P. Comparative effects of indomethacin, acetylenic acids, 15-HETE, nordihydroguaiaretic acid and BW755c on the metabolism of arachidonic acid in human leukocytes and platelets. *Prostaglandins Leukotrienes Med.* 13: 53–60, 1984.

35. SAMUELSSON, B., GOLDYNE, M., GRANSTROM, E., HAMBERG, M., HAMMARSTROM, S., and MALMSTEN, C. Prostaglandins and thromboxanes. *Annu. Rev. Biochem.* 47: 997–1029, 1978.

36. SETTY, B. N. Y., DUBOWY, R. L., and STUART, M. J. Endothelial cell proliferation may be mediated via the production of endogenous lipoxygenase metabolites. *Biochem. Biophys. Res. Commun.* 144: 345–351, 1987.

37. SETTY, B. N. Y., GRAEBER, J. E., and STUART, M. J. The mitogenic effect of 15- and 12-hydroxyeicosatetraenoic acid on endothelial cells may be mediated via diacylglycerol kinase inhibition. *J. Biol. Chem.* 262: 17613–17622, 1987.

38. SETTY, B. N. Y., and STUART, M. J. 15-Hydroxy-5,8,11,13-eicosatetraenoic acid inhibits

vascular cyclooxygenase. Potential role in diabetic vascular disease. *J. Clin. Invest.* 77: 202–217, 1986.

39. SHAKIR, K. M. M., REED, H. L., and O'BRIAN, J. T. Decreased phospholipase A_2 activity in plasma and liver in uncontrolled diabetes mellitus. A defect in the early steps of prostaglandin synthesis? *Diabetes* 35: 403–410, 1986.

40. SILBERBAUER, K., SCHNERNTHANER, A., SINZINGER, H., PIZA-KATZER, H., and WINTER, M. Decreased vascular prostacyclin in juvenile-onset diabetes (Letter). *N. Engl. J. Med.* 300: 366–367, 1979.

41. SPECTOR, A. A., KADUCE, T. L., HOAK, J. C., and FRY, G. L. Utilization of arachidonic and linoleic acids by cultured human endothelial cells. *J. Clin. Invest.* 68: 1003–1011, 1981.

42. STERIN-BORDA, L., BORDA, E. S., GIMENO, M. F., LAZZARI, M. A., del CASTILLO, E., and GIMENO, A. L. Contractile activity and prostacyclin generation in isolated coronary arteries from diabetic dogs. *Diabetologia* 22: 56–69, 1982.

43. STOUT, R. W. Glucose inhibits replication of cultured human endothelial cells. *Diabetologia* 23: 436–439, 1982.

44. TAKAMURA, H., KASAI, H., ARITA, H., and KITO, M. Phospholipid molecular species in human umbilical artery and vein endothelial cells. *J. Lipid Res.* 31: 709–717, 1990.

45. TAKEDA, H., MAEDA, H., FUKUSHIMA, H., NAKAMURA, N., and UZAWA, H. Increased platelet phospholipase activity in diabetic subjects. *Thrombosis Res.* 24: 131–141, 1981.

46. TESFAMARIAM, B., BROWN, M. L., DEYKIN, D., and COHEN, R. A. Elevated glucose promotes generation of endothelium-derived vasoconstrictor prostanoids in rabbit aorta. *J. Clin. Invest.* 85: 929–932, 1990.

47. THOMAS, J. M. F., CHAP, H., and DOUSTE-BLAZY, L. Calcium ionophore A23187 induces arachidonic acid release from phosphatidylcholine in cultured human endothelial cells. *Biochem. Biophys. Res. Commun.* 103: 819–824, 1981.

48. THOMAS, J. M. F., HULLIN, F., CHAP, H., and DOUSTE-BLAZY, L. Phosphatidylcholine is the major phospholipid providing arachidonic acid for prostacyclin synthesis in thrombin-stimulated endothelial cells. *Thrombosis Res.* 34: 117–123, 1984.

49. VANDERHOEK, J. Y., BRYANT, R. W., and BAILEY, J. M. Inhibition of leukotriene biosynthesis by the leukocyte product 15-hydroxy-5,8,11,13-eicosatetraenoic acid. *J. Biol. Chem.* 255: 10064–10066.

50. VANDERHOEK, J. Y., TARE, N. S., BAILEY, J. M., GOLDSTEIN, A. L., and PLUZNIK, D. H. New role for 15-hydroxyeicosatetraenoic acid. Activation of leukotriene biosynthesis in PT-18 mast/basophil cells. *J. Biol. Chem.* 261: 12191–121915, 1983.

51. WEIMANN, B. J., LORCH, E., and BAUMGARTNER. H. R. High glucose concentrations do not influence replication and prostacyclin release of human endothelial cells (Letter). *Diabetologia* 27: 62–63, 1984.

52. WEY, H. E., JAKUBOWSKI, J. A., and DEYKIN, D. Effect of streptozotocin-induced diabetes on prostaglandin production by rat cerebral microvessels. *Thrombosis Res.* 42: 527–538, 1986.

53. WEY, H. E., JAKUBOWSKI, J. A., and DEYKIN, D. Incorporation and redistribution of arachidonic acid in diacyl and ether phospholipids of bovine aortic endothelial cells. *Biochim. Biophys. Acta* 878: 380–386, 1986.

III

GLYCATION PRODUCTS AND GLYCOSOAMINOGLYCANS

11

Glycation and Autoxidation of Proteins in Aging and Diabetes

TIMOTHY J. LYONS, SUZANNE R. THORPE, AND JOHN W. BAYNES

Glycation (nonenzymatic glycosylation) of protein is the first step in a complex series of reactions that lead to the gradual browning, cross-linking, and denaturation of proteins by glucose. These reactions are known collectively as the Maillard reaction (17,25,39), in honor of Louis Camille Maillard for his work during the early part of this century, or the browning reaction because of the characteristic brown and fluorescent products formed during the reaction. In food chemistry the brown, soluble products formed during the later stages of the Maillard reaction are known as *pre-melanoidins,* and the final, insoluble products as *melanoidins* (17,25,39). In living systems the brown and fluorescent products that accumulate in long-lived proteins are more commonly referred to as *advanced glycosylation end products,* or AGE-products (8,39). Only a few melanoidins or AGE-products have been structurally characterized; however, it has been apparent for decades that the Maillard reaction is stimulated by oxygen and catalysts of oxidation reactions, such as iron and copper ions, and inhibited by reducing agents, such as bisulfite and thiol compounds (17,25,33). This chapter focuses on the significance of oxidation reactions and their role in mediating the chemical damage caused by glycation and Maillard reactions in vivo. It begins with a discussion of the nature of oxidation and autoxidation reactions, then describes several products of oxidation of glycated proteins that have been identified in vivo, and concludes with a summary of current information regarding the accumulation of these products in tissue proteins with age and in diabetes. Evidence regarding the role of autoxidative glycosylation of protein and the role of Maillard reaction products as catalysts of oxidation of adjacent molecules is also examined. Although glucose is the primary focus of the discussion, the biological significance of autoxidative modification of protein by ascorbate is also considered. We try to present a balance between knowledge and hypothesis, and to point out directions for future research. Among the new ideas to be developed is the proposal that oxidation may be the "fixative" that renders permanent the chemical modification of proteins initiated by glycation. Indeed, the only nonenzymatically formed, carbohydrate-derived products that are known to accumulate in tissue proteins with age, and at an accelerated rate in diabetes, are products of both glycation and oxidation reactions. Thus, the interplay between glycation and oxidation— i.e. "glycoxidation" of protein—may be more important than either glycation or oxidation alone. As will become clear, glycoxidation products constitute a unique group of AGE-products that are biomarkers of chemical damage to protein in aging and diabetes.

REDOX CHEMISTRY DURING THE EARLY STAGES OF THE MAILLARD REACTION

Intramolecular Redox Reactions

Rearrangements—Eneaminol and Enediol Intermediates
Balanced redox reactions require both an oxidizing agent and a reducing agent. In carbohydrate chemistry, many rearrangement reactions are, in fact, internal redox reactions in which one atom of a molecule is oxidized and another reduced. The redox phenomenon is commonplace in the Maillard reaction. Thus, even in the Amadori rearrangement of an aldimine to a ketamine (Fig. 11.1), C-1 of the sugar is reduced while C-2 is oxidized, without a change in the overall oxidation state of the carbons in the molecule. Enols, enediols, and eneaminols are common intermediates in these rearrangement reactions (17,25). Some of the enediol intermediates, known as *reductones,* are also facile reductants of metal ions and oxygen and can initiate metal-catalyzed intermolecular oxidation reactions (17,25,55).

Dehydration Reactions—Formation of Deoxyglucosones
The elimination of a molecule of water from vicinal carbons is another characteristic redox reaction in carbohydrate chemistry, equivalent to oxidation and reduction of adjacent carbon atoms. Dehydration is favored when the reaction leads to formation of a conjugated double-bond system, such as a $C=C$ double bond adjacent to an existing $C=C$, $C=O$, or $C=N$ bond. Reversible rearrangement and dehydration reactions are involved in the formation of 1- and 3-deoxyglucosones (1-DOG, 3-DOG) from Amadori products during the Maillard reaction (Fig. 11.1). The deoxyglucosones formed in these reactions are potent browning agents and have been identified as intermediates in the browning of proteins by hexoses in vitro (17,25). Kato and colleagues (34) have

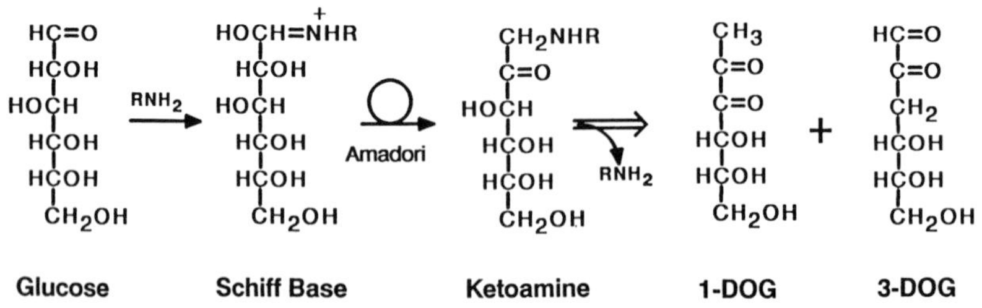

FIGURE 11.1. Nonoxidative pathway for formation of dicarbonyl sugars during the Maillard reaction. Glucose reacts initially with amino groups on proteins to form a labile Schiff base (aldimine) adduct. The Amadori rearrangement leads to formation of a relatively stable Amadori adduct (ketamine). Through a series of rearrangements and dehydration and hydrolysis reactions, the Amadori adduct yields the dicarbonyl sugars, 1- and 3-deoxyglucosone.

also shown that 3-DOG is a precursor to a fluorescent product, L_1, found in tissue proteins. The amount of L_1 in rat aortic proteins increases with age, and L_1 is also elevated in diabetic compared to nondiabetic human cataract proteins (34). In a later study (43) the same investigators observed that the level of L_1 in the nucleus of diabetic cataracts was increased primarily in patients with pre-proliferative or proliferative retinopathy, suggesting a relationship between glycation of proteins, formation of 3-DOG and L_1, and development of microangiopathy in diabetes. Knecht et al. (38) recently showed that 3-DOG is present at trace levels ($\sim$10 μg/liter) in human plasma. The low level of 3-DOG probably results from its low rate of formation, combined with its high intrinsic reactivity. There are also endogenous mechanisms for oxidative or reductive inactivation of 3-DOG to 2-keto-3-deoxygluconate (32) or 3-deoxyfructose (35), respectively. Knecht et al. (38) observed that 3-deoxyfructose is also present in human urine and plasma ($\sim$50 μg/liter in plasma), and that its concentration is increased in diabetes, suggesting increased production and metabolism of 3-DOG in diabetes and supporting the role of 3-DOG as a precursor to L_1 and other Maillard products in tissue proteins. Less is known about 1-DOG, since its metabolites or products formed on reaction with protein are unknown.

Reverse Aldol Reactions—Fragmentation of the Carbon Chain of Sugars
Aldol condensation and reverse aldol reactions are internal redox reactions that are catalyzed by amines and that provide a mechanism for the reversible anaerobic cleavage of C—C bonds in sugars. An active site lysine residue in aldolase participates in the reversible interconversion of fructose-1,6-diphosphate to dihydroxyacetone-P and glyceraldehyde-3-P during glycolysis. As illustrated in Figure 11.2, similar, but nonenzymatic, retroaldol reactions may be involved in the fragmentation of Schiff base and Amadori adducts to protein during the Maillard reaction. Because of their smaller size, both the aldose sugars released as split products and the fragments remaining bound to the protein would exist to a greater extent in their acyclic, carbonyl conformations, rather than the less reactive hemiacetal and hemiketal conformations characteristic of glucose and its Schiff base and Amadori adducts to protein. Because of the greater reactivity of the acyclic compounds, reverse aldol reactions would accelerate protein browning and cross-linking reactions by glucose. The fragments remaining bound to protein could also dissociate reversibly to form reactive compounds, such as formaldehyde and glyoxal. At this time, however, there is no evidence that reverse aldol reactions actually occur during the Maillard reaction in vivo since the split products formed in the reaction would only slightly affect the pool of intermediary metabolites in the cell, while cross-links formed from the fragments remaining attached to proteins have not been identified.

Biological Relevance of Internal Redox Reactions of Glucose and Its Adducts with Protein In Vivo
Internal redox reactions (rearrangement, dehydration, and reverse aldol reactions) provide a number of possible mechanisms for enhancing the reactivity of glucose with protein. These reactions, which lead to the formation of reactive deoxyglucosones (Fig. 11.1) and fragmentation of the carbon skeleton of glu-

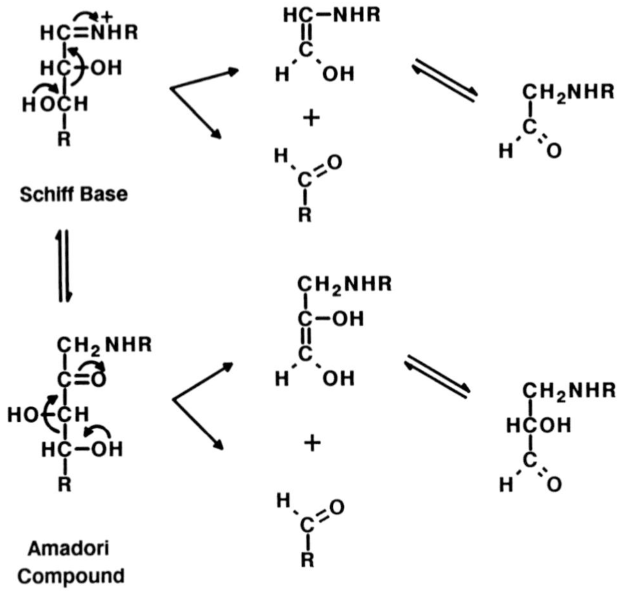

FIGURE 11.2. Nonoxidative fragmentation of carbohydrates by reverse aldol reactions. Rearrangements of both Schiff bases and Amadori compounds may release shorter chain sugars from glycated proteins, leaving reactive carbonyl adducts attached to protein. In effect, two more reactive carbonyl compounds are produced from the original sugar, stimulating the browning and cross-linking of proteins.

cose (Fig. 11.2) to yield smaller, more reactive aldoses and ketoses, are known to occur in Maillard reaction systems in vitro (17,25,39). Because they occur at lower temperature and greater dilution in biological systems, it may be difficult to detect the same Maillard reaction intermediates in vivo. Detection is also limited by the presence of endogenous mechanisms for inactivation or metabolism of the intermediates. Thus, it will probably be necessary to focus on the identification of metabolites, such as 3-deoxyfructose, or the characterization of trace amounts of end products, such as L_1, to gain insight into the primary pathways of the Maillard reaction in vivo. Knowledge of the metabolic pathways for detoxification of Maillard intermediates is scarce, but especially important since these studies should yield critical information on the biological mechanisms for limiting potential damage from the Maillard reaction in long-lived species. Differences in the levels of defensive metabolic pathways may also explain individual variation in susceptibility to development of pathophysiology in aging and diabetes and could suggest pharmacological approaches for enhancing defense mechanisms.

Autoxidative Reactions

The Nature of Autoxidation
Autoxidation is defined as the oxidation of a compound by molecular oxygen, e.g., the spontaneous oxidation of iron (formation of rust) or peroxidation of lipids (formation of lipid hydro- and endo-peroxides). The oxidizing species in

autoxidation reactions is some activated form of oxygen, including excited states of oxygen (singlet, triplet), oxygen radicals (superoxide, hydroxyl), and redox metal complexes, such as the ferryl or perferryl radical. Because of the high redox potential of oxygen, autoxidative reactions are often, like the formation of rust, essentially irreversible processes. Thus, living systems have had to develop various mechanisms for limiting cumulative damage from autoxidation reactions.

The transition metal ions, iron and copper, are potent catalysts of autoxidation reactions, and for this reason autoxidation reactions are often referred to as metal-catalyzed oxidation reactions. Strong chelators, such as diethylenetriaminepentaacetic acid, phytic acid, and desferrioxamine are efficient inhibitors of metal-catalyzed autoxidation reactions in vitro. The iron binding protein, transferrin, performs a similar inhibitory function in vivo by limiting the concentration of free iron in extracellular fluids to the sub-micromolar range. Excess iron is also sequestered intracellularly as a complex in the protein, ferritin. The copper protein, ceruloplasmin, through its ferroxidase activity, maintains traces of free iron in the ferric state, which promotes its binding to transferrin. Extracellular copper is also sequestered by binding to albumin. However, despite the efficiency of chelation of redox metals in vivo, trace amounts of free metal ions are constantly being released into the extracellular milieu, e.g. during cell death, phagocytosis, and inflammation. When this occurs, the enzymes superoxide dismutase, catalase, and glutathione peroxidase provide an additional line of defense against the spread of autoxidative damage. These enzymes limit the accumulation of superoxide radical and hydrogen peroxide, which are precursors of stronger oxidizing species, such as hypochlorous acid and the hydroxyl radical. There are also potent oxygen radical scavengers, such as vitamins C (ascorbate) and E (tocopherol), glutathione, and uric acid, which quench reactive radicals and limit damage to biomolecules. Despite this armory of defense mechanisms, products of autoxidation of lipids, proteins, carbohydrates, and nucleic acids are readily detected in tissues and urine.

There is no evidence that autoxidative damage, once it occurs, may be reversed by chemical or enzymatic reduction of the oxidized species back to the native form. In the case of DNA, repair enzymes act by excision and replacement of the modified base or nucleotide. For most proteins, lipids, saccharides, and RNA, metabolic turnover appears to be the critical factor limiting the accumulation of damaged molecules. However, in long-lived, unrepairable protein molecules, such as crystallins, collagens, and elastin and myelin proteins, products of oxygen radical reactions may accumulate with time. Thus, long-lived proteins provide a unique sensor for exposure to oxidative stress and a convenient source for identification of products formed on oxidative modification of proteins. As will be discussed later, the accumulation of autoxidation products also causes alterations in protein structure and function and may lead to the development of pathology.

Involvement of Amadori Compounds in Autoxidation Reactions
The compounds N^ε-(carboxymethyl)lysine (CML) and 3-(N^ε-lysino)-lactic acid (Fig. 11.3) have been identified as products of autoxidation of the Amadori

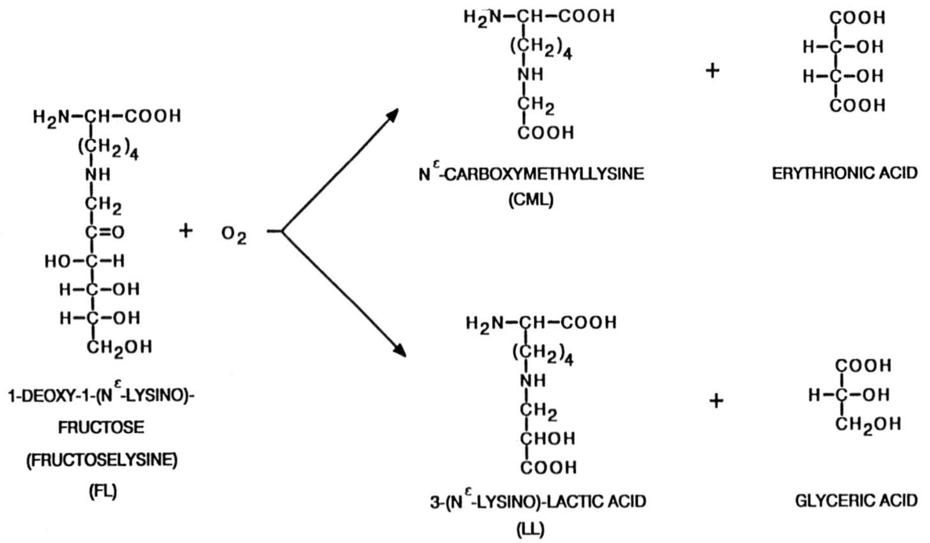

FIGURE 11.3. Pathways for oxidative cleavage of fructoselysine in metal catalyzed oxidation reaction. Erythronic and glyceric acid have been identified among the split products.

compound, fructoselysine [FL; (1,2)]. These compounds are formed from FL by metal-catalyzed oxidation reactions in vitro (1,2), and have been detected in human lens crystallin (15), skin collagen (14), and urine (1,2,37,58). The CML analog, N^ε-(carboxymethyl)hydroxylysine (CMhL), formed by oxidation of glycated hydroxylysine, has also been detected in human skin collagen (14). While the oxidation of Amadori compounds could be initiated by reactive oxygen species generated from other autoxidation reactions in vivo, it is possible that the Amadori compound itself reacts directly with metals and oxygen and functions as an initiator of autoxidation reactions. Studies with rapidly autoxidized sugars, such as glyceraldehyde, indicate that the enolate anion of the sugar is capable of reducing oxygen to superoxide, either directly or via the semidione radical formed from the enolate on reduction of a redox active metal ion [(55); Fig. 11.4]. Indeed, the ability of the Amadori compound to mediate the reduction of molecular oxygen is the basis for the fructosamine assay, one of the newer methods for measuring the extent of glycation of plasma proteins (28). This assay depends on reduction of a dye, such as nitroblue tetrazolium, by Amadori adducts on plasma proteins. Based on inhibitory effects of superoxide dismutase, the reaction mechanism involves the superoxide radical as the reduced oxygen intermediate, which directly reduces the tetrazolium dye (31). Although autoxidation of sugars and Amadori compounds is favored at high pH (the fructosamine assay is usually conducted at about pH 10), similar reactions occur, although at slower rates, at physiological pH.

The products of oxidation of Amadori adducts in the fructosamine assay have not been identified, but they might be reactive with protein and, if formed spontaneously in vivo, could exacerbate the chemical damage resulting from glycation of protein. Sakurai and Tsuchiya (45) have proposed, however, that the inert compound, CML, is formed in this reaction (Fig. 11.3). In either case, the simultaneous reduction of molecular oxygen to superoxide would provide a mechanism for the propagation of autoxidative reactions. Hicks et al. (24) and Azevedo and colleagues (3) have shown, in fact, that spontaneous autoxidation of glycated proteins or Maillard reaction intermediates under physiological conditions can initiate oxidative damage to bystander molecules, causing, for example, peroxidation of lipids and cleavage or cross-linkage of protein. The products of oxidation of the Amadori compound were not measured in these studies, but whether the formation of CML is the result of spontaneous autoxidation of FL or of autoxidation initiated by reactive oxygen generated in other reactions, the total concentration of CML in tissue proteins and urine should serve as a useful index of exposure of proteins to oxidative damage in vivo. This hypothesis deserves attention since, as discussed below, there are limitations to current methods for assessing oxidative stress and the extent of oxidative damage to biomolecules.

Autoxidative Glycosylation

Wolff and colleagues (26,62) have proposed that, in addition to products of autoxidation of Amadori compounds, products of autoxidation of sugars may also be directly involved in the glycation of proteins in vivo; thus the term *autoxidative glycosylation*. The proposed intermediates in this reaction are glucosones, produced by autoxidation of reducing sugars (Fig. 11.4). Glucosones are distinct from the deoxyglucosones (1-DOG, 3-DOG) produced by internal redox reactions (Fig. 11.1); however, their reactivity with proteins should be similar. As shown in Figure 11.4, the initial adduct of glucosones (or deoxyglucosones) to primary amino groups in protein would be a ketimine (keto-imine), rather than an aldimine (Fig. 11.1) formed from the parent sugar. Ketimines are more reactive toward autoxidation than either hexoses or Amadori compounds (25) and would set the stage for propagating further chemical modifications of proteins.

The significance of autoxidation glycosylation in vivo, and particularly its role in modification of proteins by glucose in diabetes, is a topic of some controversy (22,61). The proposed ketimine intermediate or other unique products of autoxidative glycosylation have not yet been identified in glycation reactions, either in vitro or in vivo. To complicate matters, an effort to trap the ketimine by reduction with $NaBH_4$ would yield products chemically identical to the hexitollysines obtained on reduction of Amadori adducts, so that initial products of conventional (nonoxidative) glycation and autoxidative glycosylation could not be distinguished. Because sugar autoxidation products may rap-

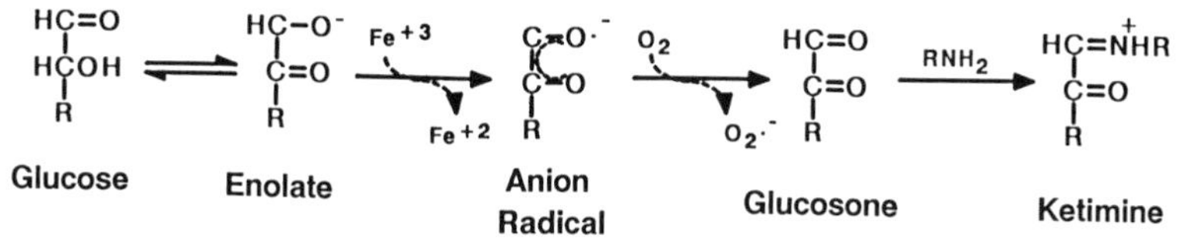

FIGURE 11.4. Proposed pathway for autoxidative glycosylation of protein. Autoxidation of glucose yields dicarbonyl sugars, which react to form ketimine adducts to protein. [Modified from Hunt et al. (26).]

idly react with protein, or rearrange or be metabolized to less reactive products, it may be difficult to determine the role of autoxidative glycosylation in vivo unless unique metabolites or end products can be identified. One indirect indication that autoxidative glycosylation may be relevant is the experimental finding that both aspirin and salicylate inhibit the reaction of glucose with collagen in vitro (64) and that in vivo salicylates and nonsteroidal anti-inflammatory agents (NSAIDs) also inhibit the increase in tail collagen cross-linking in the diabetic rat, as measured by changes in thermal rupture time (65). In the in vivo experiments, however, the salicylates and NSAIDs inhibited the diabetes-induced changes in collagen without an effect on the level of the Amadori adducts. These results suggest that salicylates and NSAIDs may be functioning as inhibitors of autoxidation reactions, either primarily by inhibition of autoxidative glycosylation or secondarily by inhibition of the oxidation of Amadori adducts or other intermediates in the Maillard reaction. In most cases the assays used to measure the effects of these compounds on glycation, such as incorporation of radioactive glucose into protein, identification of products by phenylboronic acid affinity chromatography, or assay of glycated protein by the thiobarbituric assay lack the specificity to distinguish between products of nonoxidative glycation and those resulting from autoxidation of sugar adducts to protein or autoxidative glycosylation of protein. It is also possible that the salicylates and NSAIDs inhibit the advanced stages of the Maillard reaction indirectly by inhibition of nonenzymatic autoxidation of lipids or of enzymatic pathways of lipid peroxidation involved in the biosynthesis of prostaglandins and leukotrienes. In these cases it is assumed that metal-catalyzed decomposition of lipid peroxides may initiate adventitious autoxidation of Maillard reaction products, just as the autoxidation of sugars may initiate the peroxidation of lipids (24). Thus, autoxidation reactions of lipids, reducing sugars and carbohydrate adducts to proteins and lipids, may propagate oxidative damage to proteins by reinforcing cyclic and auto-catalytic mechanisms. Clearly, more research is needed to determine whether autoxidative glycosylation occurs in vivo and, if so, whether anti-inflammatory agents limit this process, as well as the spontaneous autoxidation of Amadori compounds. Depending on the significance of autoxidation reactions, therapy with anti-inflammatory agents may provide a novel approach for limiting tissue damage via the Maillard reaction.

Autoxidative Glycosylation by Ascorbate

We have recently observed that CML is formed on reaction of ascorbic acid with protein under autoxidative conditions (12). Ascorbic acid exists naturally as a cyclic lactone and contains an internal enediol structure. In aerobic, aqueous solution and in the presence of traces of transition metal ions such as iron or copper, ascorbate is rapidly autoxidized to the dicarbonyl sugar, dehydroascorbate. Kinetics studies show that oxidation of ascorbate to dehydroascorbate precedes the formation of CML, and that the pathway to formation of CML from dehydroascorbate under autoxidizing conditions proceeds by decomposition of dehydroascorbate to threose, the reaction of threose with lysine to form the Amadori adduct, threuloselysine, and then oxidation of threuloselysine to CML (Fig. 11.5). This pathway was confirmed by the identification of threose

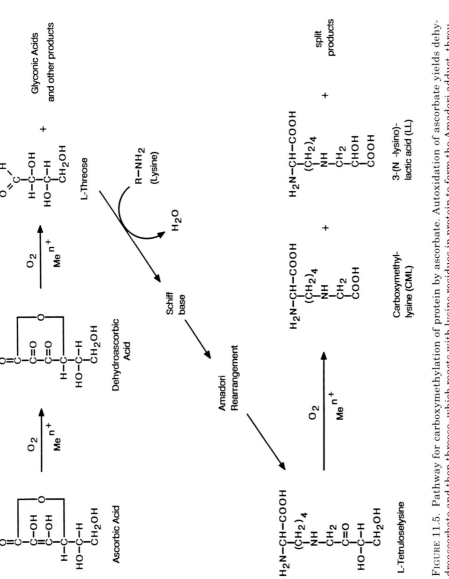

FIGURE 11.5. Pathway for carboxymethylation of protein by ascorbate. Autoxidation of ascorbate yields dehydroascorbate and then threose, which reacts with lysine residues in protein to form the Amadori adduct, threuloselysine. Like fructoselysine, threuloselysine is oxidative cleaved to form CML.

205

as a major product of autoxidative degradation of both ascorbate and dehydroascorbate, and by the rapid kinetics of synthesis of CML from threose and lysine. Incubation of proteins with ascorbic acid under physiological conditions in vitro also yielded CML in protein. The formation of threuloselysine (and CML) in protein by this pathway represents the first clear example of autoxidative glycosylation of a protein in vitro, i.e. glycation of a protein by threose, a product of autoxidation of ascorbate. In this case, however, the further oxidation of the Amadori adduct, threuloselysine, leads to the formation of CML in the protein. Thus, carboxymethylation of the protein by ascorbate is the result of both autoxidative glycosylation and autoxidation of an Amadori adduct to protein. The biological relevance of ascorbate-mediated autoxidative glycosylation of protein is uncertain, since ascorbate's primary role in vivo appears to be as an antioxidant, rather than as a pro-oxidant compound (6,18). However, decreased total ascorbate concentration and increased dehydroascorbate concentration in tissues and plasma, such as occurs in diabetes (9,40,51), may promote autoxidative glycosylation by ascorbate. The high ratio of CML to FL concentration observed in lens proteins, compared to skin collagen (12), also suggests that ascorbate, rather than FL, may be the primary source of CML in the lens. The presence of threuloselysine in tissue proteins would be indicative of ascorbate-mediated autoxidative glycosylation, but we were unable to detect this compound in lens proteins or urine, using a sensitive, selected ion monitoring, gas chromatography–mass spectrometry assay for tetritollysines, the acid-stable products formed on reduction of threuloselysine by $NaBH_4$. This may be the result of either the low concentrations of dehydroascorbate in tissues or high rates of spontaneous autoxidation of threuloselysine to CML. Studies on the effect of ascorbate depletion and supplementation on tissue and urinary CML concentration may yield insight into the nonenzymatic pro-oxidative metabolism of ascorbate in vivo, but regardless of the source of CML in tissue proteins—i.e. from glucose by autoxidation of FL (Fig. 11.3) or from ascorbate by a more complicated pathway (Fig. 11.5)—CML and related compounds (Fig. 11.3) are products of autoxidative reactions and should be useful as indicators of carbohydrate-mediated oxidative modification of proteins. It is impossible at this time to distinguish between autoxidative damage derived from autoxidation of sugars and subsequent autoxidative glycosylation reactions versus damage derived from nonoxidative glycation followed by autoxidation of carbohydrate adducts to protein. Thus, the relative importance of these two autoxidative pathways in vivo cannot be discerned. The experiments with ascorbic acid in vitro suggest, however, that the two processes are likely to occur simultaneously in vivo and provide complementary mechanisms for extending the damage to proteins resulting from their exposure to reducing sugars.

INVOLVEMENT OF OXYGEN IN LATER STAGES OF THE MAILLARD REACTION

Cross-Linking of Protein by Dicarbonyl Compounds

Although browning and caramelization reactions of sugars proceed spontaneously at extremes of pH and temperature, amines perform an important

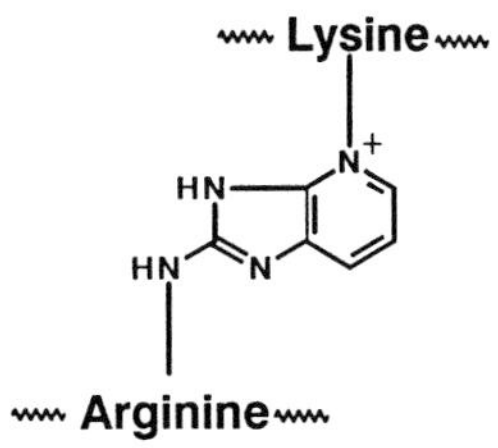

Pentosidine

FIGURE 11.6. Pentosidine, the major fluorescent cross-link formed between lysine and arginine residues during glycation of protein (49,50).

function both as stoichiometric reagents and as catalysts of the Maillard re-action at physiological pH and temperature. The stoichiometric role is to act as a co-substrate for formation of Schiff base and Amadori adducts, while the catalytic role is to act as catalyst for sugar rearrangement, dehydration, and fragmentation reactions. Among the products of these reactions are the dicar-bonyl sugars, 1-DOG and 3-DOG (Fig. 11.1) and fragmentation products (Fig. 11.2), which are much more reactive in browning reactions than their parent compounds (17,25). In addition, in the presence of oxygen, there is an alter-native autoxidative route to the formation of glucosones, as illustrated in Fig-ure 11.4. Although the browning of proteins by glucose proceeds in the absence of oxygen, Ortwerth and colleagues (44) have shown that glycation and brown-ing of protein by ascorbate is inhibited by glutathione, which prevents the ox-idation of the enediol in ascorbate to the vicinal dicarbonyls in dehydroascor-bate. Autoxidation of similar enediol intermediates derived from glucose (or Amadori adducts) would also generate reactive dicarbonyl compounds, either free in solution or bound to protein. Thus, the antioxidant status of cells, as measured by the concentration of reduced glutathione or other radical scav-engers, may indirectly modulate the chemical modification of proteins by glu-cose in vivo.

While the parent aldoses and ketoses appear to react exclusively with pri-mary amino groups in protein, dicarbonyl sugars may also react with arginine residues. In fact, dicarbonyl compounds, such as butanedione (diacetyl), phen-ylglyoxal (41), and phenanthrenequinone (63), are commonly used for chemical modification or titration of arginine residues in protein. Notably, pentosidine [Fig. 11.6; (4,13,49,50)], the only well-characterized cross-link formed in Mail-lard reactions of sugars with protein under physiological conditions,[1] contains arginine and requires oxygen for its synthesis from aldoses, suggesting its for-mation by an autoxidative route involving dicarbonyl compounds. It is also possible that oxygen may be required for formation of the fluorescent com-pound L_1 by reaction of 3-DOG with protein (34), and that L_1 may contain

---

1. In references 4 and 13, Baynes and colleagues identified the compound named Maillard Fluorescent Product #1 (MFP-1) as a glucose-derived fluorescent cross-link formed during browning reactions of glucose with protein. Using NMR spectroscopy and mass spectrometry, MFP-1 has recently been shown to be iden-tical to pentosidine, characterized earlier by Sell and Monnier (49,50) as a product of reaction of pentoses with protein. While there is some debate about whether pentosidine is derived from glucose (4,13), pentoses (49,50), and/or other sugars, the term *pentosidine* is used in further reference to this compound.

arginine. The involvement of oxygen may be either in the autoxidative activation of sugars or sugar adducts to protein or in the oxidative maturation of
fluorescent precursors in protein, suggesting a variety of routes by which the
interplay between glycation and oxidation could be involved in the irreversible
chemical modification of proteins via the Maillard reaction.

PRESENCE AND ACCUMULATION OF GLYCOXIDATION PRODUCTS IN
TISSUE PROTEINS

There is some evidence that Maillard reaction products accumulate in tissue
proteins with age and that their accumulation is accelerated in diabetes. In
this discussion, the terms *glycation* and *glycative* are used in a general sense
to refer to products formed by reaction between proteins and reducing sugars.
Similarly, the terms *glycoxidation* and *glycoxidative* are used to refer specifically to chemical modifications of protein resulting from sequential glycation
and oxidation reactions, in either order. Table 11.1 summarizes the results of
studies on the accumulation of Maillard reaction products in human skin collagen. It should be noted that CML, CMhL, and pentosidine are the only Maillard reaction products known to accumulate with age in tissue protein and at
an accelerated rate in diabetes. In addition, they are all glycoxidation products,
formed by sequential glycation and oxidation reactions. Each increases 5–
10fold in collagen between the ages of 10 and 80, while the concentration of
the Amadori product, FL, is relatively constant with age (14). All three of these
compounds could be derived from oxidation of hexose, pentose, ascorbate, and
perhaps other sugar adducts to proteins, but the increases in their concentrations in diabetic tissue proteins and urine [(36,50); unpublished observations]
suggests their origin, at least in part, from glucose. In diabetes the increase in
glycoxidation products in lens proteins and skin collagen is typically less than
twofold, compared to age-matched nondiabetic protein, despite 2–5-fold or
larger increases in the extent of glycation of protein. The smaller increase in
these products is explained, however, by the fact that diabetes-dependent in-

TABLE 11.1. Accumulation of glycoxidation products in collagen

Compound	Concentration units	Amount		Effect of diabetes
		Age 10	Age 80	
CML[a]	mmol/mol Lys	0.15	1.4	Increased
CMhL[a]	mmol/mol HyLys	0.5	4.7	Increased
Pentosidine[b]	μmol/mol Lys	3	32	Increased
Pentosidine[c]	μmol/mol Lys	22	126	Variable[d]

[a]Dunn et al. (13).

[b]Dyer et al. [(16); unpublished observations].

[c]Sell and Monnier (49,50).

[d]The pentosidine concentration in skin collagen was increased primarily in diabetic patients with complicating renal disease (50).

creases are additive to age-dependent levels of the glycoxidation products and that the increment due to diabetes would vary with age of onset, duration, and severity of disease. Thus, despite significantly higher levels of protein glycation in a young diabetic patient in poor glycemic control, the overall extent of modification of collagen by CML, CMhL, and pentosidine may still be significantly less than that observed in an older, nondiabetic person. In effect, the accumulation of these and probably other related compounds in long-lived proteins with age suggests a role for glycoxidation in the chemical aging of tissue proteins, while the accelerated rate of their accumulation in diabetes provides a rational basis for describing diabetes as a disease of accelerated aging of tissue proteins.

STATUS OF OXIDATIVE STRESS IN DIABETES

Introduction

There is considerable controversy about the role of oxidative stress in the development of vascular disease in diabetes [for current reviews, see Wolff (60), Godin and Wohaieb (20) and Oberly (42)]. The term *oxidative stress* refers to the rate of oxidative damage to biomolecules, but it is unfortunately a "catch-all" term, referring to damage derived from a variety of sources (singlet oxygen, superoxide, hydroxyl, and nitroxide radicals) and directed at a variety of substrates (lipids, proteins, DNA, saccharides, and metabolic intermediates) in different environments (blood plasma, cell membranes, intracellular organelles, basement membranes). Oxidative stress may also vary significantly among various tissues in the body, since it is affected by the local balance between oxygen radical production and scavenging systems. It is greatly increased, for example, at sites of inflammation or ischemia. Because of the complexity of biological systems, it is difficult to derive one universal measure of the status of oxidative stress or of cumulative damage from oxidation reactions. However, the measurement of products of oxygen radical reactions in specific biomolecules and in selected tissues should provide insight into the level of stress, and, where more than one product can be measured, there may be some agreement with respect to the extent of oxidative damage.

Evidence from Studies of Lipid Peroxidation

Measurements of lipid peroxidation products in plasma by the thiobarbituric acid assay suggest that oxidative stress is increased in diabetic patients with complicating vascular disease (46), including occlusive arterial (54) and cerebrovascular disease (47) and retinopathy (56). Stringer et al. (54) concluded, however, that the increase in plasma lipid peroxides was associated with the atherosclerotic process rather than with diabetes per se. A major deficiency of the thiobarbituric acid assay is that it does not distinguish between nonenzymatically generated lipid autoxidation products and lipid peroxides derived from enzymatic reactions, e.g. prostaglandins and other arachidonate metabolites (21). Thus the increase in plasma lipid peroxides may result from an increase in enzymatically derived products resulting from inflammatory processes in the vascular wall, and, indeed, treatment with aspirin may cause a decrease in thiobarbituric acid reactive substances in plasma (23). Jennings et al. (27) introduced a spectrophotometric assay for lipid autoxidation based on measurement of the plasma concentration of diene conjugates, which are non-peroxide products of lipid peroxidation and do not react with TBA. In agreement with conclusions based on the thiobarbituric acid assay (46,47,54,56), these authors reported an increase in diene conjugates in plasma from diabetic patients with microangiopathy (retinopathy $\pm$ nephropathy), but not in patients without complications. The increase in diene conjugates was observed whether the levels were normalized to plasma volume or to triglyceride content. Like the thiobarbituric acid assay, however, the diene conjugate assay also has limited specificity, since it is based on measurements of the absorbance of a crude organic extract of plasma and interference by other lipid species is not rigorously excluded. Thus, in later studies using an HPLC assay for a specific conjugated diene derived from linoleic acid, normalized to the total linoleate concentration in plasma, Collier et al. (10) found a decrease in diene conjugates in plasma from insulin-dependent diabetic patients, regardless of the presence of microangiopathy. These authors concluded that oxidative stress was actually decreased in diabetes, even in patients with retinopathy and poor glycemic control. In contrast, Collier et al. (11) reported more recently that oxidative stress may be increased in diabetes, based on an increase in plasma thiols and decreased erythrocyte superoxide dismutase in a group of diabetic patients without complications. However, the argument was weakened by the observation that erythrocyte thiol concentration was not increased in these patients (despite the decrease in superoxide dismutase), nor was plasma ceruloplasmin concentration altered. Jones et al. (30) also concluded that oxidative stress was increased in diabetes, based on increases in serum transferrin, total iron binding capacity, and ceruloplasmin in diabetic serum. However the increases were modest (20%–25%) and did not distinguish between patients with or without retinopathy. Furthermore, C-reactive protein, a sensitive indicator of an acute phase response, was not altered in either group of patients. In summary, studies on plasma lipid peroxidation products, antioxidant enzymes, and metalloproteins have failed to provide a consistent assessment of the status of oxidative stress in diabetes, and in those studies that do show an increase in indicators of oxidative stress, the role of diabetes as a causative agent has not been convincingly established. In instances in which oxidative stress appears to be increased, the role of enzymatic versus nonenzymatic sources of autoxidative stress will have to be clarified. The distinction is not merely of academic interest, since different therapeutic approaches may be warranted for dealing with different sources of oxidants.

Glycoxidation Products as Biomarkers of Oxidative Stress and
Damage in Diabetes

Although the glycoxidation products CML, CMhL, and pentosidine are present in only trace concentrations, their measurement in long-lived tissue proteins may provide a useful alternative for assessing changes in oxidative stress in aging and diabetes. Because of the relatively rapid turnover of plasma and membrane lipids and, conversely, the metabolic stability of long-lived proteins, measurement of lipid peroxidation may be more appropriate as an index of ongoing oxidative stress, while the accumulation of glycoxidation products in long-lived proteins should provide a better index of cumulative oxidative damage. Increases in glycoxidation products in tissue proteins should occur in parallel, and there is, in fact, a strong correlation between the concentrations of CML, CMhL, and pentosidine in skin collagen in both the diabetic and nondiabetic population, as well as between levels of these compounds and the visible wavelength fluorescence [yellow-blue; Ex = 325 nm, Em = 375 nm) of the collagen (unpublished observations)]. However, while levels of CML, CMhL, pentosidine, and fluorescence correlate strongly with age, their tissue concentrations are more strongly correlated with one another than with age [(14,16); unpublished observations]. Thus, the concentration of these compounds in tissue proteins provides a consistent measure of cumulative glycoxidative damage, while differences among individuals and/or tissues are consistent with individual variability in rates of oxidative stress and aging.

In recent studies we have determined that although levels of CML and CMhL are increased in diabetic, compared to nondiabetic skin collagen, the increase in these glycoxidation products is only about 50% that predicted based on age, duration of disease, and the extent of glycation of lysine residues in collagen. The general observation is that while both glycation, as measured by FL, and glycoxidation, as measured by CML and CMhL, are increased in skin collagen in diabetes (Table 11.1), the fractional ratio of CML to FL is lower than expected. This suggests a decreased rate of oxidation of FL to CML, and thus that oxidative stress to protein, as measured by the ratio of CML to FL, is decreased in diabetes. Although this conclusion must be considered cautiously because of uncertainty regarding effects of diabetes on the turnover of proteins, the analysis of CML and FL in urine yields similar results. Thus, while there is a significant correlation between the concentration of CML and FL in diabetic urine (37), the concentration of CML increases less than that of FL, and the ratio of CML to FL decreases significantly. It is important to emphasize, however, that regardless of how the rate of oxidative damage to protein is affected by diabetes, the overall extent of glycoxidative damage is actually increased, as measured by the increase in the absolute concentrations of CML, CMhL, and pentosidine in diabetic skin collagen. Thus, despite a possible decrease in oxidative stress in diabetes, there is an increase in the extent of modification of protein by glycoxidation reactions.

PATHOPHYSIOLOGICAL SIGNIFICANCE OF GLYCOXIDATION OF PROTEINS IN DIABETES

Evidence that glycation, oxidation, or glycoxidation, either of collagen or of other proteins, is of pathological significance in diabetes is still controversial (5). At this point the argument for pathophysiology resulting from accumulation of these products is weak on quantitative grounds, since CML, CMhL, and pentosidine are present in hardly more than trace amounts in collagen (Table 11.1). Even in diabetes, CML, and CMhL together account for modification of ~1% of the total lysine residues in collagen, and, since CML and CMhL are not involved in cross-linking, they are unlikely to contribute significantly to the alterations in elasticity, tensile strength, or collagenase digestibility of collagen, which occur with age and in diabetes. In comparison to CML and CMhL, the concentration of pentosidine in collagen is much lower, on the order of 10^{-3} to 10^{-2} mol pentosidine/mol of triple-stranded collagen in skin. However, in recent studies we have learned that this concentration is comparable to that of pentosidine in lysozyme or ribonuclease dimers prepared by long-term incubation of the proteins with glucose under physiological conditions; i.e. that the fluorescent cross-link, pentosidine, accounts for only about 0.1%–1% of the glucose-derived intermolecular cross-links in the protein dimer. Thus, there must be $\geqslant 100$ additional glucose-derived cross-links per mole of pentosidine in the protein dimers to account for 1 mol cross-link/mol dimerized protein. The nature of the major cross-links in the glucose-dimerized proteins is still unknown, even in these model systems, indicating that there is much to be learned about the mechanisms of glucose-dependent cross-linking of protein. However, if one extrapolates the general observation from model systems to skin collagen, then the concentration of glucose-derived cross-links in skin collagen could also be as high as 1 mol cross-link/mol triple-stranded collagen, a value comparable to the level of enzymatically derived cross-links in collagen and clearly sufficient to cause significant changes in the physical properties of the molecule. Vater et al. (57) have shown that introduction of as little as 0.1 mol of a cross-link/mol of triple-stranded collagen can have a remarkable effect on collagenase susceptibility and thus, presumably, on other structural properties the protein.

While the nature of the majority of the cross-links formed in proteins during the Maillard reaction is unknown, it is possible that a range of cross-links, structurally unrelated to glucose, i.e. not containing the carbon skeleton of glucose, could be formed by secondary oxidation reactions. For example, in Figure 11.4, the superoxide and metal ions formed on oxidation of glucose could initiate oxidative damage to adjacent protein molecules, including fragmentation and polymerization of the protein. Wickens et al. (59) and Jones and Lunec (29) have noted that the fluorescence generated during glycation of proteins in vitro is indistinguishable from that found in free radical damaged proteins, and Fujimori (19) has shown that glycation enhances the fluorescence generated in proteins exposed to autoxidizing conditions. Thus, it is possible that much of the increase in protein fluorescence and protein cross-linking observed in diabetes is the result of a nonspecific glycation-enhanced sensitivity of the protein to metal-catalyzed free radical damage. The nature of these autoxidation (metal-catalyzed oxidation) products in protein are just beginning to be explored (52), and analysis for these products in control and diabetic skin collagen should be especially helpful for understanding the relationship between glycation and oxidation reactions. In the meantime, despite their low concentrations in proteins, the glycoxidation products, CML, CMhL, and pentosidine, appear to be the most useful biomarkers for comparative measurements of age- and diabetes-dependent, glycative and oxidative damage to proteins.

The observation that all of the structurally characterized products of glycation known to accumulate in proteins with age and in diabetes are glycoxidation products suggests that oxidation may have a unique role as a fixative for damage to tissue molecules via the Maillard reaction. As illustrated in Figure 11.7, the interplay between glycation and oxidation may be more significant than either process alone in determining the pathophysiological effects of the Maillard reaction. While nonoxidative products of the Maillard reaction may also accumulate in tissue protein, it is the irreversibility of oxidation reactions which, in effect, may make oxygen, via autoxidation, a fixative of chemical damage to proteins and other biological molecules. The correlation between the CML, CMhL, and pentosidine concentrations and total fluorescence in skin collagen suggests that all three of the compounds and other uncharacterized fluorescent products are being produced in response to similar environmental stresses, and the accumulation of these compounds in tissue proteins supports a unique role for the oxidative arm of the Maillard reaction in the chemical aging of tissue proteins.

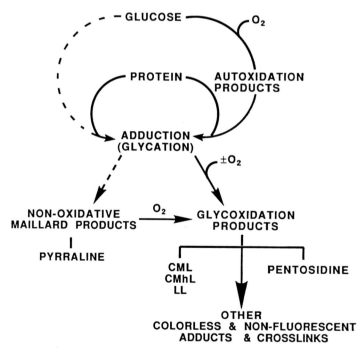

FIGURE 11.7. Possible pathways for glycoxidation of protein, illustrating the role of oxygen as a fixative for chemical modification of protein by reducing sugars via the Maillard reaction. Oxygen may be involved in oxidation of free sugar and Amadori adducts or in the maturation of products formed in later stages of the Maillard reaction. The eventual glycoxidation products include CML, CMhL, and pentosidine, the latter being involved in the cross-linking of protein. These compounds are present at trace levels in proteins and are viewed as biomarkers of more extensive glycative and/or oxidative damage to proteins.

GLYCOXIDATION AND VASCULAR DISEASE

The focus of this chapter has been on the nature of glycative and glycoxidative damage to skin collagen. Skin was chosen for these initial studies because it is obviously a more convenient source of control and diabetic collagen than the aorta or other vascular tissues. There is every reason to believe, however, that the chemical changes in skin are mirrored in the vascular collagens, based on the similarity in physical and chemical changes observed in all collagens with age and in diabetes. Future studies on the role of glucose in the aging of collagen should be directed not only at the collagens in the major vasculature and microvasculature, but also to the analysis of other proteins in the extracellular matrix, particularly the elastins and laminin, which determine the viscoelastic properties and integrate the assembly of matrix components. It will be important to confirm the degree to which changes in skin collagen are reflected in collagens and other proteins in other tissues, so that the overall impact of glycoxidative damage and differences in the susceptibility of tissues can be assessed. There is also increasing evidence that autoxidation of circulating lipoproteins may be a factor in the development of vascular disease in diabetes (53), and several studies already cited (46,47,54,56) emphasize the association between increased perixodation of plasma lipoproteins and the development of diabetic vascular disease. The extent to which glycation of lipoproteins may catalyze the autoxidation of blood lipids and lipoproteins has not been adequately explored, but it should provide a unique insight into the role of glycoxidation of lipoproteins in the development of vascular complications in diabetes. In addition to further studies on extracellular matrix proteins and plasma lipoproteins, it will be necessary to continue with the characterization of other glycation and glycoxidation products formed in model reaction systems and to explore the variety of noncarbohydrate products that might be formed in metal-catalyzed autoxidative reactions initiated by carbohydrates and their adducts to proteins. Only when the chemistry of glycation and oxidation is better understood will it be possible to assess the extent to which these nonenzymatic reactions contribute to the development of pathophysiology in diabetes.

ACKNOWLEDGMENT

Work in the authors' laboratories was supported by Research Grant DK-19971 from the National Institute of Diabetes and Digestive and Kidney Diseases.

REFERENCES

1. AHMED, M. U., THORPE, S. R., and BAYNES, J. W. Identification of N^ϵ-(carboxymethyl)lysine as a degradation product of fructoselysine in glycated protein. *J. Biol. Chem.* 261: 4889–4894, 1986.
2. AHMED, M. U., DUNN, J. A., WALLA, M. D., THORPE, S. R., and BAYNES, J. W. Oxidative degradation of glucose adducts to protein: formation of 3-(N^ϵ-lysino)-lactic acid from model compounds and glycated proteins. *J. Biol. Chem.* 263: 8816–8821, 1988.
3. AZEVEDO, M. S., RAPOSO, J., FALCAO, J., FONTES, G., and MANSO, C. Oxygen radical generation by Maillard compounds. *J. Diabetes Complic.* 2: 19–21, 1988.
4. BAYNES, J. W., DUNN, J. A., DYER, D. G., KNECHT, K. J., AHMED, M. U., and THORPE, S. R.

Role of glycation in development of pathophysiology in diabetes and aging. In: *Gly-cated Proteins in Diabetes Mellitus*, edited by R. G. Ryall. Adelaide, Australia: Adelaide University Press, 1990, pp. 221–236.

5. BAYNES, J. W., WATKINS, N. G., FISHER, C. I., HULL, C. J., PATRICK, J. S., AHMED, M. U., DUNN, J. A., and THORPE, S. R. The Amadori product on protein: structure and reactions. In: *The Maillard Reaction in Aging, Diabetes and Nutrition*, edited by J. W. Baynes and V. M. Monnier. New York: Alan R. Liss, 1989, pp. 43–67.

6. BENDICH, A., MACHLIN, A. L., and SCANDURRA, O. The antioxidant role of vitamin C. *Adv. Free Rad. Biol. Med.* 2: 419–444, 1986.

7. BLACK, C. T., HENNESSEY, P. J., FORD, E. G., and ANDRASSY, R. J. Protein glycosylation and collagen metabolism in normal and diabetic rats. *J. Surg. Res.* 47: 200–202, 1989.

8. BROWNLEE, M., CERAMI, A., and VLASSARA, H. Advanced products of nonenzymatic glycosylation and the pathogenesis of diabetic vascular disease. *Diabetes/Metab. Rev.* 4: 437–451, 1988.

9. CHATTERLEE, I. B., and BANERJEE, A. Estimation of dehydroascorbic acid in blood of diabetic patients. *Anal. Biochem.* 98: 368–374, 1979.

10. COLLIER, A. M., JACKSON, M., DAWKES, R. M., BELL, D., and CLARKE, B. F. Reduced free radical activity detected by decreased diene conjugates in insulin-dependent diabetic patients. *Diabetic Med.* 5: 737–749, 1988.

11. COLLIER, A., WILSON, R., BRADLEY, H., THOMSON, J. A., and SMALL, M. Free radical activity in type 2 diabetes. *Diabetic Med.* 7: 27–30, 1990.

12. DUNN, J. A., AHMED, M. U., MURTIASHAW, M. H., RICHARDSON, J. M., WALLA, M. D., THORPE, S. R., and BAYNES, J. W. Reaction of ascorbate with lysine and protein under autoxidizing conditions: formation of N^ϵ-(carboxymethyl)lysine by reaction between lysine and products of autoxidation of ascorbate. *Biochemistry* 29: 10964–10970, 1990.

13. DUNN, J. A., DYER, D. G., KNECHT, K. J., THORPE, S. R., MCCANCE, D. R., BAILIE, K., SILVESTRI, G., LYONS, T. J., and BAYNES, J. W. Accumulation of Maillard reaction products in tissue proteins. In: *The Maillard Reaction in Food Processing, Human Nutrition and Physiology*, edited by P. A. Finot, H. U. Aeschbacher, R. F. Hurrell, and R. Liardon. Basel: Birkhäuser Verlag, 1990, pp. 379–384.

14. DUNN, J. A., MCCANCE, D. R., THORPE, S. R., LYONS, T. J., and BAYNES, J. W. Age-dependent accumulation of N^ϵ-(carboxymethyl)lysine and N^ϵ-(carboxymethyl)hydroxylysine in human skin collagen. *Biochemistry* in press.

15. DUNN, J. A., PATRICK, J. S., THORPE, S. R., and BAYNES, J. W. Oxidation of glycated proteins: age-dependent accumulation of N^ϵ-(carboxymethyl)lysine in lens proteins. *Biochemistry* 28: 9464–9468, 1989.

16. DYER, D. G., BLACKLEDGE, J. A., KATZ, B. M., HULL, C. J., ADKISSON, H. D., THORPE, S. R., LYONS, T. J., and BAYNES, J. W. The Maillard reaction *in vivo*. *J. Nutr. Sci.*, in press.

17. ELLIS, G. P. The Maillard reaction. *Adv. Carbohyd. Chem.* 14: 63–133, 1959.

18. FREI, B., ENGLAND, L., and AMES, B. N. Ascorbate is an outstanding antioxidant in human blood plasma. *Proc. Natl. Acad. Sci. USA* 86: 6377–6381, 1989.

19. FUJIMORI, E. Cross-linking and fluorescence changes of collagen by glycation and oxidation. *Biochim. Biophys. Acta* 998: 105–110, 1989.

20. GODIN, D. V., and WOHAIEB, S. A. Reactive oxygen radical processes in diabetes. In: *Oxygen Radicals in the Pathophysiology of Heart Diseases*, edited by P. K. Singal. Boston: Kluwer Academic Publishers, 1988, pp. 303–322.

21. GUTTERIDGE, J. M. C., and HALLIWELL, B. The measurement and mechanism of lipid peroxidation in biological systems. *Trends Biochem. Sci.* 15: 129–135, 1990.

22. HARDING, J. J., and BESWICK, H. T. The possible contribution of glucose autoxidation to protein modification in diabetes. *Biochem. J.* 249: 617–618, 1988.

23. HAYAISHI, O., and SHIMIZU, T. Metabolic and functional significance of prostaglandins in lipid peroxide research. In: *Lipid Peroxides in Biology and Medicine*, edited by K. Yagi. New York: Academic Press, 1982, pp. 41–53.

24. HICKS, M., DELBRIDGE, L., YUE, D. K., and REEVE, T. S. Catalysis of lipid peroxidation by glucose and glycosylated proteins. *Biochem. Biophys. Res. Commun.* 151: 649–655, 1990.

25. HODGE, J. E. Dehydrated foods: chemistry of browning reactions in model systems. *J. Agr. Food. Chem.* 1: 928–943, 1953.

26. HUNT, J. V., DEAN, R. T., and WOLFF, S. P. Hydroxyl radical production and autoxidative glycosylation: glucose autoxidation as a cause of protein damage in experimental glycation models of diabetes mellitus and ageing. *Biochem. J.* 256: 205–212, 1988.

27. JENNINGS, P. E., JONES, A. F., FLORKOWSKI, C. M., LUNEC, J., and BARNETT, A. H. Increased diene conjugates in diabetic subjects with microangiopathy. *Diabetic Med.* 7: 27–30, 1990.

28. JOHNSON, R. N., METCALF, P. A., and BAKER, J. R. Fructosamine: a new approach to estimation of serum glycosyl protein. *Clin. Chim. Acta* 127: 87–95, 1982.

29. JONES, A. F., and LUNEC, J. Protein fluorescence and its relationship to free radical activity. *Br. J. Cancer* 55(Suppl. VIII): 60–65, 1987.

30. JONES, A. F., WINKLES, J. W., JENNINGS, P. E., FLOWKOWSKI, C. M., LUNEC, J., and BARNETT, A. H. Serum antioxidant activity in diabetes mellitus. *Diabetes Res.* 7: 89–92, 1988.

31. JONES, A. F., WINKLES, J. W., THORNALLEY, P. A., LUNEC, J., JENNINGS, P. E., and BARNETT, A. H. Inhibitory effect of superoxide dismutase on fructosamine assay. *Clin. Chem.* 33: 147–149, 1987.

32. JELLUM, E. Metabolism of the ketoaldehyde, 2-keto-3-deoxyglucose. *Biochim. Biophys. Acta* 165: 357–363, 1969.

33. KAANANE, A., and LABUZA, T. P. The Maillard reaction in foods. In: *The Maillard Reaction in Aging, Diabetes and Nutrition,* edited by J. W. Baynes and V. M. Monnier. New York: Alan R. Liss, 1989, pp. 301–327.

34. KATO, H., HAYASE, F., SHIN, D. B., OIMOMI, M., and BABA, S. 3-Deoxyglucosone, an intermediate product of the Maillard reaction. In: *The Maillard Reaction in Aging, Diabetes and Nutrition,* edited by J. W. Baynes and V. M. Monnier. New York: Alan R. Liss, 1989, pp. 68–83.

35. KATO, H., LIANG, Z. Q., NISHIMURA, T., SHIN, H. S., and HAYASE, F. 2-Oxoaldehyde-metabolizing enzymes in animal and plant tissues. In: *The Maillard Reaction in Food Processing, Human Nutrition and Physiology,* edited by P. A. Finot, H. U. Aeschbacher, R. F. Hurrell, and R. Liardon. Basel: Birkhäuser Verlag, 1990, pp. 379–384.

36. KITAOKA, S., and ONODERA, K. Oxidative cleavages of 2,3-diaminosugars and their significance in the mechanism of the amino-carbonyl reactions. *Agr. Biol. Chem.* 27: 572–580, 1962.

37. KNECHT, K. J., DUNN, J. A., THORPE, S. R., MCFARLAND, K. F., MCCANCE, D. R., LYONS, T. J., and BAYNES, J. W. Oxidative degradation of glycated proteins: effect of diabetes and aging on carboxymethyllysine levels in urine. *Diabetes* (in press).

38. KNECHT, K. J., FEATHER, M. F., LYONS, T. J., MCCANCE, D. R., and BAYNES, J. W. Detection of 3-deoxyglucosone in human plasma: evidence for intermediate stages of the Maillard reaction *in vivo. FASEB J.* 5: A912, 1991.

39. LEDL, F., and SCHLEICHER, E. New aspects of the Maillard reaction in foods and in the human body. *Angew. Chim. Int. Ed. Engl.* 29: 565–594, 1990.

40. MCLENNAN, S., YUE, D. K., FISHER, E., CAPOGRECO, C., HEFFERNAN, S., ROSS, G. R., and TURTLE, J. R. Deficiency of ascorbic acid in experimental diabetes: relationship with collagen and polyol pathway abnormalities. *Diabetes* 37: 359–361, 1988.

41. MEANS, G. E., and FEENEY, R. E. *Chemical Modification of Protein.* San Francisco: Holden-Day, 1971, pp. 194–198.

42. OBERLY, L. W. Free radicals in diabetes. *Free Rad. Biol. Med.* 5: 113–124, 1988.

43. OIMOMI, M., MAEDA, Y., BABA, S., IGA, T., and YAMAMOTO, M. Relationship between levels of advanced-stage products of the Maillard reaction and the development of diabetic retinopathy. *Exp. Eye Res.* 49: 317–320, 1989.

44. ORTWERTH, B. J., FEATHER, M. F., and OLESEN, P. R. Glutathione inhibits the glycation and crosslinking of lens protein by ascorbate. *Exp. Eye Res.* 47: 155–168, 1988.

45. SAKURAI, T., and TSUCHIYA, S. Superoxide production from nonenzymatically glycated protein. *FEBS Lett.* 236: 406–410, 1988.

46. SATO, Y., HOTTA, N. SAKAMOTO, N., MAUSUOKA, S., OHISHI, N., and YAGI, K. Lipid peroxide level in plasma of diabetic patients. *Biochem. Med.* 21: 104–107, 1979.

47. SATOH, K. Serum lipid peroxide in cerebrovascular disorders determined by a new colorimetric method. *Clin. Chim. Acta* 90: 37–43, 1978.

48. SCHNEIR, M., RAMAMURTHY, N., and GOLUB, L. Skin collagen metabolism in the streptozotocin-induced diabetic rat: enhanced catabolism of collagen formed both before and during the diabetic state. *Diabetes* 31: 426–431, 1982.

49. SELL, D. R., and MONNIER. V. M. Structure elucidation of a senescence cross-link from human extracellular matrix: implication of pentoses in the aging process. *J. Biol. Chem.* 264: 21597–21602, 1989.

50. SELL, D. R., and MONNIER, V. M. End-stage renal disease and diabetes catalyze the formation of a pentose-derived crosslink from aging human collagen. *J. Clin. Invest.* 85: 380–384, 1990.

51. SOM, S. BASU, S., MUKHERJEE, D., DEB, S., CHOUDHURY, P. R., MUKHERJEE, S., CHATTERJEE, S. N., and CHATTERJEE, I. B. Ascorbic acid metabolism in diabetes mellitus. *Metabolism* 30: 572–577, 1981.

52. STADTMAN, E. R. Metal ion catalyzed oxidation of proteins: biochemical mechanism and biological consequences. *Free Rad. Biol. Med.* 9: 315–325, 1990.

53. STEINBERG, D., PARTHASARATHY, S., CAREW, T. E., KHOO, J. C., and WITZTUM, J. L. Beyond cholesterol: modification of low density lipoprotein that increase its atherogenicity. *N. Engl. J. Med.* 320: 915–924, 1989.

54. STRINGER, M. D., GÖRÖG, P. G., FREEMAN, A., and KAKKAR, V. V. Lipid peroxides and atherosclerosis. *Br. Med. J.* 298: 281–284, 1988.

55. THORNALLEY, P. J. Monosaccharide autoxidation in health and disease. *Environ. Health Perspec.* 64: 297–307, 1985.

56. UZEL, N., SIVAS, A., UYSAL, M., and ÖZ, H. Erythrocyte lipid peroxidation and glutathione peroxidase activities in patients with diabetes mellitus. *Horm. Metab. Res.* 19: 89–90, 1987.

57. VATER, C. A., HARRIS, E. D., and SIEGEL, R. C. Native cross-links in collagen fibrils induce resistance to human synovial collagenase. *Biochem. J.* 181: 639–645, 1979.

58. WADMAN, S. K. DEBREE, P. K., VAN SPRANG, F. J., KAMERLING, J. P., HAVERKAMP, J., and VLIEGENTHART, J. F. G. N^{ε}-(carboxymethyl)-lysine, a constituent of normal urine. *Clin. Chim. Acta* 59: 313–320, 1975.

59. WICKENS, D. G., NORDEN, A. G., LUNEC, J., and DORMANDY, T. L. Fluorescence changes in human gamma-globulin induced by free-radical activity. *Biochim. Biophys. Acta* 742: 607–616, 1983.

60. WOLFF, S. P. The potential role of oxidative stress in diabetes and its complications: novel implications for theory and therapy. In: *Diabetic Complications,* edited by M. J. C. Crabbe. New York: Churchill Livingstone, 1987, pp. 167–220.

61. WOLFF, S. P., and DEAN, R. T. Aldehydes and dicarbonyls in non-enzymic glycosylation of proteins. *Biochem. J.* 249: 618–619, 1988.

62. WOLFF, S. P., and DEAN, R. T. Glucose autoxidation and protein modification: the potential role of "autoxidative glycosylation" in diabetes. *Biochem. J.* 245: 243–250, 1987.

63. YAMADA, S., and ITANO, H. A. Phenanthrenequinone as an analytical reagent for arginine and other monosubstituted guanidines. *Biochim, Biophys. Acta* 130: 538–540, 1966.

64. YUE, D. K. MCLENNAN, S., HANDELSMAN, D. J., DELBRIDGE, L., REEVE, T., and TURTLE, J. R. The effect of salicylates on nonenzymatic glycosylation and thermal stability of collagen in diabetic rats. *Diabetes* 33: 745–751, 1984.

65. YUE, D. K., MCLENNAN, S., HANDELSMAN, D. J., DELBRIDGE, L., REEVE, T., and TURTLE, J. R. The effects of cyclooxygenase and lipoxygenase inhibitors on the collagen abnormalities of diabetic rats. *Diabetes* 34: 74–78, 1985.

12

Nonenzymatic Glycosylation of Macromolecules: Prospects for Pharmacologic Modulation

HANS-PETER HAMMES AND MICHAEL BROWNLEE

The primary factor associated with the development of most diabetic complications is prolonged exposure to hyperglycemia (7). The extent and rate of progression of retinopathy, nephropathy, and neuropathy correlate closely with the magnitude and duration of target tissue exposure to abnormally high levels of blood glucose. Data from ongoing prospective studies of selected diabetic populations also indicate a clear association with diabetic macrovascular complications. Current evidence suggests that a particular diabetic individual's clinical course is also influenced by genetic determinants of tissue susceptibility and independent accelerating factors such as hypertension.

The exclusive mechanistic paradigm for hyperglycemic damage to diabetic tissues has involved excessive glucose flux through a variety of metabolic pathways in cells not dependent on insulin for glucose transport, with resultant toxic alterations in substrate concentrations. Excessive polyol pathway activity, altered redox state of pyridine nucleotides, decreased *myo*-inositol levels in selected subcellular pools, and an increased rate of de novo diacylglycerol synthesis and protein kinase C activation have all been associated with increased intracellular levels of glucose and its derivatives (8).

By definition, all known and yet-to-be-discovered examples of this paradigm involve transient changes in metabolite concentrations induced by increased glucose flux. When increased glucose flux is normalized, these abnormalities are rapidly reversed. The development of severe retinopathy in histologically normal eyes of diabetic dogs exclusively during a 2.5 yr period of euglycemia cannot be explained by this mechanistic paradigm, however (14). Rather than implicating acutely abnormal levels of toxic metabolites in the pathogenetic process, this observation strongly suggests that antecedent hyperglycemia induced *irreversible* pathogenic changes in long-lived microvascular molecules that persisted in the absence of continued hyperglycemia.

FORMATION AND ACCUMULATION OF ADVANCED GLYCOSYLATION PRODUCTS

In chemical terms, irreversible pathogenetic changes in long-lived molecules induced by antecedent metabolic abnormalities must mean that transient ab-

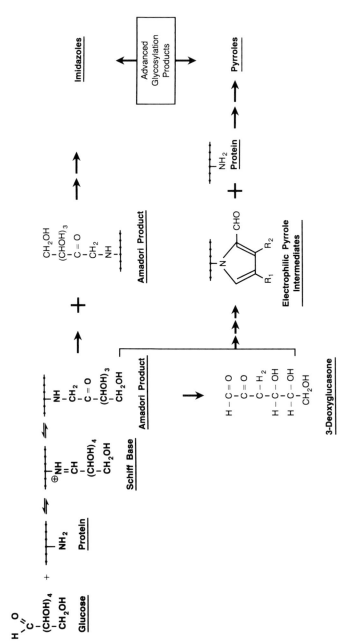

FIGURE 12.1. Schematic outline of advanced glycosylation product formation from glucose.

normalities in glucose or glucose-derived metabolite concentration covalently modify long-lived extracellular and/or intracellular constituents in a cumulative fashion. The most well-characterized and best-understood example of this mechanistic paradigm is the formation and accumulation of advanced glycosylation products (6). Glucose and glycolytic intermediates react rapidly with nucleophiles, electron-rich donors such as epsilon amino groups of lysine and amino groups of selected nucleotides, to form unstable Schiff base products at a rate proportional to glucose concentration and duration of exposure (Fig. 12.1). These Schiff base adducts quickly rearrange to form more stable glycohemoglobin-like Amadori products, which reach equilibrium levels over a period of several weeks. Both types of early glycosylation products are completely reversible.

These chemically reversible early glycosylation products undergo a slow, complex series of chemical rearrangements over a period of years on long-lived extracellular matrix proteins, and probably also on DNA in terminally differentiated cells, forming a variety of irreversible adducts called advanced glycosylation products (AGPs) or advanced glycosylation end products (AGEs) that accumulated as a function of both time and Amadori product concentration. To date, two general classes of AGPs have been described. One class is formed by the condensation of two Amadori products, and resembles the heterocyclic imidazole derivative, 2-furoyl-4(5)-(2-furanyl)1-H-imidazole. The second class of AGPs appears to form from the reaction of an Amadori product with Amadori-derived fragmentation products, resulting in the formation of heterocyclic pyrrole-based structures. Arginine, as well as lysine, contributes to the formation of some of these products (1). (For more detailed information about these reactions, see Chapter 11.)

The level of these products in diabetic vascular tissues is four or more times that found in nondiabetic specimens (25). This level reflects the net effect of both the rate of AGP formation and the rate of AGP removal. Since the rate of AGP formation is greater than first order with respect to the ambient glucose concentration (i.e. it is not simply proportional to [glucose concentration]), even modest elevations of blood glucose could result in significant AGP accumulation.

Recent evidence suggests that the rate of AGP formation can be markedly increased by products of lipid peroxidation (18). Interactions between hyperglycemia and other diabetes-associated metabolic abnormalities may thus help explain some of the variance in complications severity seen among patients with similar hyperglycemic histories.

ADVANCED GLYCOSYLATION PRODUCT ACCUMULATION AND DIABETIC PATHOLOGY

The presence and severity of clinical manifestations of a number of diabetic complications have been correlated with the magnitude of AGP accumulation. How might excessive AGP accumulation contribute to the pathogenesis of these lesions? Three main consequences of AGP formation have been extensively investigated in vitro: cross-linking of extracellular proteins; altered cell–matrix interactions; and modification of DNA structure and function (Table 12.1).

TABLE 12.1. Pathologic effects of AGPs

Extracellar matrix	Cell–matrix interactions	DNA/nuclear proteins
↓ BM component interactions	↑ Growth-promoting cytokine secretion	↑ Nucleotide modification
↑ Protein deposition	↑ Endothelial surface coagulation activity	↑ AP sites
↓ Susceptibility to degradation	↓ Endothelial cell adhesion	↑ DNA breaks
↓ EDRF effect	↓ Neurite out growth	↑ Genetic mutations

Cross-Linking of Extracellular Proteins

The progressive occlusion of diabetic vessels involves extraluminal accumulation of both plasma proteins and extracellular matrix components. Short-lived plasma proteins such as low density lipoprotein (LDL) and IgG are chemically bound by reactive AGP precursors on matrix proteins (3,4). Once immobilized, these cross-linked plasma proteins themselves serve as additional substrate for AGP formation.

The formation of AGPs on specific matrix proteins interferes with the precise, geometrically ordered self-assembly process involving site-specific interactions among various matrix protein components that are critical for maintaining normal basement membrane structure and function.

Formation of AGP cross-links on laminin causes decreased polymer self-assembly, decreased binding of type IV collagen, and decreased binding of heparan sulfate proteoglycan (11). Formation of AGP cross-links on collagen also causes decreased ultrastructural assembly, and in addition, markedly reduces the susceptibility of this basement membrane component to proteolytic degradation (31,24). X-ray diffraction studies of type I collagen demonstrate that AGPs also cause increased intermolecular spacing, as well as increased cross-linking (29). The irreversible vascular leakiness seen in long-term diabetics may reflect both AGP-induced fixed increases in intermolecular pore size and permanent loss of bound anionic heparan sulfate proteoglycan due to decreased binding properties of laminin and collagen.

AGP-induced loss of proteoglycan-binding capacity may also stimulate the overproduction of other matrix components that occurs in diabetic vessels, since heparan sulfate proteoglycans are thought to downmodulate the proliferative activity of adherent cells (28,21). The increased synthesis of fibronectin, laminin, and collagen by these cells, together with decreased degradation due to AGP-cross-linking, could explain the observed diabetes-induced changes in basement membrane metabolism that result in characteristic basement membrane thickening. Aspects of AGP cross-linking are considered in greater detail in Chapter 14.

In addition to decreasing luminal area and blood flow directly, matrix accumulation of AGPs may further impair blood flow to ischemic areas in long-term diabetics by blunting the effect of vasodilatory factors. Endothelium-derived relaxing factor (NO) is quenched by AGPs in a dose-dependent fashion, and in diabetic animals, defects in the vasodilatory response to NO correlate well with the level of accumulated AGPs (9).

AGP accumulation on laminin also inhibits neurite outgrowth (Lawrence, D., Brownlee, M., and Federoff, H., in preparation) and AGP formation on axonal cytoskeletal proteins is associated with the induction of axonal atrophy (Brownlee, M., et al. unpublished).

Altered Cell–Matrix Interactions

Extracellular matrix provides much more than simple structural support to cells. It also provides feedback information about the structural protein environment through specific cell membrane receptors, which serves to modulate a variety of cellular functions. Pathologic alterations in cell function occur when matrix proteins are modified by AGPs.

Monocytes and macrophages were the first cells on which high-affinity receptors specific for AGPs and the potentially pathologic effects of AGP interactions with these receptors were identified. These cells secrete tumor necrosis factor alpha (TNF), interleukin-1 (IL-1), and insulin-like growth factor 1 (IGF-1) when they interact with AGP-containing proteins, in concentrations that have been shown to stimulate glomerular synthesis of type IV collagen and the proliferation of endothelial, mesangial, and smooth muscle cells (33,20). This receptor has been isolated and partially purified, and has an apparent M_r of 90,000 daltons (27).

Endothelial cells also bind AGPs through specific receptors. This ligand–receptor interaction induces two additive procoagulatory changes in the endothelial surface (15). First, there is a rapid reduction in thrombomodulin activity, which prevents activation of the anticoagulant protein C pathway. At the same time, there is increased tissue factor activity, which activates coagulation factors IX and X through factor VIIa binding. TNF released from AGP-stimulated macrophages amplifies this effect, and the factor Xa generated, along with thrombin, stimulates endothelial cell release of mitogenic platelet-derived growth factor–like activity. Recently, the endothelial AGP receptor has been isolated and its gene partially cloned (Stern, D., personal communication). Additional details about these receptors are provided in Chapter 13.

AGPs on matrix also modify cellular properties by altering normal interactions of transmembrane receptors with their specific matrix ligands. Modification of the cell-binding domains of type IV collagen causes decreased endothelial cell adhesion (32), while modification of mesangial cell matrix has no effect on adhesion, but decreases cell proliferation by 50% (12). AGP accumulation on laminin inhibits neurite outgrowth by 55%–65%.

Modification of DNA Structure and Function

It has long been known that diabetes induces increased basement membrane collagen production in vivo (2). The recent observation that endothelial cells cultured in high glucose-containing media increase their production of mRNA for a variety of matrix components, independent of extracellular matrix changes (10), suggests that intracellular modifications affecting gene transcription may play a direct role in this process.

In the nucleus of cells from diabetic patients, Amadori products have been identified histologically (19). Also, it has been shown that glucose-6-phosphate can react with amino groups of both DNA nucleotides and histones in vitro (1).

The formation of AGPs on DNA is associated with structural changes, mutations, and altered gene expression. In one study, the mutation rate in a transfected plasmid was shown to be proportional to the degree to which glucose-6-phosphate was elevated in *Escherichia coli* mutants that accumulate this sugar (22). Similarly, when human endothelial cells are cultured in 30 m*M* glucose, there is an increase in single strand breaks and an increase in DNA repair synthesis (23). Increased single strand breaks in DNA also occur in lymphocytes from chronically hyperglycemic diabetic patients.

The mechanisms by which hyperglycemia induces DNA damage and altered transcription have only recently begun to be elucidated. In order to define chemically the nature of this damage, studies have been carried out with supercoiled plasmid DNA. Using a sensitive gel electrophoresis assay, it has been determined that the following classes of damage occur: loss of superhelicity, strand breakage, and loss of purine bases. Products formed from glucose-6-phosphate and glyceraldehyde-3-phosphate have been purified by FPLC, and each of these AGP peaks induces DNA damage. Using class I and class II apurinic endonuclease digestion, the majority of DNA damage by AGPs has been shown to occur by two mechanisms: specific alteration of nucleotide base structure, and creation of apurinic sites (Fig. 12.2).

How does such random AGP-induced DNA damage result in the specific abnormalities of gene expression that characterize diabetic vascular cells? One hypothesis currently being evaluated involves the random DNA damage signal transduction pathway. This pathway recognizes DNA damage caused by a variety of unrelated agents, and then specifically activates the expression of a coordinated set of growth-associated and angiogenesis-associated genes. Continued stimulation of this pathway by AGP-modified DNA may be one mechanism involved in the "memory" effect observed in the development of post-hyperglycemic retinopathy.

Prospects for Pharmacologic Modulation

Pharmacologic agents that inhibit AGP formation were developed to evaluate the pathologic consequences of AGPs accumulated in vivo, (5). Aminoguanidine HCl was selected as the prototype compound because of its low toxicity ($LD_{50} = 1800$ mg/kg) and its preferential localization to matrix-containing structures. Aminoguanidine HCl effectively inhibits AGP formation without interfering with normal lysyl oxidase–dependent cross-links, although the exact mechanism by which this occurs has only recently become clear.

Using ribonuclease A and derived peptides as a model, four mechanistic possibilities have been investigated. These were the possibility (*1*) that aminoguanidine directly reduces ambient glucose concentration; (*2*) that aminoguanidine destabilizes the conversion of labile Schiff bases to the Amadori product; (*3*) that aminoguanidine reacts with Amadori fragmentation products such as 3-deoxyglucasone in solution; and (*4*) that aminoguanidine reacts with Amadori products directly. Using fast atom bombardment mass spectrometry, reaction with Amadori-derived fragmentation products in solution was shown to be the primary mechanism of aminoguanidine action. The data further suggest that all Amadori products are not equally capable of undergoing the sub-

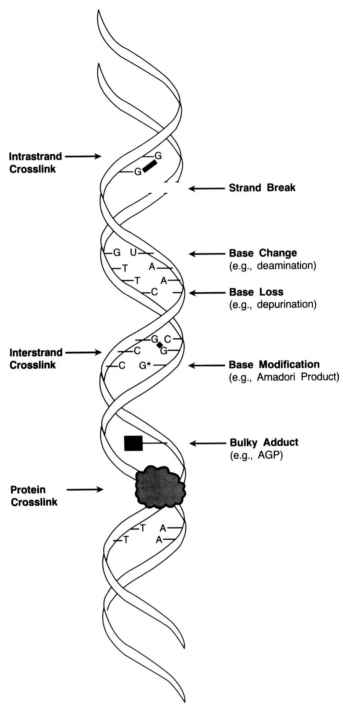

Intrastrand Crosslink

Strand Break

Base Change
(e.g., deamination)

Base Loss
(e.g., depurination)

Interstrand Crosslink

Base Modification
(e.g., Amadori Product)

Bulky Adduct
(e.g., AGP)

Protein Crosslink

FIGURE 12.2. Mechanisms of glycosylation product-induced DNA damage. [Modified from Bohr, V. A., et al., 1989. *Lab Invest.* 61: 143–161.]

sequent reactions involved in AGP formation (Edelstein, D., and Brownlee, M., *Diabetes,* in press).

In vitro, aminoguanidine effectively inhibits AGP-induced cross-linking of collagen and prevents cross-link–induced defects of heparin binding to collagen/fibronectin. In addition, aminoguanidine prevents AGP-induced defects in laminin structure and self-assembly (11). AGP-matrix–induced defects in endothelial cell adhesion and mesangial cell proliferation are also prevented (32,12).

In vivo, aminoguanidine treatment prevents (Table 12.2) the increases in retinal vascular permeability (30), AGP formation, and the subsequent intercapillary deposition of extravasated proteins in long-term diabetic rats. In addition, there is a significant reduction in the diabetes-induced PAS-positive deposits at branching sites of precapillary arterioles in aminoguanidine-treated animals. Overall, these findings suggest that AGP accumulation precedes the occurrence of vascular damage and capillary occlusion (16,17). In keeping with this conclusion, pathologic development of retinal microaneurysms and an 18-fold increase in acellular capillaries are dramatically reduced by aminoguanidine in long-term diabetic rats, and the endothelial/pericyte cell ratio, which is increased in untreated diabetic animals, remains nearly normal (16).

Aminoguanidine treatment also reduces the AGP content in the aortic wall, decreases the quantity of plasma protein cross-linked to diabetic matrix, and diminishes the excessive cross-linking of aortic matrix protein itself in diabetic rats (5).

In the kidney of diabetic mice and rats, aminoguanidine treatment decreases glomerular basement membrane AGP content (26) and reduces matrix susceptibility to degradation by proteases. Because of this, the pathognomonic basement membrane thickening and mesangial expansion of diabetes does not occur [(13,35); Brownlee, M. et al., unpublished]. The functional corollary of this structural normalization in diabetic kidneys is a concomitant reduction of the 4–10-fold increase in diabetic urinary albumin excretion to near-normal values (34,36).

In peripheral nerve of diabetic rats, axonal atrophy, motor and sensory nerve conduction velocities, and vasa nervorum blood flow are normalized by treatment with aminoguanidine (37).

From these positive studies, it may be concluded that aminoguanidine and its analogues have a potential therapeutic role in the prevention and treatment of chronic diabetic complications. However, only from well-designed clinical studies will the actual therapeutic place of such compounds in the treatment of diabetic patients become clear.

TABLE 12.2. Effects of aminoguanidine treatment on diabetic complications

Retina	Kidney	Nerve
↓ Intercapillary protein deposits	↓ Urinary albumin excretion	↓ Axonal atrophy
↓ Microaneurysms	↓ Basement membrane thickening	↑ MNCV*
↓ Acellular capillaries	↓ Mesangial expansion	↑ SNCV†

*Motor nerve conduction velocity
†Sensory nerve conduction velocity

SUMMARY

In tissues that develop diabetic complications, excessive amounts of irreversible advanced glycosylation products (AGPs) accumulate on long-lived extracellular matrix proteins and intracellular constituents, due to chronically elevated plasma glucose concentrations. Abnormalities in extracellular protein cross-linking, cell–matrix interactions, and DNA structure have been demonstrated in vitro, and inhibitors of AGP formation have been developed. Administration of the prototype compound, aminoguanidine, to long-term diabetic animals prevents pathology in retinal capillaries, the renal glomerulus, and peripheral nerve. The therapeutic potential of glycosylation inhibitor use in diabetic patients is being evaluated.

ACKNOWLEDGMENTS

Work from this laboratory was facilitated by the Albert Einstein NIH Diabetes Research and Training Center grant. Grant support to M.B. from the Juvenile Diabetes Foundation, the American Diabetes Association, the Diabetes Research and Education Foundation, Inc., and the National Institutes of Health (RO1H37979-04, RO1DK33861-05, and RO1DK41457-01) contributed to the studies described.

REFERENCES

1. BAYNES, J. W., and MONNIER, V. M. (eds.). *The NIH Conference on the Maillard Reaction in Aging, Diabetes and Nutrition*. New York: Alan R. Liss, 410 pp, 1989.
2. BROWNLEE, M., and SPIRO, R. G. Glomerular basement membrane metabolism in the diabetic rat: in vivo studies. *Diabetes* 28: 121–125, 1979.
3. BROWNLEE, M., PONGOR, S., and CERAMI, A. Covalent attachment of soluble proteins by nonenzymatically glycosylated collagen. *J. Exp. Med.* 158: 1739–1744, 1983.
4. BROWNLEE, M., VLASSARA, H., and CERAMI, A. Nonenzymatic glycosylation products on collagen covalently trap low-density lipoprotein. *Diabetes* 34: 938–941, 1985.
5. BROWNLEE, M., VLASSARA, H., KOONEY, T., ULRICH, P., and CERAMI, A. Aminoguanidine prevents diabetes-induced arterial wall protein cross-linking. *Science* 232: 1629–1632, 1986.
6. BROWNLEE, M., VLASSARA, H., and CERAMI, A. Advanced glycosylation endproducts in tissue and biochemical basis of complications. (Beth Israel Seminar in Medicine). *N. Engl. J. Med.* 318: 1315–1321, 1988.
7. BROWNLEE, M., and SHERWOOD, L. M. (eds.). *Diabetes Mellitus and Its Complications: Pathogenesis and Treatment*. Philadelphia: Hanley & Belfus, pp. 1–300, 1990.
8. BROWNLEE, M., WILLIAMSON, J. R., and RUDERMAN, N. B. Hyperglycemia, diabetes and the vascular wall. *FASEB J.* (in press).
9. BUCALA, R., TRACEY, K., and CERAMI, A. *Diabetes* 39: 30A, 1990 (abstr.).
10. CAGLIERO, E., ROTH, T., SAYON, R., and LORENZI, M. Characteristics and mechanisms of high-glucose-induced overexpression of basement membrane components in cultured human endothelial cells. *Diabetes* 40: 102–110, 1991.
11. CHARONIS, A. S., REGER, L. A., DEGE, J. E., KOUZII-KOLIAKOS, K., FURCHT, L. T., et al. Laminin alteration after in vitro nonenzymatic glucosylation. *Diabetes* 39: 807–814, 1990.
12. CROWLEY, S., BROWNLEE, M., EDELSTEIN, D., SATRIANO, J., MORI, T., et al. Effect of nonenzymatic glycation of mesangial matrix on proliferation of mesangial cells. *Diabetes* 40: 540–547, 1990.
13. ELLIS, E. N., and GOOD, B. H. Prevention of glomerular basement membrane thickening by aminoguanidine in experimental Diabetes Mellitus. *Metabolism* 40: 1016–1019, 1991.
14. ENGERMAN, R. L., and KERN, T. S. Progression of incipient diabetic retinopathy during good glycemic control. *Diabetes* 36: 808–812, 1987.
15. ESPOSITO, C., GERLACH, H., BRETT, J., STERN, D., and VLASSARA, H. Endothelial receptor-mediated binding of glucose-modified albumin is associated with increased mono-

layer permeability and modulation of cell surface coagulant properties. *J. Exp. Med.* 170: 1387–1407, 1989.

16. HAMMES, H. P., MARTIN, S., FEDERLIN, K., GEISEN, K., and BROWNLEE, M. Aminoguanidine treatment inhibits the development of experimental diabetic retinopathy. *Proc. Natl. Acad. Sci. USA* 88: 11555–11558, 1991.

17. HAMMES, H. P., FEDERLIN, K., and BROWNLEE, M. Aminoguanidine treatment inhibits advanced glycosylation product accumulation in diabetic retinal vessels. International Diabetes Federation Congress, 1991 (abstr.).

18. HICKS, M., DELBRIDGE, L., YUE, D. K., and REEVE, T. S. Increase in crosslinking of nonenzymatically glycosylated collagen induced by products of lipid peroxidation. *Arch. Biochem. Biophys.* 268: 249–254, 1989.

19. KELLY, S. B., OLERUD, J. E., WITZTUM, J. L., CURTIS, L. K., GOWN, A. M., et al. A method for localizing the early products of nonenzymatic glycosylation in fixed tissue. *J. Invest. Dermatol.* 93: 327–331, 1989.

20. KIRSTEIN, M., ASTON, C., and VLASSARA, H. *Diabetes* 39: 182A, 1990 (abstr.).

21. KLAHR, S., SCHREINER, G., and ICHIKAWA, I. The progression of renal disease. *N. Engl. J. Med.* 318: 1657–1666, 1988.

22. LEE, A. T., and CERAMI, A. Elevated glucose 6-phosphate levels are associated with plasmid mutations in vivo. *Proc. Natl. Acad. Sci. USA* 84: 8311–8314, 1987.

23. LORENZI, M., MONTISANO, D. F., TOLEDO, S., and BARRIEUX, A. High glucose and DNA damage in endothelial cells. *J. Clin. Invest.* 77: 322–325, 1986.

24. LUBEC, G., and POLLAK, A. Reduced susceptibility of nonenzymatically glucosylated glomerular basement membrane to proteases. *Renal. Physiol.* 3: 4–8, 1980.

25. MAKITA, Z., RADOFF, S., RAYFIELD E., and CERAMI, A. *Diabetes* 39(Suppl. 1): 29A, 1990 (abstr.).

26. NICHOLLS, K., and MANDEL, T. E. Advanced glycosylation end-products in experimental murine diabetic nephropathy: effect of islet isografting and aminoguanidine. *Lab. Invest.* 60: 486–493, 1989.

27. RADOFF, S., VLASSARA, H., and CERAMI, A. Characterization of a solubilized cell surface binding protein on macrophages specific for proteins modified nonenzymatically by advanced glycosylated end products. *Arch. Biochem. Biophys.* 263: 418–423, 1988.

28. ROHRBACH, D. H., HASSEL, J. R., KLEINMAN, H. K., and MARTIN, G. R. Alterations in basement membrane (heparan sulfate) proteoglycan in diabetic mice. *Diabetes* 31: 185–188, 1982.

29. TANAKA, S., AVIGAD, G., BRODSKY, B., and EIKENBERRY, E. F. Glycation induces expansion of the molecular packing of collagen. *J. Mol. Biol.* 203: 495–505, 1988.

30. TILTON, R. G., CHANG, K., OSTROW, E., ALLISON, W., and WILLIAMSON, J. R. Aminoguanidine reduces increased ^{131}I albumin permeation of retinal and uveal vessels in streptozotocin diabetic rats. *Invest. Ophthalmol.* 31: 342, 1990.

31. TSILIBARY, E. C., CHARONIS, A. S., REGER, L. A., WOHLHUETER, R. M., and FURCHT, L. T. The effect of nonenzymatic glucosylation on the binding of the main noncollagenous NCl domain to type IV collagen. *J. Biol. Chem.* 263: 4302–4308, 1988.

32. TSILIBARY, E. C., and CHARONIS, A. S. The effect of nonenzymatic glucosylation on cell and heparin binding microdomains from type IV collagen and laminin. (abstr.). *Diabetes* 39: 194A, 1990.

33. VLASSARA, H., BROWNLEE, M., MONOGUE, K., DINARELLO, C. A., and PASAGIAN, A. Cachectin/TNF and IL-1 induced by glucose-modified proteins: role in normal tissue remodeling. *Science* 240: 1546–1548, 1988.

34. YAMASHITA, N., YOSHIKAWA, C., et al. Glycation of glomerular basement membrane (GBM) type IV collagen (IVC) and proteinuria. (abstr.). *Diabetes* 38: 25A, 1989.

35. SOULES-LAPARATA T., COOPER M., PAPAZOGLOU D., CLARKE B., and JERUMS G. Retardation by aminoguanidine of development of albuminuria mesangial expansion and tissue fluorescence in streptozotocin induced diabetic rat. *Diabetes* 40: 1328–1335, 1991.

36. EDELSTEIN D. and BROWNLEE M. Aminoguanidine ameliorates albuminuria in diabetic hypertensive rats. *Diabetologia* 35: 96–97, 1992.

37. KIHARA M., SCHMELZER J. D., PODUSLO J. F., CURRAN F. F., NICKANDER K. K., LOW P. A. Aminoguanidine effect on nerve blood flow, vascular permeability, electrophysiology, and oxygen free radicals. *Proc. Natl. Acad. Sci. USA* 88: 6107–6111, 1991.

13

Cell-Mediated Interactions of Advanced Glycosylation End Products and the Vascular Wall

HELEN VLASSARA

Thickening of the arterial wall in atherosclerosis is associated with abnormal basement membrane and subintimal collagen deposition, and the focal proliferation of vascular smooth muscle cells leads to an increase in peripheral resistance. Related events include increases in endothelial cell permeability and leakage, and the deposition of serum proteins, such as albumin, cholesterol esters, and fibrin. These pathological changes are believed to contribute to the pathogenesis of both the atherosclerotic and the thrombotic vasculopathies associated with aging and chronic diabetes (1,14,18,28).

Over many years we have been studying the biochemical basis of these vascular complications. In particular we have been evaluating the hypothesis that exposure of structural proteins to glucose leads, over time, to alterations that could explain many of the pathological changes (4,6,7,8,10). Work from numerous laboratories has demonstrated that the aldehyde- or keto-groups of reducing sugars are capable of reacting with amino groups of amino acids or nucleic acids to form Schiff bases, which can then rearrange to the more stable Amadori-type early glycosylation products (23,25). The formation of these early glycosylation products is both reversible and proportional to the glucose levels; thus their concentration rises in hyperglycemia and falls with restoration of normoglycemia (9–23).

These early glycosylation products when forming on proteins with long half-lives, do not dissociate but undergo a slow, complex series of chemical rearrangements to become irreversible advanced glycosylation end products (AGEs). AGEs are a heterogenous group of structures characterized by a yellow-brown color, fluorescence, and a propensity to form cross-links to and between proteins (8). Analysis of the structure of a minor fluorescent-protein adduct, 2-furoyl-4[5]-[2-furanyl]-1-H-imidazole, has revealed that cross-linking may occur by means of a heterocyclic condensation of two glucose molecules and two lysine-derived amino groups, suggesting the importance of free amino groups on the protein and reactive moieties on the hexose for their formation (32). The presence of this adduct in vivo is currently being challenged (29,40); however, further insight into its character has been obtained by the isolation of a formed intermediate in vitro, 1-alkyl-2-formyl-3,4-diglucosyl-pyrrole

(AFGP) (13), a pyrraline detected in albumin from diabetic subjects (20), and in a pentosidine identified in human extracellular matrix (30).

The potential of AGEs to perturb the vessel wall is suggested by studies showing that their presence on long-lived molecules in the vessel wall increases both as a function of age (27,31) and the presence of diabetes (26,27). Reactive AGEs alter structural properties of the matrix by inducing collagen-to-collagen cross-linking (5), and by causing thickening and rigidity. In addition they result in trapping of plasma proteins such as low-density lipoproteins (LDL) and IgG (2,3). These changes in the matrix could be responsible for some of the pathologic features characteristically observed in the subendothelium of vasculature in the aged and in patients with diabetes. Recent information obtained with the use of an AGE-specific sensitive radioreceptor assay suggests that AGE-proteins are present in sera in greater concentrations in diabetics than in normal individuals, and that they reach very high levels in diabetics with end-stage renal failure (25). Given the abundance of AGEs in tissue and in the circulation, and their direct contact with various cellular elements, e.g. monocyte/macrophages and endothelial cells, we have recently begun to examine such interactions.

MACROPHAGES AND MONOCYTES HAVE A DISTINCT SURFACE RECEPTOR FOR AGES

Given the central role attributed to monocyte-derived macrophages in the turnover of extracellular matrix proteins and the ubiquitous presence of tissue AGEs, we first examined the interaction of these cells with AGEs. We have identified and purified a membrane-associated macrophage receptor that specifically recognizes proteins to which AGEs are bound (42,43). This receptor selectively binds AGEs, has an affinity constant of 1.75×10^7/mole for the ligand, and appears to be distinct from the mannose-fucose receptor involved in glycoprotein uptake, and from previously described scavenger receptors, such as those for modified LDL and formaldehyde-treated albumin (41). This putative AGE-receptor, now isolated from the transformed macrophage cell line RAW 264.7, is a polypeptide that consists of a 90 kD binding unit [Fig. 13.1; (33,34)].

In addition to internalizing AGE-modified soluble proteins, macrophages can recognize intact cells that have AGEs chemically attached to their outer membrane (Fig. 13.2). Thus AGE-modified erythrocytes are removed from the circulation more rapidly than unmodified cells (44). Such studies suggest that accumulation of AGEs on the surface of long-lived cells could be responsible in part for the normal turnover of erythrocytes and other cells as they age.

REGULATORY ROLE OF MACROPHAGE AGE-RECEPTOR: EFFECT OF AGES ON TISSUE TURNOVER

Following the interaction of AGE-modified proteins with the macrophage receptor, uptake and degradation of AGEs occurs, and the synthesis and release

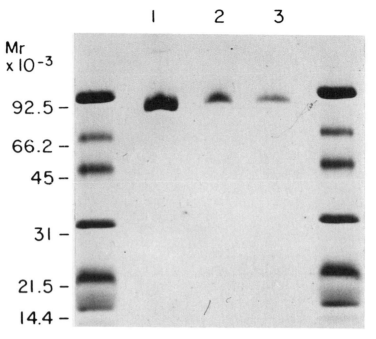

FIGURE 13.1. SDS-PAGE of purified AGE-receptor protein isolated from a macrophage-like cell line, RAW 264.7, following affinity chromatography, and FPLC analysis (33,34). The receptor is shown as a 90 kD protein at three different concentrations (lanes 1–3).

of growth-promoting mediators cachectin/TNF and interleukin-1 are stimulated (45). These cytokines have been shown to stimulate the recruitment of cells of mesenchymal derivation, which can then be triggered to synthesize and release degradative enzymes, such as collagenase and other extracellular proteases (24), and new matrix proteins. The AGE-mediated release of factors with known growth-promoting activity may represent a mechanism by which macrophages signal to nearby cells to remove and replace senescent proteins. It has also been hypothesized that the monocyte–macrophage interaction with AGEs may induce insulin-like growth factor-1 (IGF-1), a potent growth factor for a variety of mesenchymal cells, including fibroblasts and smooth muscle cells (15). Recently obtained data indicated that normal freshly isolated human monocytes express both IGF-1 mRNA and protein in response to AGE-modified matrix (fibronectin) or soluble (albumin) proteins (22). These findings lend further support to the notion that AGEs, abundant in most tissues and fluids, play a role in tissue remodeling by inducing cytokines and growth-promoting substances.

Since the effectiveness of this repair process is dependent on the efficient removal of modified proteins, we examined the ability of endogenous mediators such as insulin (46), cachectin/TNF, IFN-τ, and IL-1 to regulate the rate of uptake and elimination of AGE-proteins by monocyte–macrophages (47). Macrophages from hypoinsulinemic, alloxan-induced, or genetically diabetic animals exhibited a modest twofold increase in AGE-receptor number, accompa-

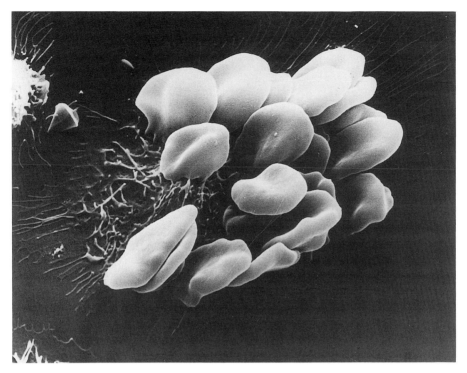

FIGURE 13.2. AGE-modified (by using the synthetic model compound FFI) human erythrocytes bound by human peripheral monocytes. [Electron scanning micrograph by David M. Phillips of the Population Council, New York.]

nied by a 25%–30% increase in its degradation rate. In contrast, macrophages from hyperinsulinemic C57B1/6J (db/db) mice displayed a distinct reduction in both number of AGE-receptors and binding affinity, along with a 50% reduction in AGE degradation (46). These observations suggest that the AGE-receptor may be modulated in vivo by high or low insulin concentrations. Downregulation of AGE-receptors in certain non-insulin-dependent diabetes mellitus (NIDDM) patients with elevated peripheral insulin levels could have important clinical implications. In particular, it could be a key determinant of the amount and rate of accumulation of hyperglycemia-accelerated glucose-modified protein in the blood vessel walls.

In contrast to insulin, cachectin/TNF was shown to induce a severalfold enhancement of the binding, endocytosis, and degradation of AGE-modified albumin by both murine and human macrophage–monocytes in vitro. In addition, it enhanced the rate of disappearance of AGE-erythrocytes in vivo [Fig. 13.3; (47)]. Interestingly, IL-1 and IFN-τ did not stimulate AGE-receptor activity (47). The upregulation of the AGE-receptor by cachectin/TNF appears to occur through an autocrine pathway (45). Since this cytokine is released in response to AGE-protein uptake, it may provide a mechanism through which the receptor system adapts to local demands as tissue AGEs accumulate.

Macrophages thus appear to have an important role in the host-response

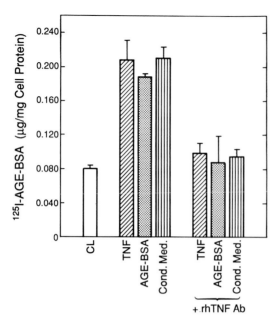

FIGURE 13.3. AGE-receptor up-regulation after preincubation with cachectin/TNF, AGE (FFI)-BSA, or FFI-BSA-conditioned medium, in the presence and absence of rhTNF antibody (47).

to the deposition of AGEs in the vessel wall. In turn, the ever-present AGEs may represent important signals that normally, through macrophage AGE-specific receptors, direct and coordinate tissue protein turnover and repair. The normal balance may be disturbed in such conditions as chronic diabetes and aging, where accelerated AGE formation prevails.

Finally, the influence of aging on the murine peritoneal macrophage AGE-receptor function was investigated, using soluble AGE-protein as the ligand and macrophages from young (6 mo) and old (2.5 yr) mice. A significant reduction (> 2-fold) in both receptor number and binding affinity was noted in cells from the old mice as compared to the young group (19). The evidence suggests that aging in itself may compound tissue damage by adversely influencing AGE-receptor efficiency and preventing the removal of deleterious AGE-modified molecules.

EFFECT OF AGES ON THE MIGRATION OF HUMAN MONOCYTES

Infiltration of the vascular wall by monocytes is thought to be an early pathogenetic event observed in atherosclerosis (16,36). Once in the subendothelium, monocyte/macrophages can secrete multiple products that directly, or indirectly via the attraction of other cells, lead to reorganization of the intima and profoundly alter surrounding tissues. An important missing link in previous studies has been the recognition of a specific stimulus that selectively induces monocytes to cross endothelial monolayers.

In an attempt to provide the missing link, we recently hypothesized that AGEs forming with time on normal vascular wall proteins may target circulating monocytes to sites of AGE accumulation for their subsequent removal (21). The results follow.

1. In vitro glycosylated proteins, such as AGE-albumin, and AGE-LDL [under conditions of optimal protection against oxidation (38)], are selectively chemotactic for monocytes. Thus modified LDL has almost 60% of the activity of the highly chemotactic molecule FMLP, whereas unmodified control LDL does not exhibit such activity (Fig. 13.4A, B). LDL was selected for testing, because accumulation of extravasated LDL in the arterial subintima is central to the development of atherosclerosis (36). In this context, LDL has been shown to be covalently cross-linked to wall AGE-matrix proteins (2). There it can be glycosylated, thus becoming an additional migratory signal for monocytes.

2. In vivo glycosylated proteins from nonvascular tissue, such as peripheral nerve myelin proteins, which, unlike native collagen, lack inherent che-

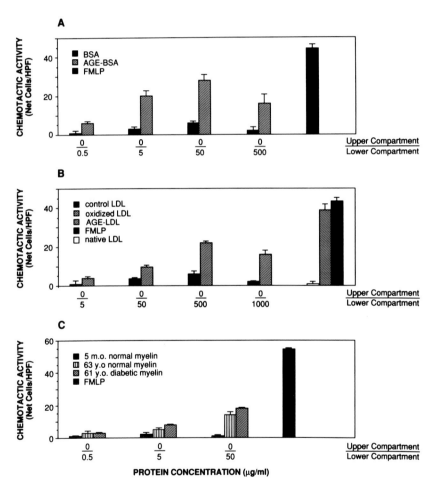

FIGURE 13.4. Monocyte chemotaxis to AGE-proteins assayed in a modified Boyden chamber, and using FMLP (10 nM) as a positive control (38). A: in vitro glycosylated AGE-BSA glycosylated (80 AFU/100 µg), vs unmodified BSA (4 AFU/100 µg). B: In vitro glycosylated AGE-low density lipoprotein (LDL; 30 AFU/100 µg), vs unmodified BSA (9 AFU/100 µg), both prepared in the presence of antioxidants BHT (20 µM), and EDTA (500 µM) under a N2 blanket in sealed tubes, vs oxidized LDL. C: In vivo glycosylated diabetic/aged human peripheral nerve myelin (156 AFU/100 µg) vs normal/young myelin (14 AFU/100 µg).

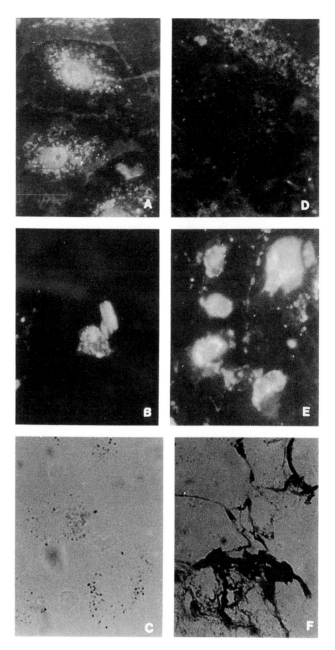

FIGURE 13.5. Effect of AGEs on endothelial cell–monocyte interaction. *A, D:* Confluent monolayer on normal (*A*), and AGE-containing matrix (*D*) is visualized by an FITC-conjugated lectin.
B, E: Same fields as *A* and *D*, respectively, showing PH26-stained monocytes below the monolayer and in normal (*B*), or AGE-containing (*E*) subendothelial matrix. *C, F:* Same fields as *A*
and *D*, respectively, showing localization of gold-conjugated normal (*C*) and AGE-modified (*E*)
matrix.

motactic activity, are also chemotactic for monocytes. Myelin proteins isolated from a 61-year-old diabetic, a 63-year-old normal individual, and a 5-month-old normal infant, were tested (Fig. 13.4C). Myelin from both the diabetic and the age-matched normal individual were found to be severalfold more chemotactic than myelin from the 5-month-old child, and, as expected, the myelin of the diabetic was more chemotactic than that of the age-matched control (25%–30%).

"Checkerboard analysis" data have demonstrated that the locomotive response of monocytes to AGE-ligands was due to chemotaxis and not enhanced random cell migration (chemokinesis). In experiments using AGE-BSA as the model ligand and specific fluorescence as an AGE indicator, the chemotaxis to AGE-protein was shown to correlate with the amount of AGEs formed on the protein (21). These studies suggested that in vivo AGE-formation could mediate monocyte recruitment from the circulation, possibly by inducing monocytes to move through normal endothelium and aggregate on sites of excessive AGE accumulation. They also raised the possibility that AGE-induced covalent trapping of lipoproteins and other plasma proteins could be responsible for their increased pressure in the diabetic or aged vessel wall. We have tested this possibility in the studies described below.

When human monocytes were incubated with intact endothelial monolayers grown on a substrate containing AGE-BSA (1:1 mixture of AGE-BSA and collagen IV), they were induced to cross the endothelial cell monolayers; at least three times as many monocytes were demonstrable in the matrix beneath the endothelial cell when it contained monolayers on the AGE substrate rather than unmodified BSA (Fig. 13.5). Monocytes crossed intact, confluent endothelial monolayers, and could be visualized in close association with matrix deposits of AGE-BSA. Figure 13.5 shows monocytes that have migrated through an endothelial cell monolayer to the subendothelial space in proximity to AGE-BSA-gold particles. In contrast, polymorphonuclear leukocytes did not display enhanced AGE-induced migration across endothelial cell monolayers.

The potential significance of these results is emphasized by the observation that monocytes incubated with an AGE-containing matrix become activated. For instance, they produce much more platelet-derived growth factor (PDGF) than do monocytes incubated with normal matrix (21). This leads to the hypothesis that subendothelial AGEs attract monocytes in the presence of an overlying endothelial cell monolayer, and that this sets in motion processes leading to monocyte migration through the endothelium and their subsequent deposition in the matrix, where they endocytose AGEs and become activated.

BOVINE AND HUMAN ENDOTHELIAL CELL AGE-SPECIFIC RECEPTORS

Endothelial cells constitute a dynamic barrier that regulates vascular permeability, interaction of the vessel wall with circulating cells, and multiple hemostatic processes. In a continuous layer of viable endothelium, abnormal metabolites, cytokines, and other factors can trigger pathological reactions, even in the absence of endothelial cell death or desquamation (17,37,39). In this context, AGEs are normally found in the plasma, as well as in the vascular basement membrane, and their quantity is significantly increased in sera and tissues in the aged and in patients with diabetes (4,6–8,25,27). Furthermore, their presence is closely correlated with advanced vascular lesions in the vessel wall.

These considerations led us to speculate that specific interactions with AGEs may influence endothelial cell function, and that this contributes to some of the principal features of vascular disease in the elderly and in the diabetic. At the outset, our intention was to determine whether endothelium expresses specific binding sites for AGE that might mediate their uptake from the plasma and facilitate their subsequent deposition within the subendothelial matrix. In addition, we speculated that interaction with either plasma-derived and/or matrix-associated AGEs, would cause disturbances in the endothelial cell properties, resulting in impairment of its barrier function, and altered coagulant activity. To test these hypotheses, binding studies were carried out using AGE-BSA as a model AGE-modified ligand (12) and cultured bovine aortic endothelium. At 4°C, binding was localized to the cell surface; specifically bound material could be eluted with an heparin-containing buffer or brief exposure of cultures to a low concentration of trypsin. Studies with AGE-BSA conjugated to colloidal gold particles demonstrated surface binding that could be inhibited by excess AGE-BSA not bound to gold (12). Binding to the cell surface was time-dependent and reversible. Equilibrium binding studies showed that AGE-endothelial cell binding was half-maximal at ≈ 100 nM and, at saturation, there were $\approx 2.6 \times 10^6$ molecules bound/cell. Similar results were observed with human umbilical vein and bovine capillary endothelial cells, demonstrating that this type of AGE-endothelial interaction occurs in all the major types of blood vessels and in humans, as well as experimental animals.

The results also indicated that endothelial cells express specific binding sites for glucose-modified albumin which selectively recognizes the AGE adduct of the molecule. We further established that AGE adducts of other proteins, such as AGE-ribonuclease, and AGE-hemoglobin, competed effectively for occupancy of these binding sites (12). However, FFI, a chemically defined AGE shown previously to bind to macrophage AGE-receptors, did not appear to compete for the binding of [^{125}I]AGE-BSA to the endothelial cell. These data suggest that there might be important differences between the AGE receptor on macrophages and other cell types, such as endothelium. Further competitive binding studies indicated that the endothelial cell AGE-BSA binding site was distinct from the mannose-fucose receptor(s), as well as from the scavenger receptor(s) for acetylated and other forms of modified LDL.

EFFECTS OF AGE-PROTEINS ON ENDOTHELIAL CELL PERMEABILITY

In view of the association of AGEs with vascular complications, in which increased vascular permeability is often evident, perturbation of endothelial cell barrier function by AGE-BSA was examined (12). Confluent endothelial cell monolayers on filters form a barrier that restricts the passage of macromolecules and lower molecular weight solutes. Using this experimental system, we found that cultures incubated with AGE-BSA demonstrated an increase in their permeability (Fig. 13.6A). After ≈ 24 h of incubation with AGE-BSA there

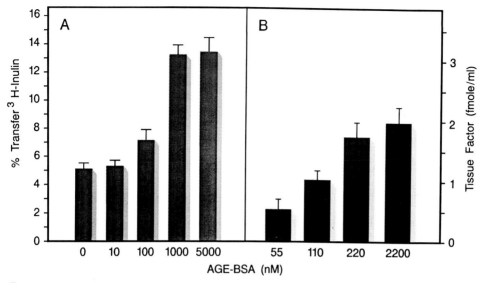

FIGURE 13.6. Effect of AGEs on endothelial cell function: *A:* Effect of AGE-BSA on endothelial cell permeability, as a function of ligand concentration, following a 48 h incubation, as assessed by inulin transfer (12). *B:* Effect of AGE-BSA on EC tissue factor activity, as a function of ligand concentration, at 48 h incubation (12).

was a time- and dose-dependent increase in the diffusion of [³H]inulin and other tracers across these monolayers. Concomitant with the AGE-BSA–induced perturbation of monolayer barrier function, there was an alteration in cell shape/cytoskeletal organization (12).

Thus, in contrast to the transcytosis of AGE-BSA, which occurs as soon as the ligand binds to the surface of an intact monolayer, longer exposure of the monolayer to AGE-BSA causes changes in cell architecture, with the appearance of gaps that permit paracellular (binding site independent) escape of solutes.

EFFECTS OF AGE-PROTEINS ON ENDOTHELIAL CELL COAGULANT FUNCTION

Alterations in vascular permeability are closely linked to perturbation of the coagulation mechanism. Conversely, activation of coagulation on the endothelial cell surface leads to the formation of proteases and fibrin, which can alter endothelial cell shape and increase vascular permeability. These considerations led us to examine whether exposure of endothelium to AGE-BSA could alter certain cell surface anticoagulant and procoagulant properties.

AGE-MEDIATED INCREASE OF TISSUE FACTOR ACTIVITY AND SUPPRESSION OF THROMBOMODULIN

Exposure of endothelium to AGE-BSA augmented "tissue factor"–dependent endothelial cell procoagulant activity (12). A significant dose-dependent induction of tissue factor occurred steadily over several days (Fig. 13.6*B*). This is different from TNF-induced or IL-1–induced increases in endothelial tissue factor, which disappear within 24 h.

Since the anticoagulant protein C/protein S pathway is closely linked to endothelium, we examined the modulation by AGE-BSA of thrombomodulin, the cofactor promoting thrombin-mediated formation of activated protein C (11). The activity of thrombomodulin decreased during incubation of endothelial cell cultures with AGE-BSA (12). Suppression of thrombomodulin activity on intact endothelial cell cultures was evident by 1 h, reached a maximum by 20 h, and persisted up to the longest time points tested (48 h). This effect was concentration dependent, being half-maximal at 70–100 nM AGE-BSA (12). In contrast, native BSA did not depress thrombomodulin activity. To examine the mechanism of AGE-induced suppression of thrombomodulin, radioimmunoassays for cellular thrombomodulin antigen were performed. Total thrombomodulin antigen remained unchanged during the incubation with AGE-BSA (unlike the decrease induced by LPS and cachectin/TNF on thrombomodulin) (12), but expression on the cell surface declined, as observed from measurement of indirect immunofluorescence and functional assays in intact cells [(12); Fig. 13.7]. AGE-BSA had no direct effect on the activity of purified thrombomodu-

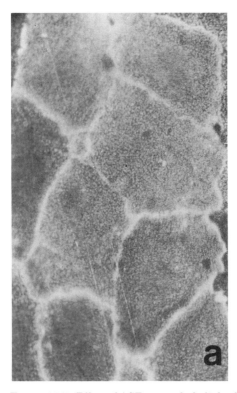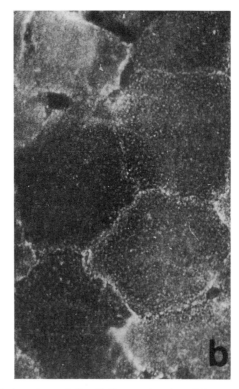

FIGURE 13.7. Effect of AGEs on endothelial cell thrombomodulin. Cells were incubated in normal (*A*) or AGE-BSA containing medium (*B*) for 48 h, and thrombomodulin was visualized by immunofluorescence (12), showing reduced intensity in AGE-treated cells compared to controls.

lin. These data suggest that sequestration of thrombomodulin at an inaccessible site, probably in an intracellular location, could be responsible for AGE-induced thrombomodulin suppression.

ADVANCED GLYCOSYLATION END PRODUCTS ARE PRESENT IN
ARTERIAL WALL TISSUES AND IN SERA OF BOTH NORMAL AND
DIABETIC INDIVIDUALS

In our hypothesis we have speculated that vascular endothelium can interact both with subendothelial and circulating AGEs. However, with the exception of the measurements of relative fluorescence and collagen solubility, no direct methodology has accurately estimated the extent of AGE-modification in human tissues or sera. Because of the relatively short life-span of most circulating proteins and the expectation that tissue AGE degradation products reaching the plasma are rapidly cleared by the kidneys, serum AGE levels have been thought to be below the detection limits of existing assays. It was important, therefore, to develop a precise and sensitive method to measure serum and tissue AGE levels, and to establish differences between the normal and diabetic state.

Based on our earlier identification of a major AGE-specific binding site on the murine macrophage-like tumor cell line RAW 264.7 (33,34), we have now constructed a new radio-receptor assay for quantitation of AGE in tissues and sera (25). Using intact cells, [^{125}I]AGE-BSA as the ligand, and unlabeled AGE-BSA as the competitor, a standard curve is produced with each assay. One unit of AGE is defined as the amount of AGE required to inhibit 50% of [^{125}I]AGE-BSA binding (22 μg AGE-BSA). Intra- and inter-assay precision were assessed to be less than 10% at 1 U of AGE/ml (c.v. 6.2% and 8.9%, respectively). Using this assay, we determined the AGE content in human collagenase-digested arterial wall tissue from 16 diabetic (mean age 67 $\pm$ 10) and 23 age-matched normal (mean age 63 $\pm$ 12.9) people. Diabetic arteries contained four times more AGE than arteries from normal people ($P < 0.001$). Difference in fluorescence were less significant ($P < 0.05$). To determine whether circulating AGEs are indeed measurable by this assay, sera from eight normal people, 12 diabetic patients without renal failure (RF), 6 diabetics on hemodialysis, and 10 nondiabetic patients on hemodialysis were tested. Sera were ultrafiltered through a Centriprep-10 to separate large (>10K) from low (<10K) molecular weight proteins, concentrated, and tested. Low molecular weight serum ultrafiltrates from diabetic individuals contained almost twice as much AGE as the filtrates from normal patients [$P < 0.05$; (Fig. 13.8)]. Interestingly, the sera from the diabetics undergoing dialysis showed a nearly ninefold increase in AGE ($P < 0.001$). This significant serum AGE elevation in diabetics, and particularly in those with end-stage renal disease, supports the previously proposed association of advanced glycosylation with accelerated complications. Finally, the pronounced increase observed in diabetic dialysis patients could be indicative of inefficient clearance. Whatever the mechanism, this finding raises the possibility that uncleared recirculating AGEs are available for excessive interaction with the vascular endothelium, and they may accelerate ongoing pathology. In

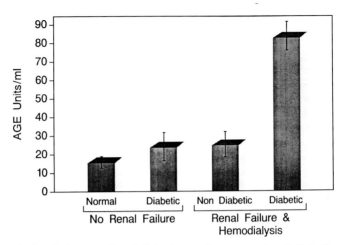

FIGURE 13.8. AGE levels in normal and diabetic sera from normal and diabetic patients with and without renal failure. Low molecular weight (<10 K) proteins were tested using an AGE-specific radioreceptor assay system (25).

keeping with this speculation, diabetics with end-stage renal disease are known to succumb to cardiovascular complications at an exceedingly high rate.

REFERENCES

1. BLOODWORTH, J. M. B., JR., and GREIDER, M. H. *Endocrine Pathology, General and Surgical,* 2nd ed. Baltimore: Williams and Wilkins, 1982, p. 556.
2. BROWNLEE, M., VLASSARA, H., and CERAMI, A. Nonenzymatic glycosylation products on collagen covalently trap low density lipoprotein. *Diabetes* 34: 938–941, 1985.
3. BROWNLEE, M., VLASSARA, H., and CERAMI, A. Trapped immunoglobulins on peripheral nerve myelin from patients with diabetes mellitus. *Diabetes* 35: 999–1003, 1986.
4. BROWNLEE, M., CERAMI, A., and VLASSARA, H. Advanced glycosylation end products in tissue and the biochemical basis of diabetic complications. *N. Engl. J. Med.* 318: 1315–1321, 1988.
5. BROWNLEE, M., PONGOR, S., and CERAMI, A. Covalent attachment of soluble proteins by nonenzymatically glycosylated collagen: role in the *in situ* formation of immune complexes. *J. Exp. Med.* 158: 1739–1744, 1983.
6. BROWNLEE, M., CERAMI, A., and VLASSARA, H. Advanced products of nonenzymatic glycosylation and the pathogenesis of diabetic vascular disease. *Diabetes/Metab. Rev.* 4: 437–451, 1988.
7. BROWNLEE, M., VLASSARA, H., and CERAMI, A. Nonenzymatic glycosylation and the pathogenesis of diabetic complications. *Ann. Intern. Med.* 101: 527–537, 1984.
8. BROWNLEE, M., VLASSARA, H., and CERAMI, A. The pathogenetic role of nonenzymatic glycosylation in diabetic complications. In *Diabetic Complications: Scientific and Clinical Aspects,* edited by M. J. C. Crabbe. London: Pitman, pp. 94–139, 1987.
9. BUNN, H. F., GABBAY, K. H., and GALLOP, P. M. The glycosylation of hemoglobin: relevance to diabetes mellitus. *Science* 200: 21–27, 1978.
10. CERAMI, A., VLASSARA, H., and BROWNLEE, M. Role of nonenzymatic glycosylation in atherogenesis. In *Perspectives in Inflammation, Neoplasia and Vascular Cell Biology. Proceedings of The UCLA Symposia on Molecular and Cellular Biology,* edited by T. Edgington, R. Ross, and S. Silverstein. New York: Alan R. Liss, pp. 105–114, 1986. *J. Cell. Biochem.* 30: 111–120, 1986.
11. ESMON, C. The regulation of natural anticoagulant pathways. *Science* 235: 1348–1352, 1987.
12. ESPOSITO, C., GERLACH, H., BRETT, J., STERN, D., and VLASSARA, H. Endothelial receptor-mediated binding of glucose-modified albumin is associated with increased mono-

layer permeability and modulation of cell surface coagulant properties. *J. Exp. Med.* 170: 1387–1407, 1989.

13. FARMAR, J. G., ULRICH, P. C., and CERAMI, A. Novel pyrroles from sulfite-inhibited Maillard reactions: insight into the mechanism of inhibition. *J. Organic Chem.* 53: 2346–2349, 1988.

14. FLEG, J. L. Alterations in cardiovascular structure and function with advancing age. *Am. J. Cardiol.* 57: 33C–44C, 1986.

15. FROESCH, E. R., SCHMID, CHR., SCHWANDER, J., and ZAPF, J. Actions of insulin-like growth factors. *Annu. Rev. Physiol.* 47: 443–467, 1985.

16. GERRITY, R. G. The role of the monocyte in atherogenesis: I. Transition of blood-borne monocytes into foam cells in fatty lesions. *Am. J. Pathol.* 103: 181–190, 1981.

17. GIMBRONE, M. (ed). *Vascular Endothelium in Hemostasis and Thrombosis.* Edinburgh: Churchill Livingstone, 1986.

18. GREENE, D. A. Acute and chronic complications of diabetes mellitus in older patients. *Am. J. Med.* 80(5A): 39–53, 1986.

19. HARRISON, D., and VLASSARA, H. Receptor-mediated binding of advanced glycosylation endproducts to murine macrophages: effects on aging. (submitted).

20. HAYASE, F., NAGARAJ, R. H., MIYATA, S., NJOROGE, F. G., and MONNIER, V. M. Aging of proteins: immunological detection of a glucose derived pyrrole formed during Maillard reaction in vivo. *J. Biol. Chem.* 264: 3758–3764, 1989.

21. KIRSTEIN, M., BRETT, J., RADOFF, S., OGAWA, S., STERN, D., and VLASSARA, H. Advanced protein glycosylation induces selective transendothelial human monocyte chemotaxis and secretion of PDGF: role in vascular disease of diabetes and aging. *Proc. Natl. Acad. Sci. USA* 87: 9010–9014, 1990.

22. KIRSTEIN, M., ASTON, C., and VLASSARA, H. Normal human monocytes express insulin-like growth factor-1 (IGF-1) in response to matrix glycation: role in tissue remodelling. *FASEB J.* 4: A1759, 1990.

23. KOENIG, R. J., and CERAMI, A. Synthesis of hemoglobin A_{1c} in normal and diabetic mice: potential model of basement membrane thickening. *Proc. Natl. Acad. Sci. USA* 72: 3587–3691, 1975.

24. LE, J. M., WEINSTEIN, D., GUBLER, U., and VILCEK, J. Induction of membrane-associated interleukin by tumor necrosis factor in human fibroblasts. *J. Immunol.* 138: 2137–2142, 1987.

25. MAKITA, Z., RADOFF, S., RAYFIELD, E. J., YANG, Z., SKOLNIK, E., FRIEDMAN, E. A., CERAMI, A., and VLASSARA, H. Advanced glycosylation endproducts in patients with diabetic nephropathy. *N. Eng. J. Med.* 325: 836–842, 1991.

26. MONNIER, V. M., VISHWANATH, V., FRANK, K. E., ELMETS, C. A., DAUCHOT, P., and KOHN, R. R. Relation between complications of type I diabetes mellitus and collagen-linked fluorescence. *N. Engl. J. Med.* 314: 403–408, 1986.

27. MONNIER, V. M., KOHN, R., R., and CERAMI, A. Accelerated age-related browning of human collagen in diabetes mellitus. *Proc. Natl. Acad. Sci. USA* 81: 583–587, 1984.

28. NATIONAL DIABETES DATA GROUP. *Diabetes in America.* Washington, DC: U.S. Government Printing Office, NIH Publication No. 85-1468, 1985.

29. NJORGE, F. G., FERNANDES, A. A., and MONNIER, V. M. Mechanism of formation of the putative advanced glycosylation endproduct and protein crosslink 2-(2-furoyl)-4(5)-(2-furanyl)-1H-imidazole. *J. Biol. Chem.* 263: 10646–10652, 1988.

30. NJOROGE, F. G., SAYRE, L. M., and MONNIER, V. M. Detection of D-glucose-derived pyrrole compounds during Maillard reaction under physiological conditions. *Carbohydr. Res.* 167: 211–220, 1987.

31. OIMOMI, M., MAEDA, Y., HATA, F., KETAMURA, Y., MATSUMOTO, S., HATANAKA, H., and BABA, S. A study of the age-related acceleration of glycation of tissue protein in rats. *J. Gerontol.* 43: B98–101, 1988.

32. PONGOR, S., ULRICH, P. C., BENCSATH, F. A., and CERAMI, A. Aging of proteins: isolation and identification of a fluorescent chromophore from the reaction of polypeptides with glucose. *Proc. Natl. Acad. Sci. USA* 81: 2684–2688, 1984.

33. RADOFF, S., VLASSARA, H., and CERAMI, A. Characterization of a solubilized cell surface binding protein on macrophages specific for proteins modified non-enzymatically by advanced glycosylated endproducts. *Arch. Biochem. Biophys.* 263: 418–423, 1988.

34. RADOFF, S., CERAMI, A., and VLASSARA, H. Isolation of a surface binding protein specific for advanced glycosylation endproducts from the murine macrophage-derived cell line RAW 264.7. *Diabetes* 39: 1510–1518, 1990.

35. REYNOLDS, T. M. Chemistry of nonenzymatic browning. *Adv. Food Res.* 12: 1–52, 1963.

36. ROSS, R., and GLOMSET, J. A. The pathogenesis of atherosclerosis. *N. Engl. J. Med.* 295: 369–377, 1976.

37. SIMIONESCU, M., and SIMIONESCU, N. *Endothelial Cell Biology*. New York: Plenum Press, 1987.

38. STEINBRECHER, U. P., PARTHASARATHY, S., LEAKE, D. S., WITZTUM, J. L., and STEINBERG, D. Modification of low density lipoprotein by endothelial cells involves lipid peroxidation and degradation of low density lipoprotein phospholipids. *Proc. Natl. Acad. Sci. USA* 81: 3883–3887, 1984.

39. STERN, D., and NAWROTH, P. (eds). *Vessel Wall. Semin. Thromb. Hemostas.*, 1987.

40. TAKATA, K., HORIUCHI, S., ARAKI, N., SHIGA, M., and SAITOH, M. Endocytic uptake of non-enzymatically glycosylated proteins is mediated by a scavenger receptor for aldehyde-modified proteins. *J. Biol. Chem.* 263: 14819–14825, 1988.

41. VLASSARA, H., BROWNLEE, M., and CERAMI, A. Novel macrophage receptor for glucose-modified proteins is distinct from previously described scavenger receptors. *J. Exp. Med.* 164: 1301–1309, 1986.

42. VLASSARA, H., BROWNLEE, M., and CERAMI, A. High-affinity-receptor-mediated uptake and degradation of glucose-modified proteins: a potential mechanism for the removal of senescent macromolecules. *Proc. Natl. Acad. Sci. USA* 82: 5588–5592, 1985.

43. VLASSARA, H., BROWNLEE, M., and CERAMI, A. Accumulation of diabetic rat peripheral nerve myelin by macrophages increases with the presence of advanced glycosylation endproducts. *J. Exp. Med.* 160: 197–207, 1984.

44. VLASSARA, H., VALINSKY, J., BROWNLEE, M., CERAMI, C., NISHIMOTO, S., and CERAMI, A. Advanced glycosylation endproducts on erythrocyte cell surface induce receptor-mediated phagocytosis by macrophages: a model for turnover of aging cells. *J. Exp. Med.* 166: 539–549, 1987.

45. VLASSARA, H., BROWNLEE, M., MANOQUE, K. R., DINARELLO, C., and PASAGIAN, A. Cachectin/TNF and IL-1 induced by glucose-modified proteins: role in normal tissue remodelling. *Science* 240: 1546–1548, 1988.

46. VLASSARA, H., BROWNLEE, M., and CERAMI, A. Specific macrophage receptor activity for advanced glycosylation end products inversely correlates with insulin levels in vivo. *Diabetes* 37: 456–461.

47. VLASSARA, H., MOLDAWER, L., and CHAN, B. Macrophage/monocyte receptor for non-enzymatically glycosylated proteins is up-regulated by cachectin/tumor necrosis factor. *J. Clin. Invest.* 84: 1813–1820, 1989.

14

Effects of Nonenzymatic Glycation on Molecular Interactions of Basement Membrane Molecules

ARISTIDIS S. CHARONIS, EFFIE C. TSILIBARY, AND LEO T. FURCHT

Nonenzymatic glycation of proteins is considered one of the major pathogenetic processes responsible for diabetic microangiopathy. The basement membrane of the microvasculature is thought to undergo important structural and functional alterations in diabetes mellitus. In this chapter, the structural characteristics of the macromolecular components of the basement membrane are briefly described; the focus is on the intrinsic basement membrane components that are thought to be the building blocks for this structure. It should be emphasized that the current list of well-characterized basement membrane macromolecules is a partial one, and certainly other components will soon be added.

The interactions between and among basement membrane macromolecules is reviewed later in this chapter. Although most of our knowledge comes from in vitro systems, it is important to review these studies in order to appreciate the complexity of these interactions and to begin to understand how starting from a mixture of macromolecules, the final product, the complex heteropolymer called *basement membrane,* is built. Finally, the effect of nonenzymatic glycation on the structure and the functional properties of the basement membrane macromolecules is reviewed. Limited information is available so far, exclusively from the in vitro systems. These studies suggest that nonenzymatic glycation may severely compromise the ability of basement membrane components to interact with each other.

BASEMENT MEMBRANE MACROMOLECULES

The term *basement membrane* refers to a very specialized area of extracellular matrices. Basement membranes are found either at the basal surface of cells exhibiting polarity (epithelial, mesothelial, or endothelial cells) or surrounding specific cell types (muscle cells, Schwann cells, or fat cells). In the vascular wall the basement membrane provides a continuous acellular layer underlying the endothelium. The continuity of this layer is interrupted only in terminal lymphatics and in the liver, in the space of Disse. At the level of the microvasculature, where most exchanges between the blood circulation and the interstitium take place (gasses, small nutrients, macromolecules, cells) the wall of

243

the vessel consists mainly of two layers: the endothelium and the underlying basement membrane.

To be able to study the structure and the functional significance of the basement membranes (especially in the critical events that are mediated by the microvascular wall) it was imperative to isolate and characterize the macromolecules that are intrinsic components of the basement membranes. This was a very difficult task because of the low solubility of these molecules due to extensive cross-linking, which led to extremely low yields (22). Some information has been gained by using enzymatic digestion in various steps of the extraction procedure, but it was soon realized that these protocols resulted in truncated forms of basement membrane components. This issue is particularly important for basement membrane molecules due to their multidomain structure. In the late seventies, the development of model systems that produced high amounts of basement membrane macromolecules allowed detailed structural analysis of these proteins. The most widely used among these model systems is the murine—Engelbreth-Holm-Swarm (EHS)—tumor (36). The study of the structure of basement membrane components and their interactions was also considerably advanced by electron microscopic observation, using the technique of rotary shadowing (19,51). This technique has proved very useful for studying these macromolecules because of their complex, multidomain, and elongated structure. In this method, a dilute solution containing basement membrane macromolecules is sprayed on freshly cleaved mica. The solution is allowed to dry, and under extremely high vacuum, metal (usually a mixture of platinum and carbon) is evaporated and coats the macromolecules. In this way, a replica showing the fine structural details of every molecule is obtained and can be examined at very high magnification using a transmission electron microscope.

As of now, there are four major basement membrane macromolecules that have been isolated and characterized: type IV collagen, laminin, entactin/nidogen, and heparan sulfate proteoglycan. This list will undoubtedly grow larger. We will now review the main structural characteristics of these macromolecules. Figure 14.1 is a schematic representation of these macromolecules and their most frequently used fragments.

Type IV Collagen

Type IV collagen has a molecular weight of slightly over 500,000 and consists of three polypeptide chains that form a rod, which along most of its length is a triple helix. It is a heterotrimer, composed of two identical $\alpha1(IV)$ chains and one $\alpha2(IV)$ chain (56); these two chains are different gene products, showing absence of homology in the triple helical portions of the rod. Type IV collagen differs significantly from other interstitial collagens. First, it has no homology (except for the presence of glycine in every third position of the triple helical portions) with the other collagens (2,23). Second, in both the $\alpha1$ and the $\alpha2$ chain many interruptions of the Gly-X-Y motif exist (from 2 to 11 amino acids long) (5,48,49). It is speculated that one of the major functions of these interruptions is to provide the type IV collagen molecule with flexibility not observed in the other interstitial collagens. Third, the amino- and carboxy-ter-

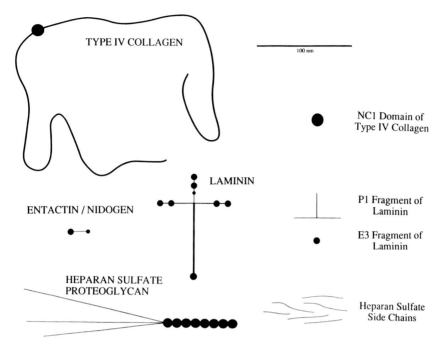

FIGURE 14.1. Diagrammatic representation of the four bona fide basement membrane macro-molecules. *Left:* The molecules are shown as they appear at the electron microscopic level in their intact form. *Right:* Fragments from these macromolecules (created by enzymatic diges-tion) are shown, with their nomenclature.

minal propeptides that are cleaved in interstitial collagens are not cleaved in type IV collagen (34). The amino terminal part of the molecule is mostly triple helical and is known as the 7S domain (57). The carboxy terminal end of the molecule forms the most prominent noncollagenous domain, known as NC1; it forms a globular compact structure and is stabilized by interchain disulfide bonds (64). Fourth, type IV collagen contains high levels of glucosyl-galactosyl groups bound to hydroxylysine in the triple helical domains (52) and also *N*-linked and *O*-linked complex oligosaccharides present in the 7S and NC1 domains (64). At the electron microscopic level, type IV collagen appears as a flexible rod with an average length of 400 nm. The EHS extracted type IV collagen is found mostly in dimeric form (66). In this case, the NC1 globule is positioned at the center of the molecule and has a diameter of 8 nm.

Laminin

Laminin is the best studied noncollagenous basement membrane glycoprotein (58). It has a molecular weight of approximately 850,000 and consists of three polypeptide chains: B1 (MW $\simeq$ 230,000), B2 (MW $\simeq$ 210,000), and A (MW $\simeq$ 400,000). These chains share significant similarities in their domain organi-zation, but they differ to a large extent in their amino acid sequence and are considered products of related but different genes (42,43,45,46,47). The tech-nique of rotary shadowing allowed visualization of the laminin molecule and appreciation of its multidomain arrangement (19). In the electron microscope, laminin appears as an asymmetric cross, with three short arms (about 35 nm in length each) and one long arm (75 nm in length). All arms exhibit substantial flexibility. The long arm appears thicker than the short arms and has a large globule at the end. The short arms exhibit two smaller globules each, one in the middle of their length and one at the end; a third small globule is sometimes observed on one of the three short arms, near the cross area. Protease digestion studies (37) and antibody studies (39) suggest that each of the short arms is made from one of the three chains (B1, B2, A), whereas the long arm contains all three chains arranged in a triple-coiled helix; the globule of the long arm is thought to be composed entirely from the A chain. In the area of intersection of the cross and near the globule of the long arm, the three chains are held together by disulfide bonds (32). Computer models from the known amino acid sequences of each chain predict a multidomain arrangement and confirm the observations at the electron microscopic level. Different functions can be mapped at various domains, but one specific function can reside in more than one domain. Laminin contains 13% carbohydrate, mainly in the form of the complex type N–linked oligosaccharide (12).

Entactin/Nidogen

Entactin/nidogen is a sulfated glycoprotein consisting of one polypeptide chain of molecular weight 158,000. It was discovered by Carlin et al. (8). Two years later, Timpl et al. (60) described an 80 kD basement membrane component which they named nidogen. It was later found that this 80 kD component was the degradation product of a protease-sensitive macromolecule that had an original molecular weight of 150 kD (17,40). Extensive cross-reactivity and high similarity in amino acid composition led to the conclusion that entactin and the intact form of nidogen are the same protein (32). In this review we are using the two names because they have both been used extensively in the literature. Entactin/nidogen is sulfated at tyrosine residues and contains about 5% sugars of the O-linked and N-linked type. At the electron microscopic level, entactin/nidogen appears as a dumbbell-shaped molecule consisting of two globular regions of diameters 6 nm and 4 nm, connected via a thin rod 16 nm long (40). The full amino acid sequence of entactin/nidogen is known (16).

Heparan-Sulfate Proteoglycan

The heparan sulfate proteoglycan macromolecule consists of a high molecular weight protein core (400,000 daltons) that is a single polypeptide chain. Three glycosaminoglycan side chains (65,000 daltons each) exhibiting the heparan sulfate type of repeated disaccharide unit are attached to it (21,29,41). Enzymatic digestion studies suggest that the attachment sites of the glycosaminoglycan side chains are clustered on one end of the protein core (29). This core is very sensitive to proteases, and it has been suggested that different forms of basement membrane–extracted heparan sulfate proteoglycan may be generated in various tissues and under various extraction conditions (25). Electron microscopic observations indicate that the protein core is a 80 nm–long macromolecule exhibiting six globular subunits of variable size, probably formed by intrachain S—S bonds. The side chains can be seen as three thin filaments 100–170 nm long that are attached to one pole of the protein core (28,41,68). The amino acid sequence of the protein core is partly known (35). One interesting feature of the protein core is the existence of domains homologous to laminin.

Another species of heparan sulfate proteoglycan of lower molecular weight has been isolated from EHS tumor matrix (20). There is controversy about whether this represents a distinct gene product (41) or it is a degradation product of the high molecular weight heparan sulfate proteoglycan (21).

Other Components

Type IV collagen, laminin, entactin/nidogen, and basement membrane heparan sulfate proteoglycan are the four well-characterized and intrinsic basement membrane macromolecules shown to be present in practically every basement membrane that has been studied. It is widely accepted that this is by no means a complete list; other macromolecules will soon be added. Basement membrane chondroitin sulfate proteoglycan may be an example. Although the current thinking is that chondroitin sulfate/dermatan sulfate proteoglycans appear to be expressed mainly in the interstitium (44), small amounts of chondroitin sulfate are found in basement membranes (30). Another possible candidate is a small protein extracted from EHS tumor matrix that has been named BM-40 (18); this macromolecule may be identical to SPARC (a protein secreted by cells in tissue culture) and osteonectin (a component found in bone) (32). The studies with model systems like EHS tumor matrix and with tissue basement membranes inevitably focus on macromolecules that exist in relatively large amounts, because the yields permit further studies of these components. It is conceivable that another category of basement membrane macromolecules might exist: those that are present in considerably lower concentrations, some of which may vary from one basement membrane to the next. These components might still be important as regulators of the assembly of the proteins mentioned above, which can be considered major structural constituents of basement membranes.

Another category of well-characterized extracellular matrix macromolecules includes molecules such as fibronectin, thrombospondin, factor VIII/von Willebrand factor, and amyloid P, among others. These macromolecules have been detected in some basement membranes by immunofluorescence and immunoelectron microscopy and may be important constituents during embryonic development or tissue repair. However, because of their presence in plasma or on cell surfaces they should not be considered intrinsic components of differentiated basement membranes (33,55).

INTERACTIONS BETWEEN BASEMENT MEMBRANE MACROMOLECULES

All basement membrane macromolecules can interact extensively with each other; they also seem to have, to a greater or lesser extent, the ability to self-assemble and form oligomers and/or polymers. These interactions are summarized in Table 14.1.

TABLE 14.1. Interactions among basement membrane macromolecules

Binding component	Substrate			
	Type IV collagen	Laminin	Entactin/nidogen	Heparan sulfate proteoglycan
Type IV collagen	Lateral association and network formation. Domain NC1 is very crucial.	At least two sites exist: one between the globules of a short arm and another on the terminal globule of the long arm.	Mainly via the carboxy terminal globule.	Not examined. Side chains may be crucial.
Laminin	At least one specific site on the collagenous portion, located $\frac{1}{3}$ of the length from domain NC1.	Oligomer and polymer formation. The terminal globules of all arms are mainly involved.	Mainly via the carboxy terminal globule.	Not examined. Side chains may be crucial.
Entactin/nidogen	Many binding sites: on domain NC1 and at least two along the length of the collagenous portion.	On one of the lateral short arms, between the cross area and the inner globule.	Aggregation has been observed but not well studied.	Not examined.
Heparan sulfate proteoglycan	Not examined. Many heparin binding sites on domain NC1 and along the length of the collagenous portion may mediate the binding to the glycosaminoglycan side chains.	Not examined. Many heparin binding sites on laminin may mediate the binding to the glycosaminoglycan side chains.	Not examined.	Dimer and oligomer formation via the pole of the protein core opposite to the origin of the side chains.

Type IV Collagen Polymerization

Type IV collagen was the first basement membrane macromolecule shown to be able to self-associate and polymerize. The process of type IV collagen polymerization is a complex one, and many aspects of it are not yet understood. The first step is apparently the formation of dimers. This occurs by the interaction of two NC1 domains, so that the two molecules are connected by their carboxy termini (59). Dimer formation seems to be an early event (intracellular?) because, as mentioned earlier, more than 90% of the extracted type IV collagen from the EHS tumor is in the form of dimers. This interaction is not thermally reversible and is resistant to mild denaturing conditions, like 2 *M* urea. However, isolated dimeric NC1 globules (created by treating type IV collagen extensively with collagenase) can be dissociated with harsher conditions, like 8 *M* urea, sodium dodecyl sulfate, or low pH [2.5–4.0; (64)]. Another association can take place at the other end of the molecule, the amino terminal 7S domain. Type IV collagen molecules can associate by overlapping their terminal triple helical portions (up to 30 nm from the end of the molecule); two, three, or a maximum of four collagen molecules have been seen to associate in this fashion with the technique of rotary shadowing and electron microscopy (59). The formation of oligomers up to tetramers was also confirmed by using velocity sedimentation and gel electrophoresis (15). This interaction is not thermally reversible, occurs at a slow rate, and is very much concentration dependent and susceptible to treatment with 2 *M* urea (66). The interaction is not mediated by pepsin-sensitive domains of type IV collagen, because pepsin-extracted collagen, which is missing the NC1 domain, is able to associate via the 7S domain to form spider-like structures visible at the electron microscopic level (59). Based on these two types of associations Timpl et al. have proposed the first model for the assembly of type IV collagen, in which associations at the carboxyl end (NC1 domain) by two molecules and at the amino end (7S domain) by four molecules could form a regular network. The polymerization of type IV collagen was studied by turbidimetric analysis, a method that detects the formation of large aggregates. A change in turbidity of type IV collagen solutions was observed that was temperature- and concentration-dependent. The phenomenon did not exhibit any appreciable lag phase and could be reversed by lowering the temperature (66). Velocity sedimentation data confirmed these data by demonstrating the formation of large aggregates of type IV collagen when incubated at 28°C, compared to 4°C (66). Examination of the polymerized material revealed an extensive semi-regular hexagonal network consisting of laterally associated type IV collagen molecules. No more than two or three triple helices were associated side by side, and intermediate forms were observed in the process of associating laterally (61,66).

Network formation is greatly reduced or totally abolished in the presence of 50% glycerol. It is also susceptible to 2 *M* urea treatment and low temperature. In this network, the NC1 domains appeared to be spaced apart at similar distances. Statistical analysis from electron microscopic images revealed that the intervals between NC1 domains were about 100 nm (61). This observation suggested an important role for the NC1 domain in the process of type IV collagen polymerization. Support for this hypothesis came from the following observations: (*1*) isolated NC1 domain can bind specifically at four sites along the length of type IV collagen spaced approximately 100 nm apart from each other; (2) antibodies against the NC1 domain can effectively block type IV collagen lateral association, and (3) the development of turbidity by type IV collagen solutions can be reduced in a concentration-dependent fashion by addition of free NC1 domain in the solution (61).

Binding of Type IV Collagen to Laminin

The interaction between laminin and type IV collagen was first suspected when laminin was observed to increase the aggregation of type IV collagen in turbidity experiments (26). Direct observation of the binding of laminin to type IV collagen was accomplished by rotary shadowing mixtures of laminin and type IV collagen. The binding exhibited one major specific site located about 140 nm or less from the NC1 domain of type IV collagen (9,27). The isolated NC1 domain did not interact with laminin; therefore the interaction is probably mediated by pepsin-resistant domains on the triple helix, because pepsin-treated type IV collagen still retained the ability to bind at this specific site (9). Electron microscopic analysis of the laminin–type IV complexes indicated that the interaction takes place preferentially via two laminin domains: the short arm(s) (27) and the terminal globule of the long arm (10). An antibody against the E3 domain of laminin, derived from the terminal globule of the long arm, could inhibit the specific binding of laminin to type IV collagen, suggesting an important role of this domain in the interaction between laminin and type IV collagen (10). Also, the major pepsin-derived fragment of laminin, P1, which lacks the terminal globules of all its arms, was found unable to bind specifically to type IV collagen. The native state of laminin was also crucial for this interaction, because heat-denatured laminin failed to bind to type IV collagen. It is interesting to note that the C1q component of complement, which contains extensive triple-helical domains without interruptions, has been observed to bind to laminin. Electron microscopic observations suggested that the binding site on laminin was on a short arm (4). These data support the original observations that two different laminin domains may participate in its interaction with type IV collagen. The molecular definition of the peptide sequences within laminin or type IV collagen responsible for these activities remains to be elucidated.

Binding of Type IV Collagen to Entactin/Nidogen

It has been proposed that the NC1 domain of type IV collagen binds to entactin/nidogen; this binding was observed in solid-phase assays using either affinity chromatography or dot blotting of constituents on nitrocellulose (17). It has recently been observed at the electron microscopic level that entactin/nidogen can interact specifically with domains located along the length of the triple helical portion of type IV collagen (1).

Binding of Type IV Collagen to Heparan Sulfate Proteoglycan

Basement membrane extracted heparan sulfate proteoglycan [the low molecular weight species; see Fujiwara et al (20)] was found to interact in affinity chromatography with type IV collagen both at the globular NC1 domain and at the triple helix. These interactions were abolished by moderate salt concentrations (0.1–0.2 M) or in the presence of various glycosaminoglycans (heparin, chondroitin sulfate, dextran sulfate), suggesting an ionic nature for this interaction (20). Binding of heparin to NC1 was also detected by velocity sedimentation in sucrose gradients.

The binding of type IV collagen to basement membrane heparan sulfate proteoglycan was also examined at the electron microscopic level, using the technique of rotary shadowing. Two sites on the collagen molecule were observed to bind specifically to heparan sulfate; these sites were localized at 82 nm and 206 nm from the NC1 domain (27). In this study, however, the heparan sulfate appeared as a collapsed, globular structure; therefore, no conclusions could be drawn regarding its domain participating in this binding. It is conceivable that specific binding sites may exist on both the glycosaminoglycan chains and the protein core.

Laminin Polymerization

The ability of laminin to polymerize and form large aggregates is documented by various techniques. In velocity sedimentation on sucrose gradients, laminin forms large aggregates when incubated at high temperature (35°C), whereas these aggregates are absent when laminin solutions are kept on ice (67). These observations were confirmed in turbidity experiments where it was found that laminin forms large aggregates in a temperature-, time-, and concentration-dependent fashion. This process could be reversed by reducing the temperature to 4°C, and cycling between high and low temperatures produced polymerized or monomeric laminin. Both sedimentation and turbidometric analysis showed an apparent critical concentration for assembly, which at 35°C was in the range of 100 µg/ml. The finding that laminin polymerization exhibits a critical concentration can be interpreted as evidence that this is a nucleation-propagation mechanism for polymerization. As a consequence, one would expect to find relatively few intermediate forms. This was shown to be the case by velocity sedimentation and rotary shadowing (67). Electron microscopic examination confirmed the presence of oligomers and large aggregates of laminin incubated at high temperature and allowed the observation that laminin polymerization was always mediated by the terminal globular domains of all four arms. A pepsin-resistant fragment from laminin (P1), which lacks all terminal globules, was not able to polymerize when examined with turbidity, velocity sedimentation, and rotary shadowing (67).

Polymer formation of laminin was also found to be divalent cation dependent. Specifically, incubation of laminin in the presence of EDTA failed to raise any turbidity and failed to produce any large aggregates in velocity sedimentation. At the electron microscopic level, laminin co-incubated with EDTA is seen to form small oligomers, but there are no large polymers formed. This inhibition of association can be reversed by addition of Ca^{2+} in concentrations above those of EDTA, which restores the ability of laminin to polymerize. In summary, it was proposed that laminin polymerization is a two-step process: the first step (nucleation?) is divalent cation-independent, whereas the second step is divalent cation-dependent (67). Part of the first step may be the formation of specific dimers. It was observed that many laminin dimers were preferentially formed by the long-to-long arm interaction. The frequency of this interaction was at least six times higher than expected if dimer formation were to be a random process (10). Using an antibody against an elastase-resistant fragment derived from the globule of the long arm, it was possible to substantially suppress laminin polymerization as examined by turbidity and rotary shadowing (10). Therefore, the terminal globule of the long arm of laminin is very important in the process of self-assembly.

Laminin–Entactin/Nidogen Interaction

Probably the strongest interaction between basement membrane macromolecules is that between laminin and entactin/nidogen; a dissociation constant of 10–20 nM has been suggested (31). Laminin and entactin/nidogen are usually extracted together, and to achieve total separation, the use of high concentrations of denaturing agents is required (40). The strength of this association can explain two early experimental observations: first, that the electrophoretic profile of purified laminin usually contained a 150 kD band that was thought to be a degradation product (39) and second, many polyclonal antisera raised against laminin exhibited extensive cross-reactivity with entactin/nidogen. From protease-resistant fragments of entactin/nidogen and of the whole complex, there is evidence that the interaction takes place via a domain located close to or at the carboxy terminal part of entactin/nidogen and that the binding occurs at the inner rod-like segment of a short arm of laminin, probably the one belonging to the B1 chain (31). Observations at the electron microscopic level confirm these data and show that entactin/nidogen is attached to laminin at the inner portion of a short arm (32).

Binding of Laminin to Heparan Sulfate Proteoglycan

Basement membrane extracted heparan sulfate proteoglycan [the low molecular weight form; see Fujiwara et al (20)] was found to bind to laminin in affinity chromatography studies. This binding could be competed by sulfated glucosaminoglycans but not with hyaluronate; it was therefore concluded that the interaction was likely ionic in nature (20). Electron microscopic observations suggested that the main domain of laminin involved in this binding was the globule of the long arm; it was not possible to identify any specific domain on heparan sulfate, because the molecule appeared collapsed in this study (27).

Entactin/Nidogen Self-Association

Entactin/nidogen fragments have been seen to aggregate at the electron microscopic level (60). However, this is not evidence of the ability of the intact molecule to self-associate, because it may be the result of "sticky ends" produced by the proteolytic cleavage. Detailed studies on the ability of intact entactin/nidogen to self-associate are missing; it is believed, however, that this interaction can take place (Dr. Albert Chung, personal communication).

Binding of Entactin/Nidogen to Heparan Sulfate Proteoglycan

It was observed that entactin/nidogen does not interact with basement membrane extracted heparan sulfate proteoglycan (17). However, in this study only the low molecular weight form of heparan sulfate proteoglycan was used. It is possible that binding to the high molecular weight proteoglycan may take place, but studies on this interaction have not been published.

Heparan Sulfate Proteoglycan Self-Association

The ability of the intact basement membrane extracted heparan sulfate proteoglycan to self-assemble was studied using velocity sedimentation and rotary shadowing (68). This macromolecule forms dimers and to a lesser extent, oligomers. The assembly is time- and concentration-dependent. At the electron microscope it is observed that the association occurs at the pole of the protein core opposite to the origin of the side chains. Dimers have a length twice that of individual molecules and oligomers appear as stellate clusters. Isolated protein cores retain the ability to self-associate; proteolytic degradation of the protein core abolishes the ability of the macromolecule to self-assemble. These data support the electron microscopic observation that the terminal domain opposite the domain of origin of the side chains is crucial for self-assembly (68).

NONENZYMATIC GLYCATION

Nonenzymatic glycation is defined as the incorporation of glucose to the free amino groups without the mediation of any enzymes (6,14). This process occurs normally in the body at low rates, but it is accelerated in hyperglycemia. Two stages of this reaction can be distinguished: a first, reversible one, where a Schiff base product and eventually an Amadori product are formed, and a second, irreversible one, where advanced glucosylation end products are formed by cross-linking. It has been suggested that the second stage of this process can be inhibited by a nucleophilic hydrazine compound, aminoguanidine (7). For more information about the action of aminoguanidine, see Chapter 12. Both stages of nonenzymatic glycation occur at very low rates. The modification occurring at free amino groups and the development of crosslinks will eventually lead to functional and structural alterations. However, because both stages of this reaction occur at extremely low rates, only macromolecules with long half-lives will be affected.

Most basement membrane macromolecules are thought to fall into this category, so it is expected that nonenzymatic glycation will modify their structure and their ability to interact. In the next section, we review the limited amount of information available regarding the effect of nonenzymatic glycation on the macromolecular interactions between basement membrane components.

Type IV Collagen Network Formation—Role of NC1 Domain

As mentioned earlier, the NC1 domain from type IV collagen plays a crucial role in network formation. Type IV collagen polymerization can be followed by turbidimetry, where an increase in turbidity is observed with time. This phenomenon was inhibited in the presence of the NC1 domain in a concentration-dependent fashion; that is, added NC1 was able to bind along the length of type IV collagen and prevent NC1 that belonged to intact type IV collagen molecules to interact and produce laterally associated macromolecules. However, when the added NC1 was previously nonenzymatically glycated in vitro in the presence of glucose, its inhibitory effect on type IV collagen polymerization was decreased. This decrease was glucose concentration–dependent; i.e. the higher the molarity of glucose to which NC1 was exposed, the less inhibition was produced. Addition of control NC1 produced a 45% decrease in the plateau value of turbidity, whereas NC1 glycated in the presence of 10 mM or 100 mM glucose produced only a 21% or 11% decrease, respectively (62).

Further confirmation of these findings was provided at the electron microscopic level. Type IV collagen network formation was examined with the technique of rotary shadowing. Semi-regular hexagonal networks were observed in 71% of the fields examined when type IV collagen was incubated alone. In the presence of BSA as a control, 73% of the fields contained type IV collagen networks. When intact NC1 was included in the incubation mixture, only 29% of the fields contained laterally associated collagen. However, nonenzymatically glycated NC1 (at 100 mM glucose) did not inhibit network formation, and 67% of the fields examined exhibited polymerized type IV collagen, as shown in Figure 14.2. Glycated NC1 domain was not able to bind along the length of intact type IV collagen (62).

To define the molecular nature of the domain on NC1 that mediates self-association of type IV collagen, several synthetic peptides have been tested. One of them, with the sequence TAGSCLRKFSTM from the α1(NC1) chain was found to bind specifically to intact type IV collagen in solid-phase assays in a concentration-dependent manner. The presence of this peptide in solution resulted in a significant inhibition of type IV collagen assembly, whereas control peptides had no effect. Therefore this peptide should represent a major recognition site for the binding of NC1 to type IV collagen and for network formation of type IV collagen molecules. Alteration of the free amino group of the lysine present in this peptide via nonenzymatic glycation may block the ability of this peptide to inhibit network formation by type IV collagen (63).

During nonenzymatic glycosylation, a minor fraction of the NC1 domain was observed to form larger aggregates. This observation was first made by measuring the perimeter of NC1 molecules after incubation under control conditions or in the presence of 100 mM glucose. The existence of such aggregates was confirmed by gel electrophoresis under reducing conditions and probably represents intermolecular cross-linking (62).

Laminin Structure-Polymerization

The effect of nonenzymatic glucosylation on the conformation of laminin was examined at the electron microscopic level with the rotary shadowing tech-

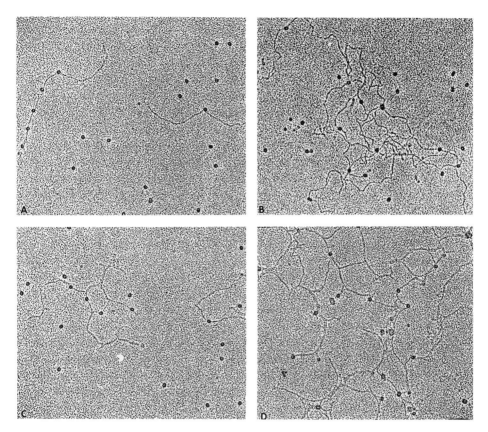

FIGURE 14.2. The NC1 domain was incubated in PBS for 17 days at 28°C in the presence of 0 and 100 mM glucose. After extensive dialysis it was coincubated (at 75 μg/ml) with intact type IV collagen (150 μg/ml) for 60 min at 35°C. The lateral association and network formation were examined at the electron microscopic level. Nonglycated domain NC1 could bind along the length of type IV collagen (A) and thus prevent network formation (B); glycated NC1 domain did not show any specific binding along the length of type IV collagen (C) and failed to inhibit network formation by intact type IV collagen molecules (D) (bar equals 100 nm).

nique. Laminin molecules incubated with relatively low glucose concentrations (50 mM) exhibited occasional shape alterations: in some instances the whole molecule, or some of the arms of laminin or parts of individual arms had globular deformations. More pronounced shape alterations in almost all laminin molecules were observed in samples incubated with higher glucose concentrations [200 mM; (11)], as shown in Figure 14.3.

To study the mechanism(s) underlying the observed changes in molecular shape after nonenzymatic glycation, the effect of aminoguanidine was examined, when present in the incubation mixture at equimolar concentrations with laminin (200 mM). Aminoguanidine has been thought to prevent the formation of advanced glycosylation end products (7). When laminin was incubated alone or in the presence of aminoguanidine, 95% of the molecules appeared normally by rotary shadowing. After incubation with glucose alone (for 6 days at 29°C), only 5% of the molecules maintained the regular cruciform structure. Incubation in the presence of both glucose and aminoguanidine substantially blocked

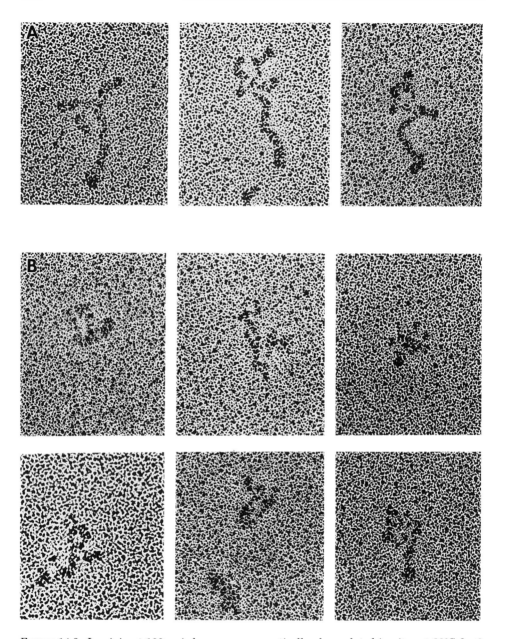

FIGURE 14.3. Laminin at 100 μg/ml was nonenzymatically glucosylated in vitro at 29°C for 6 days, in the presence of 0 or 200 mM glucose. After extensive dialysis, the material was examined at the electron microscopic level using the technique of rotary shadowing. A: Examples of laminin molecules incubated in the absence of glucose. B: Examples of laminin molecules incubated in the presence of 200 mM glucose; dramatic alteration of the shape is observed in most of them (bar equals 50 nm).

the changes in the shape of laminin, but not totally: about 70% of the examined molecules appeared intact. These findings suggest that glucose-induced intramolecular cross-links are the primary cause of the observed changes in the shape of laminin. The existence of such cross-links has been confirmed by gel electrophoresis under reducing conditions of control and glycated laminin, where after glycation a shift to lower mobilities, indicating higher molecular weight species, is observed (11).

More work is necessary to analyze in detail the effect of aminoguanidine on the nonenzymatic incorporation of glucose to proteins; possible interactions between glucose and aminoguanidine or aminoguanidine and proteins need to be explored.

The effect of nonenzymatic glucosylation on the ability of laminin to self-associate has also been examined. This complex process can be studied in vitro by a combination of techniques. One of the earliest steps in laminin assembly is the formation of specific, long-to-long arm dimers and can be studied by rotary shadowing. Under mild glucosylation conditions (50 mM glucose—6 days—29°C), most laminin molecules (>70%) do not undergo shape alterations. Quantitation of the type of dimer formed indicated that under these conditions 6.5% of the dimers were of the long-to-long arm type; under control conditions 35.0% of the dimers formed were long-to-long (11).

The later stages of laminin self-association, which result in the formation of larger polymers in vitro, can be examined by turbidimetry. Laminin was glucosylated in the presence of increasing glucose concentrations, and the development of turbidity was followed over time. Glycated laminin exhibited a decrease in the maximal turbidity developed, and this decrease was directly proportional to the concentration of glucose in the incubation mixture (11).

Interactions Between Heparin and Laminin/Type IV Collagen

Free heparin is not found in basement membranes as an integral component. However, heparan sulfate proteoglycan contains many heparin-like stretches in its side chains. These domains contain substantial amounts of negatively charged sulfate groups and are probably involved in ionic interactions between heparan sulfate and the other basement membrane glycoproteins. Therefore, heparin can be used as a model system to study such interactions with control and glycated laminin and type IV collagen.

After incubating laminin with 500 mM glucose for 1 or 3 days, the binding of laminin to saturating levels of heparin was reduced fivefold and fifteenfold respectively. Incubation of laminin with high levels of glucose for 12 days totally abolished the heparin binding. Scatchard analysis indicated that at the earlier glucosylation intervals low-affinity binding is observed, together with the high-affinity binding observed in control laminin (54).

Heparin binding to control and glycated laminin and type IV collagen mixtures was also studied. Heparin binding to laminin in the presence of type IV collagen is increased threefold, indicating a significant positive cooperativity. Glycation of type IV collagen alone reduced heparin binding to type IV collagen by 70%. Glycation of laminin alone produced an 80% reduction in heparin binding. Glycation of laminin-type IV mixtures abolished the specific binding of heparin to the mixture of laminin-type IV collagen (54). The results from the heparin binding to glycated laminin and type IV collagen suggest that glycation may affect heparin binding sites on these macromolecules. Also, the greater inhibition of heparin binding when both type IV collagen and laminin are nonenzymatically glycated would suggest that there is positive cooperativity involved in this process, which is abrogated by nonenzymatic glycation. Similar observations were made using fibronectin and either type I or type IV collagen; their nonenzymatic glycation decreased the positive cooperativity for heparin binding (53). More experiments are necessary to confirm these observations.

Many heparin binding domains from these two macromolecules have been precisely mapped to specific amino acid sequences. Most of these oligopeptides contain lysine residues; the modification of their free amino groups by nonenzymatic glycosylation might be responsible for the reduction (and eventual loss) in the ability of laminin and type IV collagen to interact with heparin and consequently with other heparin-like macromolecules.

Nonenzymatic Glycation In Vivo

The studies described above were performed with isolated macromolecules in vitro. Information about alterations of basement membranes in vivo, under hyperglycemic conditions is practically nonexistent at the moment.

Glomerular basement membranes isolated from animals made hyperglycemic after streptozotocin injection were examined for nonenzymatic addition of glucose. It was found that in diabetic animals collagen was nonenzymatically glycated more than twofold, compared to normal animals (13). Laminin and entactin/nidogen have not yet been examined after extraction from control and diabetically modified basement membranes. It should be kept in mind that the turnover rate of these two glycoproteins is not known; if their half-lives are shorter than type IV collagen, then primary or secondary modifications due to nonenzymatic glycation may not be crucial for the structure and function of basement membranes. Heparan sulfate proteoglycans are known to have a very fast turnover rate in general, on the order of a few days at most. Therefore, basement membrane heparan sulfate proteoglycans should not be altered structurally or functionally by nonenzymatic glycation. However, the interactions of heparan sulfate proteoglycans with the other basement membrane components (e.g. type IV collagen, laminin, entactin/nidogen) might be severely affected if the binding sites for heparan sulfate proteoglycans on these macromolecules were altered.

Another approach has been used in the study of basement membrane alterations under hyperglycemic conditions. Macromolecular components from basement membranes of control and diabetic animals (or humans) have been extracted and quantitated. The results from these studies suggest that under diabetic conditions the amount of collagen is relatively increased (3); the amount of laminin is relatively decreased (50); and the amount of heparan sulfate proteoglycan is dramatically decreased (50,65). Analysis of these results requires some caution because it should be kept in mind that (1) diabetic conditions can lead to differential extractability compared to control samples, and (2) diabetic conditions may lead to altered levels of basement membrane components by mechanisms other than nonenzymatic glucosylation.

Changes in the relative amounts of basement membrane macromolecules under diabetic conditions can be attributed to differential synthesis or degradation, or to interactions between these components. Metabolic labeling of proteoglycans synthesized by glomeruli isolated from control and diabetic rats led to the hypothesis that the primary reason for the decreased amount of heparan sulfate proteoglycan in diabetes may be its inability to interact with the other basement membrane macromolecules, which leads to the failure to incorporate it into the glomerular basement membrane (25). If this hypothesis is substantiated, then nonenzymatic glycation of heparan sulfate binding sites on type IV collagen, laminin, or entactin/nidogen might be the primary pathogenetic mechanism leading to reduction of heparan sulfate proteoglycan in basement membranes in diabetic conditions.

Despite the paucity of experimental data regarding macromolecular interactions between basement membrane components after nonenzymatic glycation, it is reasonable to speculate that this process may affect domains of these macromolecules crucial for their interactions and their associations to form the basement membrane network. Defective associations may lead to a "looser" network, leading eventually to higher permeability of basement membranes. Also, perturbed associations could modify the molecular composition of the glomerular basement membrane such that this causes changes in function.

ACKNOWLEDGMENTS

The authors are supported by the following NIH grants: DK-39868 (ASC); DK-39216 (ECT); CA-21463, CA-29995, and EY-06625 (LTF). The excellent technical assistance of Ms. Lorrel Reger and secretarial assistance of Ms. Carol El-Ghandour are greatly appreciated.

REFERENCES

1. AUMAILLEY, M., WIEDEMANN, H., MANN, K., and TIMPL, R. Binding of nidogen and laminin-nidogen complex to basement membrane collagen type IV. *Eur. J. Biochem.* 184: 241–248, 1989.
2. BABEL, W., and GLANVILLE, R. W. Structure of human-basement-membrane (type IV) collagen. *Eur. J. Biochem.* 143: 545–556, 1984.
3. BEISSWENGER, P. J., and SPIRO, R. G. Studies on the human glomerular basement membrane. *Diabetes* 22: 180–193, 1973.
4. BOHNSACK, J. F., TENNER, A. J., LAURIE, G. W., KLEINMAN, H. K., MARTIN, G. R., and BROWN, E. J. C1q binds to laminin: a mechanism for the deposition and retention of immune complexes in basement membrane. *Proc. Natl. Acad. Sci. USA* 82: 3824–3828, 1985.
5. BRAZEL, D., POLLNER, R., OBERBAUMER, I., and KUHN, K. Human basement membrane collagen (type IV). *Eur. J. Biochem.* 172: 35–42, 1988.
6. BROWNLEE, M., VLASSARA, H., and CERAMI, A. Nonenzymatic glycosylation and the pathogenesis of diabetic complications. *Ann. Intern. Med.* 101: 527–537, 1984.
7. BROWNLEE, M., VLASSARA, H., KOONEY, A., ULRICH, P., and CERAMI, A. Aminoguanidine prevents diabetes-induced arterial wall protein cross-linking. *Science* 232: 1629–1632, 1986.
8. CARLIN, B., JAFFE, R., BENDER, B., and CHUNG, A. E. Entactin, a novel basal lamina-associated sulfated glycoprotein. *J. Biol. Chem.* 256: 5209–5214, 1981.
9. CHARONIS, A. S., TSILIBARY, E. C., YURCHENCO, P. D., and FURTHMAYR, H. Binding of laminin to type IV collagen: a morphological study. *J. Cell. Biol.* 100: 1848–1853, 1985.
10. CHARONIS, A. S., TSILIBARY, E. C., SAKU, T., and FURTHMAYR, H. Inhibition of laminin self-

assembly and interaction with type IV collagen by antibodies to the terminal domain of the long arm. *J. Cell. Biol.* 103: 1689–1697, 1986.

11. CHARONIS, A. S., REGER, L. A., DEGE, J. E., KOUZI-KOLIAKOS, K., FURCHT, L. T., WOHLHUE-TER, R. M., and TSILIBARY, E. C. Laminin alterations after in vitro nonenzymatic gly-cosylation. *Diabetes* 39: 807–814, 1990.

12. CHUNG, A. E., JAFFE, R., FREEMAN, I. L., VERGUES, J., BRAGINSKI, J. E., and CARLIN, B. Properties of a basement membrane-related glycoprotein synthesized in culture by a mouse embryonal carcinoma-derived cell line. *Cell* 16: 277–288, 1979.

13. COHEN, M. P., URDANIVIA, E., SURMA, M., and WU, V.-Y. Increased glycosylation of glomer-ular basement membrane collagen in diabetes. *Biochem. Biophys. Res. Commun.* 95: 765–769, 1980.

14. DAY, J. F., THORPE, S. R., and BAYNES, J. W. Nonenzymatically glucosylated albumins. *J. Biol. Chem.* 254: 595–597, 1979.

15. DUNCAN, K. G., FESSLER, L. I., BÄCHINGER, H. P., and FESSLER, J. H. Procollagen IV-association to tetramers. *J. Biol. Chem.* 258: 5869–5877, 1983.

16. DURKIN, M. E., CHAKRAVARTI, S., BARTOS, B. B., LIU, S. H., FRIEDMAN, R. L., and CHUNG, A. E. Amino acid sequence and domain structure of entactin. Homology with epider-mal growth factor precursor and low density lipoprotein receptor. *J. Cell Biol.* 107: 2749, 2756, 1988.

17. DZIADEK, M., PAULSSON, M., and TIMPL, R. Identification and interaction repertoire of large forms of the basement membrane protein nidogen. *EMBO J.* 4: 2513–2518, 1985.

18. DZIADEK, M., PAULSSON, M., AUMAILLEY, M., and TIMPL, R. Purification and tissue distri-bution of a small protein (BM-40) extracted from a basement membrane tumor. *Eur. J. Biochem.* 161: 455–464, 1986.

19. ENGEL, J., ODERMATT, E., ENGEL, A., MADRI, J. A., FURTHMAYR, H., ROHDE, H., and TIMPL, R. Shapes, domain organization, and flexibility of laminin and fibronectin, two mul-tifunctional proteins of the extracellular matrix. *J. Mol. Biol.* 150: 97–120, 1981.

20. FUJIWARA, S., WIEDEMANN, H., TIMPL, R., LUSTIG, A., and ENGEL, J. Structure and inter-actions of heparan sulfate proteoglycans from a mouse tumor basement membrane. *Eur. J. Biochem.* 143: 145–157, 1984.

21. HASSELL, J. R., LEYSHON, W. C., LEDBETTER, S. R., TYREE, B., SUZUKI, S., KATO, M., KIMATA, K., and KLEINMAN, H. K. Isolation of two forms of basement membrane proteoglycans. *J. Biol. Chem.* 260: 8098–8105, 1985.

22. KEFALIDES, N. A. Structure and biosynthesis of basement membranes. *Int. Rev. Connect. Tissue Res.* 6: 63–104, 1973.

23. KILLEN, P. D., BURBELO, P., SAKURAI, Y., and YAMADA, Y. Structure of the amino-terminal portion of the murine a1(IV) collagen chain and the corresponding region of the gene. *J. Biol. Chem.* 263: 8706–8709, 1988.

24. KLEIN, D. J., BROWN, D. M., and OEGEMA, T. R. Glomerular proteoglycans in diabetes. *Diabetes* 35: 1130–1142, 1986.

25. KLEIN, D. J., BROWN, D. M., OEGEMA, T. R., BRENCHLEY, P. E., ANDERSON, J. C., DICKINSON, M. A. J., HORIGAN, E. A., and HASSEL, J. R. Glomerular basement membrane proteoglycans are derived from a large precursor. *J. Cell. Biol.* 106: 963–970, 1988.

26. KLEINMAN, H. K., MCGARVEY, M. L., HASSEL, J. R., and MARTIN, G. R. Formation of supra-molecular complex is involved in the reconstitution of basement membrane compo-nents. *Biochemistry* 22: 4969–4974, 1983.

27. LAURIE, G. W., BING, J. T., KLEINMAN, H. K., HASSEL, J. R., AUMAILLEY, M., MARTIN, G. R., and FELDMAN, R. J. Localization of binding sites for laminin, heparan sulfate proteo-glycan and fibronectin on basement membrane (type IV) collagen. *J. Mol. Biol.* 189: 205–216, 1986.

28. LAURIE, G. W., INOUE, S., BING, J. T., and HASSEL, J. R. Visualization of the large heparan sulfate proteoglycan from basement membrane. *Am. J. Anat.* 181: 320–326, 1988.

29. LEDBETTER, S. R., FISHER, L. W., and HASSELL, J. R. Domain structure of basement mem-brane heparan sulfate proteoglycan. *Biochemistry* 26: 988–995, 1987.

30. LEMKIN, M. C., and FARQUHAR, M. G. Sulfated and nonsulfated glucosaminoglycans and glycopeptides are synthesized by kidney in vivo and incorporated into glomerular basement membranes. *Proc. Natl. Acad. Sci. USA* 78: 1726–1730, 1981.

31. MANN, K., DEUTZMANN, R., and TIMPL, R. Characterization of proteolytic fragments of the laminin-nidogen complex and their activity in ligand-binding assays. *Eur. J. Biochem.* 178: 71–80, 1988.

32. MARTIN, G. R., and TIMPL, R. Laminin and other basement membrane components. *Annu. Rev. Cell. Biol.* 3: 57–85, 1987.

33. MARTINEZ-HERNANDEZ, A., and AMENTA, P. A. The basement membrane in pathology. *Lab. Invest.* 48: 656–677, 1983.

34. MINOR, R. R. CLARK, C. C., STRAUSE, E. L., KOSZALKA, T. R., BRENT, R. L., and KEFALIDES, N. A. Basement membrane procollagen is not converted to collagen in organ cultures of parietal yolk sac endoderm. *J. Biol. Chem.* 251: 1789–1795, 1976.

35. NOONAN, D. M., HORIGAN, E. A., LEDBETTER, S. R., VOGELI, G., SASAKI, M., YAMADA, Y., and HASSEL, J. R. Identification of cDNA clones encoding different domains of the basement membrane heparan sulfate proteoglycan. *J. Biol. Chem.* 263: 16379–16387, 1988.

36. ORKIN, R. W., GEHRON, P., MCGOODWIN, E. B., MARTIN, G. R., VALENTINE, T., and SWARM, R. A murine tumor producing a matrix of basement membrane. *J. Exp. Med.* 145: 204–220, 1977.

37. OTT, U., ODERMATT, E., ENGEL, J., FURTHMAYR, H., and TIMPL, R. Protease resistance and conformation of laminin. *Eur. J. Biochem.* 123: 63–72, 1981.

38. PALM, S. L., and FURCHT, L. T. Production of laminin and fibronectin by Schwannoma cells. *J. Cell Biol.* 96: 1218–1226, 1983.

39. PALM, S. L., MCCARTHY, J. B., and FURCHT, L. T. Alternative model for the internal structure of laminin. *Biochemistry* 24: 7753–7750, 1985.

40. PAULSSON, M., DEUTZMANN, R., DZIADEK, M., NOWACK, H., TIMPL, R., WEBER, S., and ENGEL, J. Purification and structural characterization of intact and fragmented nidogen obtained from a tumor basement membrane. *Eur. J. Biochem.* 156: 467–478, 1986.

41. PAULSSON, M., YURCHENCO, P. D., RUBEN, G. C., ENGEL, J., and TIMPL, R. Structure of low density heparan sulfate proteoglycan isolaged from a mouse tumor basement membrane. *J. Mol. Biol.* 197: 297–313, 1987.

42. PIKKARAINEN, T., EDDY, R., FUKUSHIMA, Y., BYERS, M., SHOWS, T., PIHLAJANIEMI, T., SARASTO, M., and TRYGGVASON, K. Human laminin B1 chain. *J. Biol. Chem.* 262: 10454–10462, 1987.

43. PIKKARAINEN, T., KOLLUNKI, T., and TRYGGVASON, K. Human laminin B2 chain. *J. Biol. Chem.* 263: 6751–6758, 1988.

44. RUOSLAHTI, E. Structure and biology of proteoglycans. *Annu. Rev. Cell Biol.* 4: 229–245.

45. SASAKI, M., and YAMADA, Y. The laminin B2 chain has a multidomain structure homologous to the B1 chain. *J. Biol. Chem.* 262: 17111–17117, 1987.

46. SASAKI, M., KATO, S., KOHNO, K., MARTIN, G. R., and YAMADA, Y. Sequence of the cDNA encoding the laminin B1 chain reveals a multidomain protein containing cysteine-rich repeats. *Proc. Natl. Acad. Sci. USA* 84: 935–939, 1987.

47. SASAKI, M., KLEINMAN, H. K., HUBER, H., DEUTZMANN, R., and YAMADA, Y. Laminin, a multidomain protein. *J. Biol. Chem.* 263: 16536–16544, 1988.

48. SCHUPPAN, D., TIMPL, R., and GLANVILLE, R. W. Discontinuities in the triple helical sequence Gly-X-Y of basement membrane (type IV) collagen. *FEBS Lett.* 115: 297–300, 1980.

49. SCHWARZ, U., SCHUPPAN, D., OBERBAUMER, I., GLANVILLE, R. W., DEUTZMANN, R., TIMPL, R., and KUHN, K. Structure of mouse type IV collagen. *Eur. J. Biochem.* 157: 49–56, 1986.

50. SHIMOMURA, H., and SPIRO, R. G. Studies on macromolecular components of human glomerular basement membrane and alterations in diabetes. *Diabetes* 36: 374–381, 1987.

51. SHOTTON, D. M., BURKE, B., and BRANTON, D. The molecular structure of human erythrocyte spectrin. Biophysical and electron microscope studies. *J. Mol. Biol.* 131: 303–329, 1979.

52. SPIRO, R. G. The structure of the disaccharide unit of the renal glomerular basement membrane. *J. Biol. Chem.* 242: 4813–4823, 1967.

53. TARSIO, J. F., REGER, L. A., and FURCHT, L. T. Decreased interaction of fibronectin, type IV collagen and heparin due to nonenzymatic glycation. *Biochemistry* 26: 1014–1020, 1987.

54. TARSIO, J. F., REGER, L. A., and FURCHT, L. T. Molecular mechanisms in basement complications of diabetes. *Diabetes* 37: 532–539, 1988.

55. TIMPL, R., and DZIADEK, M. Structure, development and molecular pathology of basement membranes. *Int. Rev. Exp. Pathol.* 29: 1–112, 1986.

56. TIMPL, R., MARTIN, G. R., BRUCKNER, P., WICK, G., and WIEDEMAN, H. Nature of the collagenous protein in a tumor basement membrane. *Eur. J. Biochem.* 84: 43–52, 1978.

57. TIMPL, R., RISTELI, J., and BÄCHINGER, H. P. Identification of a new basement membrane collagen by the aid of a large fragment resistant to bacterial collagenase. *FEBS Lett.* 101: 265–268, 1979.

58. TIMPL, R., ROHDE, H., GEHRON-ROBEY, P., RENNARD, S. I., FOIDART, J.-M., and MARTIN,

G. R. Laminin—a glycoprotein from basement membranes. *J. Biol. Chem.* 254: 9933–9937, 1979.

59. TIMPL, R., WIEDEMANN, H., VAN DELDEN, V., FURTHMAYR, H., and KÜHN, K. A network model for the organization of type IV collagen molecules in basement membranes. *Eur. J. Biochem.* 120: 203–211, 1981.

60. TIMPL, R., DZIADEK, M., FUJIWARA, S., NOWACK, H., and WICK, G. Nidogen: a new, self-aggregating basement membrane protein. *Eur. J. Biochem.* 137: 455–465, 1983.

61. TSILIBARY, E. C., and CHARONIS, A. S. The role of the main noncollagenous domain (NC1) in type IV collagen self-assembly. *J. Cell Biol.* 103: 401–410, 1986.

62. TSILIBARY, E. C., CHARONIS, A. S., REGER, L. A., WOHLHUETER, R. M., and FURCHT, L. T. The effect on nonenzymatic glucosylation on the binding of the main noncollagenous NC1 domain to type IV collagen. *J. Biol. Chem.* 263: 4302–4308, 1988.

63. TSILIBARY, E. C., REGER, L. A., VOGEL, A. M., KOLIAKOS, G. G., ANDERSON, S. S., CHARONIS, A. S., and FURCHT, L. T. Identification of a multifunctional, cell-binding peptide from the a1(NC1) of type IV collagen. *J. Cell Biol.* 111: 1583–1591, 1990.

64. WEBER, L., ENGEL, J., WIEDEMANN, H., GLANVILLE, R. W., and TIMPL, R. Subunit structure and assembly of the globular domain of basement-membrane collagen type IV. *Eur. J. Biochem.* 139: 401–410, 1984.

65. WU, V.-Y., WILSON, B., and COHEN, M. P. Disturbances in glomerular basement membrane glycosaminoglycans in experimental diabetes. *Diabetes* 36: 679–683, 1987.

66. YURCHENCO, P. D., and FURTHMAYR, H. Self-assembly of basement membrane collagen. *Biochemistry* 23: 1839–1850, 1984.

67. YURCHENCO, P. D., TSILIBARY, E. C., CHARONIS, A. S., and FURTHMAYR, H. Laminin polymerization in vitro. Evidence for a two-step assembly with domain specificity. *J. Biol. Chem.* 260: 7636–7644, 1985.

68. YURCHENCO, P. D., CHENG, Y.-S., and RUBEN, G. C. Self-assembly of high molecular weight basement membrane heparan sulfate proteoglycan into dimers and oligomers. *J. Biol. Chem.* 262: 17668–17676, 1987.

15

Effects of Diabetes on Kidney Proteoglycans

DAVID J. KLEIN

The roles played by proteoglycans (PG) in normal tissue functioning and in several disease processes, including diabetes mellitus, are being actively explored. This interest is due to recent progress in our understanding of the importance of these complex protein–polysaccharide conjugates to extracellular matrix integrity and in cell–matrix interactions. In this chapter, I describe the role played by heparan sulfate proteoglycans (HSPG) in the ability of the kidney glomerulus to restrict the filtration of charged molecules, and I summarize some important biochemical properties of PGs. I then propose several possible explanations for changes that occur in glomerular extracellular matrix composition in diabetes.

ROLE OF GLOMERULAR BASEMENT MEMBRANE HSPG
IN PLASMA ULTRAFILTRATION

An ultrafiltrate of plasma is formed by the capillary network of the glomerulus (Fig. 15.1). This filter is selective on the basis of molecular radius as well as intrinsic molecular charge (11). The structural basis for the charge barrier is thought to reside in the glomerular basement membrane (GBM), which contains regularly spaced anionic sites comprised of HSPGs (40,41). Small amounts of chondroitin sulfate (CS) PG were also present in the GBM (13). The importance of GBM HSPG to human disease was illustrated by work with kidneys from patients with the congenital nephrotic syndrome. These patients, primarily of Finnish descent, develop severe proteinuria in infancy. Vernier et al. showed by electron microscopy that GBM HSPG was present in a diminished quantity in these patients (92).

GBM HSPG may be derived from a large molecular weight precursor that is processed to several PG and glycoprotein products (48). Antibodies against basement membrane tumor (EHS) HSPG immunoprecipitated a 400 dK radiolabeled HSPG precursor from isolated rat glomeruli similar in size to tumor HSPG and reacted with several smaller glycoproteins and PGs from GBM by Western analysis. These antibodies also recognized laminin, a large cruciform molecule found in the lamina densa of the GBM, whose A chain nucleotide sequence resembles the basement membrane HSPG protein core. Laminin and other extracellular matrix components contain multiple heparin as well as cell binding sites (63,73). Noncovalent interactions between PGs and basement

263

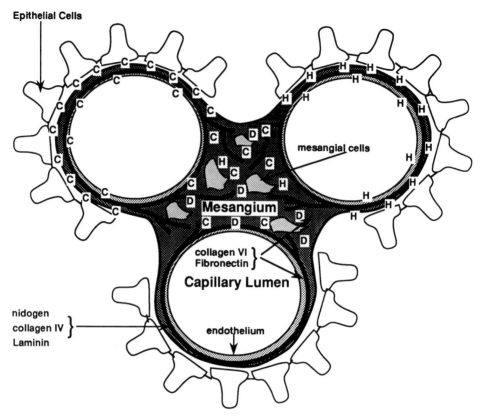

FIGURE 15.1. Distribution of proteoglycans (PG) and other extracellular matrix molecules within the glomerulus. The GBM localization of heparan sulfate PG (H) is shown in the capillary tuft on the left, while that of chondroitin sulfate PG (C) is shown on the right. H, C, as well as dermatan sulfate (D) PGs are present in the mesangium. The localization of other extracellular matrix components is shown in the lower capillary tuft.

membrane laminin, fibronectin, type IV collagen, and nidogen may be important in basement membrane assembly.

Although the GBM is thought to be the primary site of kidney filtration, the glomerular extracellular matrices form a continuum that includes both the GBM and the mesangial matrix. Therefore, it is difficult to separate the contribution of each component to the filtration barrier. In addition, three major cell types contribute to this matrix. Epithelial cells with podocytes connected by filtration slits reside on the urinary aspect of the GBM, while fenestrated endothelial cells occupy the capillary luminal surfaces. Mesangial cells are embedded in a stalk that supports the capillary network. They are smooth muscle–like in that they are contractile, contain receptors for angiotensin II, and they synthesize PGs similar to those from aorta (5,45,51,53).

It has been proposed that GBM development occurs in two stages. During the S body phase of kidney development, vascular ingrowth into the renal mesenchyma occurs. At this stage, both the ingrowing vascular cells (which eventually become endothelial and mesangial cells) and the epithelial cells contribute laminin and type IV collagen to the developing GBM. Later in development basement membrane formation is taken over mainly by epithelial cells (1,76). The involvement of basement membrane CSPG in kidney tubule formation was demonstrated in studies that showed that PG synthesis was most active at sites of ureteric bud branching and that this process was reversibly inhibited using β-D-xyloside, an agent that uncouples the addition of glycosaminoglycan (GAG) chains to the CSPG protein core (36,46,67). Epithelial cells have been proposed as the source for intestinal basement membrane HSPGs during development (83). However, little is known about the embryogenesis of GBM PGs or the relative contribution of the various cell types to the remodeling of mature GBM. The latter process may be important because of the short half-life of GBM HSPG (4–6 h), while collagens turn over more slowly (12,14).

BIOCHEMISTRY OF PROTEOGLYCANS

Before describing some of the specific characteristics of glomerular and glomerular cell PGs in normal and diabetic conditions, I will review some of the biochemical properties of PGs that led us and others to investigate their role in the pathogenesis of the diabetic nephropathy.

Proteoglycans are protein-polysaccharide conjugates containing 1–20 unbranched carbohydrate or glycosaminoglycan (GAG) side chains (reviewed in 72,36,37). Until recently, PGs were named according to the GAG chain types. Each GAG contains a characteristic repeating disaccharide unit attached via a linkage region to xylosylated serine (or threonine) residues on the protein core. Alternating N-acetyl hexosamine and glucuronic acid residues are added as individual UDP conjugates in the Golgi apparatus. Heparan sulfate contains N-acetyl glucosamine (glcNAc), while the hexosamine component of chondroitin sulfate PGs is N-acetyl galactosamine (galNAc). Heparan sulfate chain modification occurs in blocks along the carbohydrate backbone (70). This takes place via an ordered series of reactions initiated by N-deacylation of glcNAc. After this permissive step, sulfate residues are added to hydoxyl and/or amine groups via an ATP-requiring process, and glucuronic acid may be epimerized to iduronic acid.

Sulfation forms the basis by which PGs are radioactively labeled. Only a small proportion of [^{35}S]sulfate is incorporated into other glycoproteins or glycolipids. Thus, in glomerular or kidney cell culture, greater than 95% of [^{35}S]sulfate is incorporated into ^{35}S-PGs, which makes it a relatively specific labeling tool. The presence of sulfate groups also aides in PG purification by anion exchange chromatography.

Heparan sulfate is identified on the basis of its N-sulfate groups, which renders the GAG susceptible to nitrous acid deaminative cleavage at low pH (24). When heparan sulfate is highly modified it is termed *heparin*, while dermatan sulfate is a more modified version of chondroitin sulfate. Enzymes are available that specifically recognize the GAG chain configurations of CS or DS but do not recognize HS, thus allowing us to distinguish each GAG type.

Functional aspects of PGs may be directed by the protein core, by the GAGs, or by both in concert. Grouping of GAGs on a protein core may serve to

TABLE 15.1. Proteoglycan families

Proteoglycan name	GAG type	Tissue localization[a]	Function[b]	Glomerular cell[c]
Aggregan	CS/KS	Cartilage ECM	R, M, HAB, L, E	N
Versican	CS	Fibroblast	L, E	N
Biglycan	DS	ECM	M, C, F	M
Decorin	DS	ECM	M, C, F	M
Perlecan	HS	Basement membrane	Filtration, Separation	E
Syndecan	hybrid HS/CS	Cell surface	Matrix–cell interaction	E?
FGF Binding PG	HS	Cell surface	Growth factor binding	N
Serglycin	CS	Intracellular	Granule function	N

[a]ECM = extracellular matrix
[b]R = tissue resiliency; M = matrix integrity; HAB = hyaluronic acid binding; L = lectin binding; E = EGF-like repeats; C = collagen binding; F = fibrillogenesis.
[c]N = not identified. Biglycan, decorin, and perlecan mRNAs have been identified in kidney, whereas mesangial cells contain decorin mRNA. We presume that epithelial cells produce perlecan and syndecan based on structural similarities (50).

align GAG binding sites in the extracellular matrix, increasing the avidity of binding. cDNA sequence similarities, as well as cross-reactivity of anti-PG antibodies with PG protein cores from several tissues (as illustrated above for the basement membrane HSPGs), has led to the grouping of PGs into "families" [Table 15.1; (35)]. Basement membrane HSPG cDNAs recognized mRNAs in normal and diabetic kidneys (see below). In addition, protein core nucleotide sequence similarities have provided clues to other PG functions. Thus, the large CSPG aggregan and versican PG protein cores contain epidermal growth factor and lectin binding domains (6,54).

Properties of the PG protein core contribute to PG localization in compartments other than the extracellular matrix. Hydrophobic domains in the protein cores of several PGs allow for intercalation into the plasmalemma. Cell surface PGs may act as ECM receptors alternate to those on integrins, making them important in cell binding as well as in communication between the ECM and the cellular cytoskeleton (16,69,77,78,96). Intracellular PGs may be important in cellular signalling since they may be translocated from the cell surface to the nucleus (39).

Cell surface PGs may also act as growth factor receptors (20). Extracellular matrix PGs also bind growth factors, acting as reservoirs for their release and possibly modifying receptor interactions. Thus, the composition of the extracellular matrix has profound effects upon cellular functioning, and alterations that occur in diabetes or in atherosclerosis may modify cellular responses.

The extracellular matrix contains large CSPGs as well as small DSPGs. The DSPGs named *decorin* and *biglycan* show structural similarities and are the most abundant interstitial PGs (33). They also show variable binding to type I and II collagen, where they may inhibit fibrillogenesis (81,93). Decorin synthesis is controlled in a classical negative feedback manner by the growth factor TGF-β and may participate in the mesangial response to acute renal inflammatory injury (see below). The stiff GAG side chains of large cartilage and aortic CSPGs imbibe large amounts of water, allowing them to act like a coiled spring to give tissue resiliency, while collagen forms a more rigid netlike backbone. It should be apparent at this point that PGs are not just "tissue glue," but that they participate in a wide variety of cellular and extracellular processes, making them important components of the cellular signalling apparatus.

COMPOSITION OF THE GLOMERULAR EXTRACELLULAR MATRIX IN DIABETES

The structural lesion leading to diminished renal function in diabetes is expansion of the glomerular extracellular matrices (57). The enlarging mesangial matrix and thickening GBM eventually encroach upon the filtration surface of the glomerulus, leading to renal failure. Morphologic changes occur to some degree in most type I diabetics, progressing to renal failure in some 25%–30% of subjects. However, the biochemical basis for these morphologic findings is poorly understood. We hypothesize that a diminished concentration of HSPG in GBM may be the primary cause of albuminuria, the first sign of diabetic nephropathy (Fig. 15.2).

Both synthesis and deposition of most glomerular extracellular matrix components are increased in diabetes. Excess deposition of fibronectin (FN) and type IV collagen occur early in the disease (31,79). The GBM content of type VI collagen is also increased by diabetes (60). However, the content of HSPG was diminished in isolated human type I and type II diabetic GBM (66). GBM isolated from streptozotocin-induced diabetic rats after either in vitro and in vivo [^{35}S]sulfate labeling also contained less de novo synthesized heparan-^{35}SO$_4$PG than controls (12,22). In label chase experiments, not only was the GBM heparan-^{35}SO$_4$PG content diminished in streptozotocin-induced diabetic rat, but the GBM was missing a rapidly processed pool of heparan-^{35}SO$_4$ PGs (12).

Is GBM HSPG decreased in diabetes because it is not synthesized in sufficient quantities? After correcting for the decreased specific activity of [^{35}S]sulfate in diabetic sera, the total glomerular content of de novo synthesized ^{35}S PGs was not diminished by diabetes (49,84). However, it is not known whether the level of high-energy sulfated intracellular PG precursors (phosphoadenylylphosphosulfate) is directly reflected by serum sulfate levels. Abnormalities in PG reuptake and processing in diabetes may result in changes

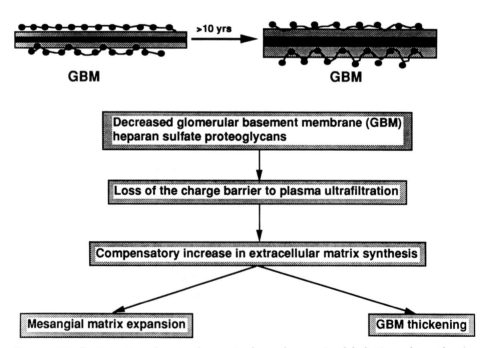

FIGURE 15.2. Participation of proteoglycans in the pathogenesis of diabetic nephropathy. An early hypothesis for the involvement of PGs in the diabetic nephropathy is depicted, where the relatively decreased concentration of GBM heparan sulfate PGs (*connected dots*) is hypothesized to be the primary signal for increased extracellular matrix synthesis, resulting in GBM thickening and mesangial matrix expansion.

in the intracellular pool size, which relies upon sulfate reutilization from GAGs degraded in lysosomes. Diabetes might also cause alterations in other tissue sulfate pools.

That diabetes does not cause decreased HSPG synthesis despite a diminished GBM content has been confirmed by several laboratories. HSPG and laminin kidney mRNA levels were not absolutely diminished in a rat model of type II diabetes when compared with controls (55). However, there was a markedly diminished ratio of HSPG and laminin to type IV collagen mRNA content. Only the altered HSPG:type IV collagen ratio correlated with the degree of albuminuria. Templeton found that anionic site staining along the GBM was reduced in streptozotocin-induced diabetic rats, but that total glomerular HSPG was not diminished (89). Again, if the PG content was expressed relative to the higher glomerular collagen content, it was decreased. Therefore, the consensus seems to be that there is a *relative* decrease in glomerular HSPG in diabetes. Loss of HSPG from a critical location such as the lamina rarae externa of the GBM, which contains only a small proportion of total glomerular PG, may result in the compensatory synthesis of other matrix components and the resultant expansion of the glomerular extracellular matrix.

Another possible cause for decreased GBM HSPG in diabetes is synthesis of PG with an altered structure. The hydrodynamic size of glomerular and GBM HSPG isolated from controls and diabetic rats labeled in vivo were similar (49). The GAGs released from these PGs were also similar in size. Since the elution profiles of PGs from gel filtration columns showed relatively broad peaks, this technique may not be sensitive enough to detect subtle changes in PG sulfation or in concentrations of various PGs, which may elute at similar elution volumes. Subsequent electrophoresis in agarose-polyacrylamide gels separated several PGs that elute under the same peak.

Heparin treatment released PGs noncovalently bound to cell surface receptors or to other extracellular matrix components (44,68,97,100). When glomeruli isolated from control and streptozotocin-induced diabetic rats were treated with heparin, glomeruli from diabetics were found to have a diminished content of a small, but significant heparin-released pool of HSPGs (40). A specific heparin-released PG identified by gel electrophoresis was present in diminished quantities in glomeruli isolated from diabetics. One possible interpretation of these results is that diabetes modifies the interactions between the cell surface and PGs. However, it is not safe to assume that heparin-released PGs are derived solely from cell surfaces since heparin may also displace PGs noncovalently associated with the extracellular matrix. Heparin-released HSPG may be diminished in diabetes because of abnormal association between PGs and extracellular matrix or cell surface receptors due to modification of either the matrix (i.e. by glycation) or the PG itself.

Changes in the periodicity of sulfate groups along the GAG chain may alter their binding abilities and thereby diminish their capacity to adhere to other GBM components. Diminished sulfation of liver (84), but not kidney (49), PGs was reported in the streptozotocin-induced diabetic rat. However, detailed analyses of each GBM GAG at the disaccharide level and by various cleavage reactions have yet to be performed.

Some questions remain unanswered concerning the ECM changes that occur in diabetes. Does mesangial cell proliferation accompany excessive matrix deposition? What is the biochemical nature of, and trigger for, mesangial matrix expansion? Is there increased deposition of all matrix components, or are they differently affected? Does one glomerular cell type contribute to a greater extent than another to the pathogenesis of the diabetic nephropathy? And finally, is progression of nephropathy the result of the abnormal metabolic milieu of diabetes or is it genetically determined?

It became apparent to us that studies of isolated glomeruli needed to be abandoned because of (1) difficulties in obtaining "pure" GBM (38); (2) the need to go through rather rigorous GBM isolation techniques that might remove PGs or activate PG degradation; (3) the presence of various cell types within the glomerulus, each of which may contribute differently to the GBM and may be affected differently by the diabetic milieu; and, (4) the yield of PGs from isolated glomeruli was insufficient for detailed studies of structure or interactions with other matrix components. The major PG synthesized by isolated glomeruli in tissue culture was a large CSPG, while HSPG was the major PG isolated after in vivo labeling. Whether this represents an in vitro artifact or whether CSPG is lost during glomerular isolation is unknown. Therefore, we have performed detailed studies of the PGs synthesized by homogeneous populations of human glomerular epithelial and mesangial cells in culture. These cells are distinguished on the basis of their morphology, growth characteristics, and the characteristic distribution of various cellular and extracellular matrix antigens (52,87,91). Once we have defined by cell culture techniques the cell of origin of each glomerular PG, as well as whether it is destined for the cell surface or extracellular matrix, it will be important to return to the in vivo models. At that point we will be able to say whether disturbances in the metabolism of an individual PG relate specifically to the effects of diabetes upon one particular cell type or to interactions within a defined cell compartment.

PROTEOGLYCANS SYNTHESIZED BY HUMAN GLOMERULAR CELLS IN CULTURE

Heparan sulfate was the predominant epithelial cell PG, while CSPG was the most abundant mesangial cell product [Fig. 15.3; (45,50)]. These results confirmed the findings of Striker et al., who studied isolated rat cell GAGs, but did not analyze intact PGs (86). Epithelial cell HSPG was similar in hydrodynamic size to that previously reported for GBM HSPG (Fig. 15.4). In addition, Stow et al. showed that antibodies to rat glomerular HSPG stained the GBM as well as the RER of epithelial cells by EM (85). Therefore, it is most likely that epithelial cells are the source for GBM HSPG. HSPG from mesangial cells was significantly larger than GBM or epithelial HSPG.

Epithelial and mesangial cell PG protein cores were studied after enzymatic removal of the HS GAGs. Epithelial cell HSPG contained core proteins of several sizes. Molecular weights were similar to those previously enumerated using antibodies to the large BM HSPG precursor (48). These data provide additional indirect evidence that epithelial cells represent a source for GBM

Epithelial Cell

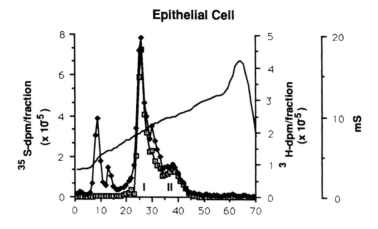

Mesangial Cell

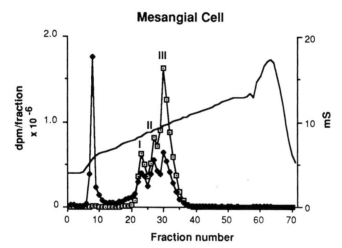

FIGURE 15.3. Human glomerular cell proteoglycans (PG); HPLC-DEAE chromatography. Dual-labeled ($[^{35}S]$sulfate, $[^{3}H]$leucine) heparan sulfate PG elutes first from anion exchange columns (peak I), while chondroitin sulfate PG elutes last. Mesangial cell dermatan sulfate PGs (biglycan and decorin) are the predominant components of peak II (*lower graph*). Heparan sulfate PG was the predominant epithelial cell product, while chondroitin sulfate was the major mesangial cell PG.

HSPG. Mesangial cell HSPG had a core protein similar in size to the larger epithelial cell core (220 kD) and therefore may be a less processed form of GBM HS PG. No studies of the relationship between glomerular cell HSPGs to the family of basement membrane HSPGs have been performed.

It is now possible to study interactions between epithelial cell HSPG and glycated and nonglycated extracellular matrix components. Interactions between PGs and matrix have been presumed on the basis of studies using a heterogenous mixture of heparin and heparin PGs, without describing interactions with intact heparan sulfate PG. Heparin PG contains more highly modified GAGs and performs a different spectrum of biological activities in vivo

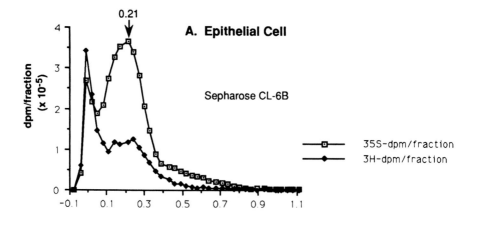

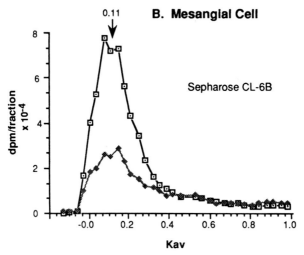

FIGURE 15.4. Glomerular cell heparan sulfate proteoglycans (HSPG). Epithelial cell HSPGs elute later from Sepharose CL-6B columns than mesangial cell HSPG.

than does HSPG. Fibronectin (FN) is comprised of an A and B chain, each containing a major heparin binding domain. Only the A chain heparin binding domain has an insert, called CS I, which contains a proteolytic site rendering it 33 kD on enzymatic digestion. The difference between the A and B chain domains allows us to distinguish whether HSPG binds to one or the other FN chain. We have demonstrated that epithelial cell HSPG binds 40 times more avidly to the A chain domain than to the B chain domain (32). This is important because the A chain domain has also been shown to be more active in cell adhesion. Therefore, HSPG may participate in the interaction of epithelial cells with basement membranes.

Descriptions of the structure and function of glomerular CS/DS PGs has been a unique interest of our laboratory. While most investigators have focused on HSPG because of its importance in GBM function, we showed that the major PG synthesized by isolated rat glomuerli in culture was a large, Sepharose CL-6B excluded, non-aggregating CSPG (47). Mesangial cell culture allowed for the purification of this PG in large quantities since it was also the predominant product of these cells (45). Early electron microscopic (EM) autoradiographic studies had also shown it to be the main mesangial PG. Label-chase experiments showed that CSPG was slowly released into the culture medium from the lipid-soluble fraction as well as the lipid-insoluble fraction, while HSPG was rapidly released. The protein core was found to be >250 kD by [^{3}H]leucine labeling. A function has yet to be attributed to mesangial CSPG, although it seems to be involved in basement membrane formation and tubulogenesis (see above). Monoclonal antibodies against Riechart's membrane CSPG stained the glomerular mesangium, indicating these cells as a possible source for basement membrane CSPGs (58). Despite their derivation from a basement membrane CSPG, these antibodies failed to stain the GBM. Thus, the epitopes may be "hidden" in GBM, or PG processing may have eliminated the antigenic site. Alternatively, GBM is unique in that it does not contain this CSPG despite its presence in other basement membranes. Further studies utilizing antibodies to glomerular mesangial PGs will be necessary to determine whether these cells might be a source for GBM PGs and whether CSPG is important in the GBM function and formation.

Biglycan is also synthesized by human fetal mesangial cells in culture (45). This PG and decorin, a PG with a very similar protein core sequence, were identified by Western analysis. Decorin cDNAs identified mRNAs in mesangial cells in culture (8). Decorin synthesis is under negative feedback control by TGF-β, pointing to the importance of growth factors in normal extracellular matrix function and reactions to disease (99).

The importance of decorin and biglycan to the pathophysiology of kidney disease was pointed out by Border and Ruoslahti in an elegant series of studies in which they showed that synthesis of decorin and biglycan, as well as FN, was greatly enhanced during the mesangial proliferative stage of acute glomerulonephritis (9,64). Since antibodies against TGF-β inhibited the increased glomerular PG as well as FN synthesis, they proposed that TGF-β mediated extracellular matrix synthesis was responsible for the acute glomerulonephritis.

TGF-β also stimulated synthesis and decreased catabolism of CSPGs by cartilage cells and nonproliferating arterial smooth muscle cells, but not endothelial cells (21,61). It increased both the rate of CSPG core protein synthesis as well as GAG chain size (7). Interestingly, TGF-β has been shown to be an inhibitor of mesangial and endothelial cell proliferation (10,82,98). Thus, TGF-β may modulate glomerular response to disease by altering extracellular matrix processing, but whether it participates directly in mesangial cell proliferative response to acute glomerular injury or in the chronic changes seen in diabetes has yet to be determined.

THE METABOLIC MILIEU MODULATES RESPONSES TO GROWTH FACTORS

Alterations in the Hormonal Milieu in Diabetes

Growth hormone (GH) action is mediated in part by its ability to stimulate insulin-like growth factor-1 (IGF-1) production by the liver. IGF-I in turn stimulates synthesis of extracellular matrix and in particular PGs, resulting in tissue growth (3,59,75). This growth factor has also been shown to stimulate proliferation of fibroblasts and mesangial cells in culture (23,25). Local production of IGF-1 may be important, as evident from the finding that kidney IGF-1 mRNA levels are increased during compensatory renal hypertrophy (30,80). In addition, mesangial cells in culture synthesize IGF-1 and contain abundant IGF-1 receptors (2,4).

Perturbations in the hormonal as well as metabolic milieu may modulate tissue responses. Mice made transgenic with GH, GHRH, and IGF-1 genes contained hypertrophied glomeruli, a morphologic change apparent in human diabetes (27). However, only mice with GH excess developed glomerulosclerosis, despite higher IGF-1 levels in the transgenic IGF-1 group (26). These results may indicate that GH itself plays a role in the pathogenesis of glomerulosclerosis. However, serum GH and IGF-1 levels were both high in these mice, while in human and animal model diabetes circulating IGF-1 levels are low. That GH levels are also low in streptozotocin-induced diabetic rats despite the fact that they develop nephropathy argues against a pathogenic role for this hormone in diabetic nephropathy. That additional factors must be operating in diabetes to decrease local IGF-1 levels was apparent from studies that showed that GH excess induced in diabetic rats by implantation of a GH producing tumor did not fully correct the effect of diabetes on kidney IGF-1 mRNA (30). Insulin treatment also failed to rectify the kidney IGF-1 mRNA deficiency.

Not only are growth factors themselves important modulators of tissue response, but one must also account for the ability of IGF-1 binding proteins (BP) to regulate, and indeed enhance the cellular response to the growth factor (28). Circulating IGF BPs 1 and 2 levels as well as tissue mRNAs are increased by diabetes, but only IGF BP 1 levels are totally corrected by insulin treatment (65,90). IGF BP 2 mRNAs are relatively high in kidney, and this BP contains arginine-glycine-aspartic acid (RGD), a peptide sequence important in adhesion to cell surface integrin receptors. Tissue response to growth factors may not only stem from binding to their own receptors, but also from interactions with other components of the cell surface. In addition, the extracellular matrix acts as a reservoir for growth factors that may be altered by disease (74).

The Metabolic Milieu May Alter the Extracellular Matrix Synthetic Response to Growth Factors (Fig. 15.5)

Now that we are beginning to understand more about the structure and function of PGs synthesized by kidney cells under physiologic conditions, it is appropriate to perturb the in vitro environment with a metabolic milieu similar to that seen in diabetes. Insulin in high concentrations stimulated both HSPG and protein synthesis by EHS sarcoma basement membrane–producing cells from diabetic mice, but not in tumor cells from controls (55). PG synthesis was stimulated to a lesser extent than was protein synthesis, causing a lower proportionate PG synthesis. The insulin-mediated stimulation of PG, but not protein synthesis was abrogated at high glucose concentrations, resulting in the accumulation of relatively PG-depleted extracellular matrix, as occurs in diabetes. That glucose itself may be an important modulator of extracellular ma-

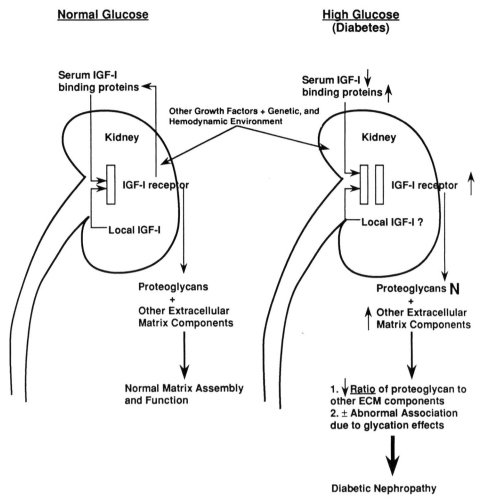

Normal Glucose

High Glucose
(Diabetes)

FIGURE 15.5. The effects of glucose and insulin-like growth factor 1 (IGF-1) on kidney proteo-glycan (PG) and protein synthesis. The control of extracellular matrix and PG synthesis by cells in normal subjects (*left*) and diabetic patients (*right*) is shown to be under control of both circulating and local growth factor production, with potential modulating influence by the hemodynamic, genetic, and metabolic milieus. The diabetic nephropathy is postulated to result from a relative decrease in proteoglycan synthesis due to a complex interaction of factors that occurs in the presence of high concentrations of glucose.

trix synthesis was also indicated by studies using human endothelial cells, which contained increased FN and type IV collagen mRNAs when incubated in high glucose concentrations (15). These changes were present in subsequent cell generations, leading these authors to postulate that tissues must have a means of "remembering" past metabolic environments (71). The organism may do this by forming advanced glycation end products. An excessively cross-linked extracellular matrix may be unable to normally assemble or interact with PGs (19,88). These changes may signal the cell to alter its synthetic patterns through matrix interactions with cell surfaces and the cytoskeleton.

We have recently reported that IGF-1 in the presence of physiologic glucose concentrations increased PG as well as protein synthesis by human fetal mesangial cells in culture (65). The PG response to IGF-1 was abrogated by glucose at high concentrations. In contrast, high concentrations of glucose enhanced the protein synthetic response to IGF-1. Thus, the ratio of newly synthesized PGs to proteins was markedly diminished in an in vitro environment mimicking the diabetic state. At the same time that high glucose concentrations relative mesangial cell PG synthesis, cell proliferation was inhibited in the presence or absence of IGF-1.

Cell proliferation is profoundly affected by the PG phenotype. Heparin or HSPG inhibited mesangial cell proliferation (17,18). Wounded, actively proliferating endothelial cells synthesized mostly CSPG, while HSPG synthesis again predominated at confluence (42). Inhibition of CSPG synthesis by β-D-xyloside results in the loss of smooth muscle cell "hillocks," while increased concentrations of CSPG are found in atherosclerotic plaques, a site of increased smooth muscle cell proliferation (34,94,95). Alterations in the PG phenotype may profoundly affect a cell's ability to proliferate by modulating interactions between extracellular matrix and cell surface receptors or through changes in the availability of growth factors stored in the matrix.

That glucose itself may affect extracellular matrix synthesis as well as cell proliferation suggests that the metabolic milieu may be an important contributor to the eventual development of the long-term complications of diabetes. These complications may result from a complex combination of effects, including changes in local and circulating hormone levels, alterations in binding protein and receptor concentrations, the genetic or hemodynamic environment, as well as the metabolic milieu. It will be important to continue to study the multifactorial control of extracellular matrix synthesis at both the translational and posttranslational levels, especially as it relates to changes found in diabetes. Research in this area will not only provide an avenue for the understanding of extracellular matrix changes in diabetes but also will contribute to our fund of knowledge in extracellular matrix biochemistry.

REFERENCES

1. ABRAHAMSON, D. R. Origin of the glomerular basement membrane visualized after in vivo labeling of laminin in newborn rat kidneys. *J. Cell Biol.* 100: 1988–2000, 1985.
2. ABRASS, C. K., RAUGI, G. J., GABOUREL, L. S., and LOVETT, D. H. Insulin and insulin-like growth factor I binding to cultured rat glomerular mesangial cells. *Endocrinology* 123: 2432–2439, 1988.
3. ADASHI, E. Y., RESNICK, C. E., SVOBODA, M. E., VAN WYK, J. J., HASCALL, V. C., and YANAGISHITA, M. Independent and synergistic actions of somatomedin-C in the stimulation of proteoglycan biosynthesis by cultured rat granulosa cells. *Endocrinology* 118: 456–458, 1986.
4. ARNQVIST, H. J., BALLERMANN, B. J., and KING, G. L. Receptors for and effects of insulin and IGF-I in rat glomerular mesangial cells. *Am. J. Physiol.* 254 (*Cell Physiol.* 23): C411–416, 1988.
5. AUSIELLO, D. A., KREISBERG, J. I., ROY, C., and KARNOVSKY, M. J. Contraction of cultured cells of apparent mesangial origin after stimulation with angiotensin II and arginine vasopressin. *J. Clin. Invest.* 65: 754–760, 1980.
6. BADLWIN, C. T., REGINATO, A. M., and PROCKOP, D. J. A new epidermal growth factor-like domain in the human core protein for the large cartilage specific proteoglycan. *J. Biol. Chem.* 264: 15747–15750, 1989.
7. BASSOLS, A., and MASSAGUE, J. Transforming growth factor beta regulates the expression

and structure of extracellular matrix chondroitin/dermatan sulfate proteoglycans. *J. Biol. Chem.* 263: 3039–3045, 1988.

8. BORDER, W. A., OKUDA, S., LANGUINO, L. R., and RUOSLAHTI, E. Transforming growth factor-β regulates production of proteoglycans by mesangial cells. *Kidney Int.* 37: 689–695, 1990.

9. BORDER, W. A., OKUDA, S., LANGUINO, L. R., SPORN, M. B., and RUOSLAHTI, E. Suppression of experimental glomerulonephritis by antiserum against transforming growth factor-β1. *Nature* 346: 371–374, 1990.

10. BOYD, F. T., and MASSAGUÉ, J. Transforming growth factor-β inhibition of epithelial cell proliferation linked to the expression of a 53-kDa membrane receptor. *J. Biol. Chem.* 264: 2272–2278, 1989.

11. BRENNER, B. M., HOSTETTER, T. H., and HUMES, H. D. Molecular basis of proteinuria of glomerular origin. *N. Engl. J. Med.* 298: 826–833, 1978.

12. BROWN, D. M., KLEIN, D. J., MICHAEL, A. F., and OEGEMA, T. R. ^{35}S-glycosaminoglycan and ^{35}S-glycopeptide metabolism by diabetic glomeruli and aorta. *Diabetes* 31: 418–425, 1982.

13. BROWN, D. M., MICHAEL, A. F., and OEGEMA, T. R. Glycosaminoglycan synthesis by glomeruli in vivo and in vitro. *Biochim. Biophys. Acta* 674: 96–104, 1981.

14. BROWNLEE, M., and SPIRO, R. G. Glomerular basement membrane metabolism in the diabetic rat. In vivo studies. *Diabetes* 28: 121–125, 1979.

15. CAGLIERO, E., MAIELLO, M., BOERI, D., ROY, S., and LORENZI, M. Increased expression of basement membrane components in human endothelial cells cultured in high glucose. *J. Clin. Invest.* 82: 735–738, 1988.

16. CAREY, D. J., and TODD, M. S. A cytoskeleton-associated plasma membrane heparan sulfate proteoglycan in Schwann cells. *J. Biol. Chem.* 261: 7518–7525, 1986.

17. CASTELLOT, J. J., FAVREAU, L. V., KARNOVSKY, M. J., and ROSENBERG, R. D. Inhibition of vascular smooth muscle cell growth by endothelial cell-derived heparan. *J. Biol. Chem.* 257: 11256–11260, 1982.

18. CASTELLOT, J. J., HOOVER, R. L., HARPER, P. A., and KARNOVSKY, M. J. Heparin and glomerular epithelial cell-secreted heparinlike species inhibit mesangial-cell proliferation. *Am. J. Pathol.* 120: 427–435, 1985.

19. CHARONIS, A. S., REGER, L. A., DEGE, J. E., KOUZI-KOLIAKOS, K., FURCHT, L. T., WOHLHUETER, R. M., and TSILIBARY, E. C. Laminin alterations after in vivo nonenzymatic glycosylation. *Diabetes* 39: 807–814, 1990.

20. CHEIFETZ, S., ANDRES, J. L., and MASSAGUÉ, J. The transforming growth factor-β receptor type III is a membrane proteoglycan. *J. Biol. Chem.* 263: 16984–16991, 1988.

21. CHEN, J-K., HOSHI, J., and MCKEEHAN, W. L. Transforming growth factor type β specifically stimulates synthesis of proteoglycan in human adult arterial smooth muscle cells. *Proc. Natl. Acad. Sci. USA* 84: 5287–5291, 1987.

22. COHEN, M. P., and SURMA, M. L. [35]S]sulfate incorporation into glomerular basement membrane glycosaminoglycans is decreased in experimental diabetes. *J. Lab. Clin. Med.* 98: 715–722, 1981.

23. CONOVER, C. A., HINTZ, R. L., and ROSENFELD, R. G. Comparative effects of somatomedin C and insulin on the metabolism and growth of cultured human fibroblasts. *J. Cell. Physiol.* 122: 133–141, 1985.

24. CONRAD, G. W., HAMILTON, L., and HAYNES, E. Differences in glycosaminoglycans synthesized by fibroblast-like cells from chick cornea, heart and skin. *J. Biol. Chem.* 252: 6861–6870, 1977.

25. CONTI, F. G., STRIKER, L. J., LESNIAK, M. A., MACKAY, K., ROTH, J., and STRIKER, G. E. Studies on binding and mitogenic effect of insulin and insulin-like growth factor I in glomerular mesangial cells. *Endocrinology* 122: 2788–2795, 1988.

26. DOI, T., STRIKER, L. J., GIBSON, C. C., AGODOA, L. Y. C., BRINSTER, R. L., and STRIKER, G. E. Glomerular lesions in mice transgenic for growth hormone and insulinlike growth factor-I. *Am. J. Pathol.* 137: 541–552, 1990.

27. DOI, T., STRIKER, L. J., QUAIFE, C., CONTI, F. G., PALMITER, R., BEHRINGER, R., BRINSTER, R., and STRIKER, G. E. Progressive glomerulosclerosis develops in transgenic mice chronically expressing growth hormone and growth hormone releasing factor but not in those expressing insulinlike growth factor-1. *Am. J. Pathol.* 131: 398–403, 1988.

28. ELGIN, G. R., BUSBY, W. H., and CLEMMONS, D. R. An insulin-like growth factor (IGF) binding protein enhances the biologic response to IGF-I. *Proc. Natl. Acad. Sci. USA* 84: 3254–3258, 1987.

29. FAGIN, J. A., and MELMED, S. Relative increase in insulin-like growth factor I messenger ribonucleic acid levels in compensatory renal hypertrophy. *Endocrinology* 120: 718–724, 1987.

30. FAGIN, J. A., ROBERTS, C. T., LeROITH, D., and BROWN, A. T. Coordinate decrease of tissue insulinlike growth factor I posttranscriptional alternative mRNA transcripts in diabetes mellitus. *Diabetes* 38: 428–434, 1989.

31. FALK, R. J., SCHEINMAN, J. I., MAUER, S. M., and MICHAEL, A. F. Polyantigenic expansion of basement membrane constituents in diabetic nephropathy. *Diabetes* 32: 34–39 (suppl 2), 1983.

32. FIORETTO, P. F., McCARTHY, J., and KLEIN, D. J., manuscript in preparation.

33. FISHER, L. W., TERMINE, J. D., and YOUNG, M. F. Deduced protein sequence of bone small proteoglycan I (Biglycan) shows homology with proteoglycan II (Decorin) and several nonconnective tissue proteins in a variety of species. *J. Biol. Chem.* 264: 4571–4576, 1989.

34. HAMATI, H. F., BRITTON, E. L., and CAREY, D. J. Inhibition of proteoglycan synthesis alters extracellular matrix deposition, proliferation, and cytoskeletal organization of rat aortic smooth muscle cells in culture. *J. Cell Biol.* 108: 2495–2505, 1989.

35. HASSELL, J. R., KIMURA, J. H., and HASCALL, V. C. Proteoglycan core protein families. *Annu. Rev. Biochem.* 55: 539–567, 1986.

36. HAY, E. (ed.) *Cell Biology of the Extracellular Matrix.* New York: Plenum, 1981.

37. HEINEGÅRD, D., and PAULSSON, M. Structure and metabolism of proteoglycans. In: *Extracellular Matrix Biochemistry,* edited by K. A. Piez and A. H. Reddi. New York: Elsevier, 1984.

38. HOUSER, M. T., SCHEINMAN, J. I., BASGEN, J., STEFFES, M. W., and MICHAEL, A. F. Preservation of mesangium and immunohistochemically defined antigens in GBM isolated by detergent extraction. *J. Clin. Invest.* 69: 1169–1175, 1982.

39. ISHIHARA, M., FEDARKO, N. S., and CONRAD, H. E. Transport of heparan sulfate into the nuclei of hepatocytes. *J. Biol. Chem.* 261: 13575–13580, 1986.

40. KANWAR, Y. S., and FARQUHAR, M. H. Presence of heparan sulfate in the glomerular basement membrane. *Proc. Natl. Acad. Sci. USA* 76: 1303–1307, 1979.

41. KANWAR, Y. S., JAKUBOWSKI, M. L., and ROSENZWEIG, L. J. Distribution of sulfated glycosaminoglycans in the glomerular basement membrane and mesangial matrix. *Eur. J. Cell Biol.* 31: 290–295, 1983.

42. KANWAR, Y. S., LINKER, A., and FARQUHAR, M. G. Increased permeability of the glomerular basement membrane to ferritin after removal of glycosaminoglycans (heparan sulfate) by enzyme digestion. *J. Cell Biol.* 86: 688–93, 1980.

43. KANWAR, Y. S., ROSENZWEIG, L. F., LINKER, A., and JAKUBOWSKI, M. L. Decreased de novo synthesis of glomerular proteoglycans in diabetes: biochemical and autoradiographic evidence. *Proc. Natl. Acad. Sci. USA* 80: 2272–2275, 1983.

44. KINSELLA, M. G., and WIGHT, T. N. Modulation of sulfated proteoglycan synthesis by bovine aortic endothelial cells during migration. *J. Cell Biol.* 102: 679–687, 1986.

45. KJELLÉN, L., BIELEFELD, D., and HÖÖK, M. Reduced sulfation of liver heparan sulfate in experimentally diabetic rats. *Diabetes* 32: 337–342, 1983.

46. KJELLÉN, L., OLDBERG, A., and HÖÖK, M. Cell surface heparan sulfate. *J. Biol. Chem.* 255: 10407–10413, 1980.

47. KLEIN, D. J., BROWN, D. M., KIM, Y. and OEGEMA, T. R. Proteoglycans synthesized by human glomerular mesangial cells in culture. *J. Biol. Chem.* 265: 9533–9543, 1990.

48. KLEIN, . J., BROWN, D. M., MORAN, A., OEGEMA, T. R., and PLATT, J. L. Chondroitin sulfate proteoglycan synthesis and reutilization of β-D-xyloside-initiated chondroitin/dermatan sulfate glycosaminoglycans in fetal kidney branching morphogenesis. *Dev. Biol.* 133: 515–528, 1989.

49. KLEIN, D. J., BROWN, D. M., and OEGEMA, T. R. Glomerular proteoglycans in diabetes. *Diabetes* 35: 1130–1142, 1986.

50. KLEIN, D. J., BROWN, D. M., and OEGEMA, T. R., JR. Partial characterization of heparan and dermatan sulfate proteoglycans synthesized by normal rat glomeruli. *J. Biol. Chem.* 261: 16636–16652, 1986.

51. KLEIN, D. J., BROWN, D. M., OEGEMA, T. R., BRENCHLEY, P. E., ANDERSON, J. C., DICKINSON, M. A. J., HORIGAN, E. A., and HASSELL, J. R. Glomerular basement membrane proteoglycans are derived from a large precursor. *J. Cell Biol.* 106: 963–970, 1988.

52. KLEIN, D. J. OEGEMA, T. R., and BROWN, D. M. Release of glomerular heparan sulfate proteoglycan by heparin from glomeruli of streptozocin-induced diabetic rats. *Diabetes* 38: 130–139, 1989.

53. KLEIN, D. J., OEGEMA, T. R., FREDEEN, T. S., VAN DER WOUDE, F., KIM, Y, and BROWN, D. M. Partial characterization of proteoglycans synthesized by human glomerular epithelial cells in culture. *Arch. Biochem. Biophys.* 277: 389–401, 1990.

54. KREISBERG, J. I., and HASSID, A. Functional properties of glomerular cells in culture. *Miner. Electrolyte Metab.* 12: 25–31, 1986.

55. KREISBERG, J. I., and KARNOVSKY, M. J. Glomerular cells in culture. *Kidney Int.* 23: 439–47, 1983.

56. KREISBERG, J. I., VENKATACHALAM, M., and TROYER, D. Contractile properties of cultured glomerular mesangial cells. *Am. J. Physiol.* 249 (*Renal Fluid Electrolyte Physiol.* 18): F457–F463, 1985.

57. KRUSIUS, T., GEHLSEN, K. R., and RUOSLAHTI, E. A fibroblast chondroitin sulfate proteoglycan core protein contains lectin-like and growth factor-like sequences. *J. Biol. Chem.* 262: 13120–13125, 1987.

58. LEDBETTER, S. R., COPELAND, E. J., NOONAN, D., VOGELI, G., and HASSELL, J. R. Altered steady-state mRNA levels of basement membrane proteins in diabetic mouse kidneys and thromboxane synthase inhibition. *Diabetes* 39: 196–203, 1990.

59. LEDBETTER, S. R., WAGNER, C. W., MARTIN, G. R., ROHRBACH, D. H., and HASSELL, J. R. Response of diabetic basement membrane-producing cells to glucose and insulin. *Diabetes* 36: 1029–1034, 1987.

60. MAUER, S. M., STEFFES, M. W., ELLIS, E. N., SUTHERLAND, D. E. R., BROWN, D. M., and GOETZ, F. C. Structural-functional relationships in diabetic nephropathy. *J. Clin. Invest.* 74: 1143–1155, 1984.

61. MCCARTHY, K. J., ACCAVITTI, M. A., and COUCHMAN, J. R. Immunological characterization of a basement membrane specific chondroitin sulfate proteoglycan. *J. Cell Biol.* 109: 3187–3198, 1989.

62. MCQUILLAN, D. J., HANDLEY, C. J., CAMPBELL, M. A., BOLIS, S., MILWAY, V. E., and HERINGTON, A. C. Stimulation of proteoglycan biosynthesis by serum and insulin-like growth factor-I in cultured bovine articular cartilage. *Biochem. J.* 240: 423–430, 1986.

63. MOHAN, P. S., CARTER, W. G., and SPIRO, R. G. Occurrence of type VI collagen in extracellular matrix of renal glomeruli and its increase in diabetes. *Diabetes* 39: 31–37, 1990.

64. MORALES, T. I., and ROBERTS, A. B. Transforming growth factor β regulates the metabolism of proteoglycans in bovine cartilage organ cultures. *J. Biol. Chem.* 263: 12828–12831, 1988.

65. MORAN, A. BROWN, D. M., KIM, Y., and KLEIN, D. J. The effects of IGF-I and hyperglycemia on protein and proteoglycan (PG) synthesis by human fetal mesangial cells in culture. *Diabetes* 40: 1346–1354, 1991.

66. NOONAN, D. M., HORIGAN, E. A., LEDBETTER, S. R., VOGELI, G., SASAKI, M., YAMADA, Y., and HASSELL, J. R. Identification of cDNA clones encoding different domains of the basement membrane heparan sulfate proteoglycan. *J. Biol. Chem.* 263: 16379–16387, 1988.

67. OKUDA, S., LANGUINO, L. R., RUOSLAHTI, E., and BORDER, W. A. Elevated expression of transforming growth factor-β and proteoglycan production in experimental glomerulonephritis. *J. Clin. Invest.* 86: 453–462, 1990.

68. OOI, G. T., ORLOWSKI, C. C., BROWN, A. L., BECKER, R. E., UNTERMAN, T. G., and RECHLER, M. M. Different tissue distribution and hormonal regulation of messenger RNAs encoding rat insulin-like growth factor-binding proteins-1 and -2. *Mol. Endocrinol.* 4: 321–328, 1990.

69. PARTHASARATHY, N., and SPIRO, R. G. Effect of diabetes on the glycosaminoglycan component of the human glomerular basement membrane. *Diabetes* 31: 738–741, 1982.

70. PLATT, J. L., BROWN, D. M., GRANLUND, K., OEGEMA, T. R., and KLEIN, D. J. Proteoglycan metabolism associated with mouse metanephric development: morphologic and biochemical effects of β-D-xyloside. *Dev. Biol.* 123: 293–306, 1987.

71. RAPRAEGER, A., and BERNFIELD, M. Cell surface proteoglycan of mammary epithelial cells. *J. Biol. Chem.* 260: 4103–4109, 1985.

72. RAPRAEGER, A., JALKANEN, M., and BERNFIELD, M. Cell surface proteoglycan associates with the cytoskeleton at the basolateral cell surface of mouse mammary epithelial cells. *J. Cell Biol.* 103: 2683–2696, 1986.

73. RODÉN, L. Structure and metabolism of connective tissue proteoglycans. In: *The Biochemistry of Glycoproteins and Proteoglycans,* edited by W. J. Lennarz. New York: Plenum Press, pp. 267–371, 1980.

74. ROY, S., SALA, R., CAGLIERO, E., and LORENZI, M. Overexpression of fibronectin induced by diabetes or high glucose: phenomenon with a memory. *Proc. Natl. Acad. Sci. USA* 87: 404–408, 1990.

75. RUOSLAHTI, E. Proteoglycans in cell regulation. *J. Biol. Chem.* 264: 13369–13372, 1989.

76. SAKASHITA, S., ENGVALL, E., and RUOSLAHTI, E. Basement membrane glycoprotein laminin binds to heparin. *FEBS Lett.* 116: 243–246, 1980.

77. SAKSELA, L., MOSCATELLI, D., SOMMER, A., and RIFKIN, D. B. Endothelial cell-derived heparan sulfate binds basic fibroblast growth factor and protects it from proteolytic degradation. *J. Cell Biol.* 107: 743–751, 1988.

78. SALMON, W. D., and DAUGHADAY, W. H. A hormonally controlled serum factor which stimulates sulfate incorporation by cartilage in vitro. *J. Lab. Clin. Med.* 49: 825–836, 1957.

79. SARIOLA, H., TIMPL, R., VON DER MARK, K. MAYNE, R., FITCH, J. M., LINSENMAYER, T. F., and EKBLOM, P. Dual origin of the glomerular basement membrane. *Dev. Biol.* 101: 86–96, 1984.

80. SAUNDERS, S., and BERNFIELD, M. Cell surface proteoglycan binds mouse mammary epithelial cells to fibronectin and behaves as a receptor for interstitial matrix. *J. Cell Biol.* 106: 423–430, 1988.

81. SAUNDERS, S., JALKANEN, M., O'FARRELL, S., and BERNFIELD, M. Molecular cloning of syndecan, an integral membrane proteoglycan. *J. Cell Biol.* 108: 1547–1556, 1989.

82. SCHEINMAN, J. I., FISH, A. J., MATAS, A. J., and MICHAEL, A. F. The immunohistopathology of glomerular antigens: II. The glomerular basement membrane, actomyosin and fibroblast surface antigens in normal, diseased and transplanted human kidneys. *Am. J. Pathol.* 90: 71–80, 1978.

83. SCHLECHTER, N. L., RUSSEL, S. M., SPENCER, E. M., and NICOLL, C. S. Evidence suggesting that the direct growth-promoting effect of growth hormone on cartilage in vivo is mediated by local production of somatomedin. *Proc. Natl. Acad. Sci. USA* 83: 7932–7934, 1986.

84. SCOTT, J. E., ORFORD, C. R., and HUGHES, E. W. Proteoglycan-collagen arrangements in developing rat tail tendon: an electron microscopical and biochemical investigation. *Biochem. J.* 195: 573–581, 1981.

85. SHIMOMURA, H., and SPIRO, R. G. Studies on the macromolecular components of human glomerular basement membrane and alterations in diabetes: decreased levels of heparan sulfate proteoglycan and laminin. *Diabetes* 36: 374–381, 1987.

86. SILVER, B. J., JAFFER, F. E., and ABBOUD, H. E. Platelet-derived growth factor synthesis in mesangial cells: induction by multiple peptide mitogens. *Proc. Natl. Acad. Sci. USA* 86: 1056–1060, 1989.

87. SIMON-ASSMANN, P., BOUZIGES, F., VIGNY, M., and KEDINGER, M. Origin and deposition of basement membrane heparan sulfate proteoglycan in the developing intestine. *J. Cell. Biol.* 109: 1837–1848, 1989.

88. SPIRO, M. J. Sulfate metabolism in the alloxan-diabetic rat: relationship of altered sulfate pools to proteoglycan sulfation in heart and other tissues. *Diabetologia* 30: 259–267, 1987.

89. STOW, J. L., SAWADA, H., and FARQUHAR, M. G. Basement membrane heparan sulfate proteoglycans are concentrated in the laminae rarae and podocytes of rate renal glomerulus. *Proc. Natl. Acad. Sci. USA* 82: 3296–3300, 1985.

90. STRIKER, G. E., KILLEN, T. D., and FARIN, F. M. Human glomerular cells in vitro: isolation and characterization. *Transplant. Proc.* XII (3):88–99, 1980.

91. STRIKER, G. E., and STRIKER, L. J. Biology of disease: glomerular cell culture. *Lab. Invest.* 53: 122–31, 1985.

92. TARSIO, J. F., WIGNESS, B., RHODE, T. D., RUPP, W. M., BUCHWALD, H., and FURCHT, L. T. Non-enzymatic glycation of fibronectin and alterations in the molecular association of cell matrix and basement membrane components in diabetes mellitus. *Diabetes* 34: 477–84, 1985.

93. TEMPLETON, D. M. Retention of glomerular basement membrane proteoglycans accompanying loss of anionic site staining in experimental diabetes. *Lab. Invest.* 61: 202–11, 1989.

94. UNTERMAN, T. G., OEHLER, D. T., and BECKER, R. E. Identification of a type 1 insulin-like growth factor binding protein (IGF BP) in serum from rats with diabetes mellitus. *Biochem. Biophys. Res. Commun.* 163: 882–887, 1989.

95. VAN DER WOUDE, F. J., MICHAEL, A. F., MULLER, E., VAN DER HEM, G. K., VERNIER, R. L., and KIM, Y. Lymphohemopoietic antigens of cultured human glomerular epithelial cells. *Br. J. Exp. Pathol.* 70: 73–82, 1989.

96. VERNIER, R. L., KLEIN, D. J., SISSON, S. P., MAHAN, J. P., OEGEMA, T. R., JR., and BROWN, D. M. Heparan sulfate-rich anionic sites in the human glomerular basement membrane: decreased concentration in congenital nephrotic syndrome. *N. Engl. J. Med.* 309: 1001–1008, 1983.

97. VOGEL, K. G., PAULSSON, M., and HEINEGÅRD, D. Specific inhibition of type I and type II collagen fibrillogenesis by the small proteoglycan of tendon. *Biochem. J.* 223: 587–97, 1984.

98. WAGNER, W. D., SALISBURY, B. G. J., and ROWE, J. A. A proposed structure of chondroitin 6-sulfate proteoglycan of human normal and adjacent atherosclerotic plaque. *Atherosclerosis* 6: 407–417, 1986.

99. WIGHT, T. N. Proteoglycan in pathological conditions: atherosclerosis. *Federation Proc.* 44: 381–385, 1985.

100. WOODS, A., HÖÖK, M., KJELLÉN, L., SMITH, C. G., and REES, D. A. Relationship of heparan sulfate proteoglycans to the cytoskeleton and extracellular matrix of cultured fibroblasts. *J. Cell Biol.* 99: 1743–1753, 1984.

101. YAMADA, K. M. Cell surface interactions with extracellular materials. In: *Annu. Rev. Biochem.*, edited by E. E. Snell, P. D. Boyer, A. Meister, and C. C. Richardson. Palo Alto, California: Annual Reviews, Inc. 52: 761–800, 1983.

102. YAMAGUCHI, Y., and RUOSLAHTI, E. Expression of human proteoglycan in Chinese hamster ovary cells inhibits cell proliferation. *Nature* 336: 244–246, 1990.

103. YAMAGUCHI, Y., MANN, D., and RUOSLAHTI, E. Negative regulation of transforming growth factor-β by the proteoglycan decorin. *Nature* 346: 281–284, 1990.

104. YANAGISHITA, M., and HASCALL, V. C. Proteoglycans synthesized by rat ovarian granulosa cells in culture. *J. Biol. Chem.* 259: 10260–10269, 1984.

Index